ACoRN: Acute Care of at-Risk Newborns

ACoRN: Acute Care of at-Risk Newborns

A Resource and Learning Tool for Health Care Professionals

SECOND EDITION

Edited by

Jill E. Boulton, MD, FRCPC
Kevin Coughlin, MD, FRCPC, MHSc
Debra O'Flaherty, RN, BScN, MSN
Alfonso Solimano, MD, FRCPC

OXFORD
UNIVERSITY PRESS

OXFORD
UNIVERSITY PRESS

Oxford University Press is a department of the University of Oxford. It furthers
the University's objective of excellence in research, scholarship, and education
by publishing worldwide. Oxford is a registered trade mark of Oxford University
Press in the UK and certain other countries.

Published in the United States of America by Oxford University Press
198 Madison Avenue, New York, NY 10016, United States of America.

First Edition published in 2005
Second Edition published in 2021

Library of Congress Cataloging-in-Publication Data
Names: E. Boulton, Jill; Coughlin, Kevin; O'Flaherty, Debra; Solimano, Alfonso, editor.
Title: ACoRN: Acute care of at-risk newborns : a resource and learning tool for
health care professionals / edited by Jill E. Boulton, MD, FRCPC
[and three others].
Description: second edition. | New York : Oxford University Press, [2021] |
Includes bibliographical references and index.
Identifiers: LCCN 2020000087 (print) | LCCN 2020000088 (ebook) |
ISBN 9780197525227 (paperback) | ISBN 9780197525241 (epub) |
ISBN 9780197525258 (online)
Subjects: LCSH: Neonatal intensive care. | Newborn infants—Medical care. |
Newborn infants—Diseases.
Classification: LCC RJ253.5 .A28 2020 (print) | LCC RJ253.5 (ebook) |
DDC 618.92/01—dc23
LC record available at https://lccn.loc.gov/2020000087
LC ebook record available at https://lccn.loc.gov/2020000088

DOI: 10.1093/med/9780197525227.001.0001

9 8 7 6 5 4 3 2 1

Printed by Integrated Books International, United States of America

Contents

About the Canadian Paediatric Society

Mission

The Canadian Paediatric Society (CPS) is the national association of paediatricians, committed to working together to advance the health of children and youth by nurturing excellence in health care, advocacy, education, research, and support of its membership.

Who We Are

Founded in 1922, the CPS is a voluntary professional association that represents more than 3,600 paediatricians, paediatric subspecialists, paediatric residents, and others who work with and care for children and youth. The CPS is governed by an elected board of directors representing all provinces and territories.

What We Do

To fulfil its mission, the CPS is active in several major areas:

- **Professional education:** The CPS supports the education needs of paediatricians and other child and youth health professionals through position statements, a peer-reviewed journal—*Paediatrics & Child Health*—and educational opportunities such as an annual conference, online education, and regional continuing medical education (CME) events. The Neonatal Resuscitation Program (NRP) and the Acute Care of at-Risk Newborns (ACoRN) Program focus on emergent care and stabilization for unwell and at-risk infants.
- **Advocacy:** The CPS works to identify gaps in care and promote improvements to public policy that affect the health of children and youth.
- **Health communication and knowledge translation:** The CPS helps parents, health professionals, and allied care providers make informed decisions about child and youth health and well-being by producing reliable and accessible health information.
- **Surveillance and research:** The CPS monitors rare diseases and conditions through the Canadian Paediatric Surveillance Program (CPSP), and ensures continued research into vaccine-associated adverse reactions and vaccine-preventable diseases through IMPACT (Immunization Monitoring Program, ACTive).

The Canadian Paediatric Society's activities and programs are funded through a wide variety of sources, including membership dues, revenue from CME events and annual conferences, publications, unrestricted grants from individuals, foundations, and corporations, as well as government grants. We collaborate with many organizations to promote the health of children and youth.

On the Internet

www.cps.ca: This is the primary online home of the CPS. Visit this site to access position statements and practice points on a wide range of health topics as well as information on professional development.

www.cps.ca/en/acorn: Find teaching and learning resources on stabilizing infants who are unwell or at risk of becoming unwell in the first few hours or days post-birth.

www.cps.ca/en/nrp-prn: The NRP website has resources for providers, instructors, and instructor trainers on resuscitating infants in the first minutes of extra-uterine life.

Preface

The transition from fetal to neonatal life is the most dramatic physiologic change in the human life cycle, and although it progresses normally most of the time, a significant number of newborns require resuscitation and/or ongoing support to survive. Being called upon to assist with the care of an ill newborn can be one of the most challenging and stressful experiences for a health care provider. The Neonatal Resuscitation Program (NRP) has been the standard of care in all facilities providing perinatal care in Canada since the 1990s. However, there was recognition among perinatal care providers and educators that there were gaps in knowledge and skill when stabilizing newborns post-NRP, especially in settings where this care was infrequent. The ACoRN textbook and educational program were developed in response to this need.

ACoRN (short for Acute Care of at-Risk Newborns) was developed by an expert group of Canadian neonatal care providers and educators. Since launching in 2005, ACoRN has been taught across Canada and internationally, in formats varying from one- to three-day local, regional, or provincial/territorial workshops to module-based learning over a period of weeks. As with many education programs, ACoRN has evolved from didactic sessions and tabletop simulations to the hands-on, simulation-based workshops utilized today. Updates to the first edition of the text were published in 2010 and 2012 to add new content (on therapeutic hypothermia, for example).

The ACoRN text describes the ACoRN process step by step, along with the essential knowledge, tools, and management principles that drive this unique approach to stabilization. The text provides the foundation for the ACoRN educational program, first by describing system-based concepts and skills for neonatal stabilization, then how to manage care along systemic pathways (sequences), and finally, when to transport infants for higher level care. ACoRN takes a uniquely systematic approach to the identification and management of ill newborns. The process applies equally to newborns needing assistance in the transition from fetal life and to newborns who become unwell or are at risk of becoming unwell over the first few hours to days after birth. ACoRN is not a resuscitation program. Before entering the ACoRN Primary Survey, practitioners must first determine whether a newborn requires resuscitative care and, if they do, are directed to follow the most current NRP sequence.

The second edition of ACoRN includes updated knowledge and clinical practices, a new Primary Survey, and revised Sequences informed by feedback from workshops and ACoRN practitioners over the past 15 years. When clinical questions arose, literature reviews were undertaken to incorporate the most recent evidence.

The basic structure of the ACoRN process has withstood the test of time and remains unchanged from the first edition. Updates in this new edition include the following:

- An introductory chapter on neonatal transition that identifies the physiologic changes occurring at birth that are central to the ACoRN approach to stabilization.
- A series of initial actions (Consolidated Core Steps) in the stabilization of unwell or at-risk newborns. These steps are completed alongside the Primary Survey.

- Reorganized chapters that present all the knowledge needed to work through each ACoRN sequence (including updated, disease-specific information) before clinical cases illustrate how they might apply in practice.
- Updated and reformatted assessment tools to guide care and decision-making.
- Revised sequence flow and structure, for consistency across system chapters and care pathways.
- A Level of Risk assessment for each chapter, based on infant condition, anticipated clinical course, and site capacity to provide and sustain care.
- An updated Cardiovascular chapter and sequence emphasizing signs and symptoms of shock and the need for urgent intervention. The response to a failed critical congenital heart disease (CCHD) screen has also been added.
- A Neurology Chapter expanded to include infants at risk for hypoxic ischemic encephalopathy (HIE) and indications for thermoregulatory management.
- Assessment and presurgical stabilization for newborns with a neural tube defect has been added to the Surgical Conditions chapter.
- The Fluid and Glucose chapter and sequence were revised collaboratively with the CPS Fetus and Newborn Committee, to align with new guidance on screening and managing infants with low blood glucose levels. Changes to the sequence include the introduction of dextrose gels, clarification of glucose thresholds, and a simplified approach to expedite the normalization of blood glucose values.
- A new Jaundice chapter and sequence, added in response to provider feedback.
- Management of newborns undergoing therapeutic hypothermia is included in the Thermoregulation sequence.
- The Infection chapter has been extensively revised to include a sepsis-scoring tool and a new sequence.

As with the first edition, the importance of providing personal support for the newborn, the family, and care providers during stabilization is an overarching theme.

Heartfelt thanks are re-extended in this book to the original editors of the 2005 edition of ACoRN. Without their determination over many years, ACoRN would not have gone through the many iterations, reformattings, and rewrites that have made the process—and program—that they are today. ACoRN has been embraced wholeheartedly by practitioners in Canada and beyond.

Thanks go to my fellow co-editors, Dr Alfonso Solimano, Ms Deborah O'Flaherty, and Dr Kevin Coughlin, for making this new edition a reality. The success of ACoRN over the past 15 years is due in great part to the dogged determination of Dr Solimano, who was responsible for the 2010 and 2012 updates and the day-to-day management of printing and sales of ACoRN materials until the program was transferred to the Canadian Paediatric Society in 2015. He was also responsible for many of the changes in this text, most notably in the management of hypoglycemia. Ms Deborah O'Flaherty has been a tireless advocate and teacher of ACoRN, bringing the program into many remote communities and offering a critical nursing perspective to the production of ACoRN materials. Dr Coughlin's passion for teaching ACoRN and his determination and hard work to complete this edition cannot be overstated.

This new edition of ACoRN would not have been possible without the involvement of many more health care practitioners, only some of whom are acknowledged specifically in the pages that follow.

Undoubtedly, practice will continue to evolve in coming years, and feedback to acorn@cps.ca from ACoRN instructors and providers is always welcome. For more information on ACoRN, visit www.cps.ca/acorn.

Jill E. Boulton, MD, FRCPC

Acknowledgments

The Canadian Paediatric Society and the ACoRN text editors extend warmest thanks to everyone involved in developing this book. We are especially grateful to the ACoRN Publication and Education Subcommittees, who have reviewed and contributed to multiple manuscript drafts. Their expertise was always a given, but their patience, forbearance, and dedication to this project—from 2015 through 2020—have been inspirational.

Each chapter of the ACoRN text was reviewed rigorously by clinical experts who stabilize newborns in a range of clinical settings. These physicians and nurses freely shared their knowledge and insights at every stage of development. Similarly, neonatologists and nurses within and outside the CPS generously gave of their time and experience, often contributing text of such quality that it now appears verbatim in these pages.

ACoRN Publication and Education Subcommittees

CO-EDITORS of this edition

Jill E. Boulton, MD, FRCPC
Neonatologist
Medical Director, Maternal Newborn Child and Youth Network, Interior Health Authority, B.C.
Medical Director, NICU, Kelowna General Hospital
Kelowna, B.C.

Kevin Coughlin, MD, MHSc, FRCPC
Neonatologist, London Health Sciences Centre
Neonatal Co-Director of Perinatal Outreach
Associate Professor, Schulich School of Medicine and Dentistry, Western University
Associate Scientist, Lawson Health Research Institute
London, Ont.

Debra O'Flaherty, RN, BScN, MSN (Ret.)
Coordinator, Neonatal Outreach, Perinatal Services B.C.
Vancouver, B.C.

Alfonso Solimano, MD, FRCPC
Neonatologist, B.C. Women's Hospital and Health Centre
Clinical Professor, Department of Paediatrics, University of British Columbia
Medical Director, B.C. RSV Program
Vancouver, B.C.

CO-CHAIRS, ACoRN Education Subcommittee

Debbie Aylward, RN, BScN, MScN (Ret.)
Perinatal Consultant
Champlain Maternal Newborn Regional Program
Ottawa, Ont.

Deepak Manhas, MHPE, MD, FRCPC, FAAP
Neonatologist, B.C. Women's Hospital and Health Centre
Clinical Assistant Professor, Department of Paediatrics
University of British Columbia
Vancouver, B.C.

Members (2015 to 2019)

Steve Arnold, MD, FRCPC
CLSC Palaqsivik,
Kangiqsualujjuaq, Que.

Khalid Aziz, MA, MEd(IT), FRCPC
Professor, Department of Paediatrics (Newborn
Medicine)
University of Alberta
Edmonton, Alta.

Roxanne R. Laforge, RN, BSN, BA, MS
Perinatal Program Coordinator—CEDN
Lecturer, Clinical instructor, College of Nursing
University of Saskatchewan
Saskatoon, Sask.

Leanne Lauzon, RN, MSc, PNC(C)
Perinatal Nurse Consultant
IWK Health Centre
Halifax, N.S.

Horacio Osiovich, MD, FRCPC
Division Head, Neonatology, B.C. Women's
Hospital and Health Centre
Clinical Professor, Department of Paediatrics,
University of British Columbia
Vancouver, B.C.

Charles 'David' Simpson, MD
Division of Neonatal-Perinatal Medicine,
IWK Health Centre
Assistant Professor, Subspecialty Program
Director
Dalhousie University, Faculty of Medicine
Halifax, N.S.

Avash Jeet Singh, MD, FRCPC
Consultant neonatologist and paediatrician
Provincial Health Services Authority
Children's and Women's Health Centre of
British Columbia
Surrey, B.C.

Elene D. Vanderpas, RN (Ret.)
Clinical Nurse Educator
Vancouver, B.C.

Susan White, RN (Ret.)
Clinical Nurse Educator
Eastern Health
St. John's, Nfld and Labrador

Jeannie Yee, RN, BN
Coordinator, Education and
Consultation
Alberta Perinatal Health Program,
Alberta Health Services
Calgary, Alta.

Manuscript reviewers and contributors (2015 to 2019)

Kirsten A. Blaine, MD
Chief of Paediatrics, Stratford
General Hospital
Adjunct Professor, Schulich School of Medicine
and Dentistry,
Western University
London, Ont.

Kim Campbell, RN, RM, MN
Faculty of Medicine, Midwifery
University of British Columbia
Vancouver, B.C.

**Roxane Carr, BSc, BSCPharm, ACPR,
PharmD, BCPS, FCSHP**
Clinical Coordinator, B.C. Women's Hospital and
Health Centre
Assistant Professor, part-time, Faculty of
Pharmaceutical Sciences
University of British Columbia
Vancouver, B.C.

Michael Castaldo, BCh, BAO, MD
Neonatologist, B.C. Women's Hospital and
Health Centre
Clinical Assistant Professor, Neonatology,
Department of Paediatrics,
Faculty of Medicine
University of British Columbia
Vancouver, B.C.

Jean-Pierre Chanoine, MD
Head, Division of Paediatric Endocrinology,
  B.C. Children's Hospital
Clinical Professor, Department of Paediatrics,
  Faculty of Medicine
Head, Division of Endocrinology and Diabetes
University of British Columbia
Vancouver, B.C.

Virginia J. Clark, MD
Family Physician
Golden, B.C.
Nancy Couto, NP–Paediatrics
Clinical Nurse Educator
London Health Sciences Centre
London, Ont.

Marion DeLand, RNC-NIC, MN
Patient Care Manager, NICU
Sunnybrook Health Sciences Centre
Adjunct lecturer, Faculty of Nursing, University
  of Toronto
Toronto, Ont.

Lynn 'Michelle' Delany, RN
Clinical Nurse Educator
Maternal Newborn Child and Youth Network,
  Interior Interior Health Authority
Kamloops, B.C.

Michael Dunn, MD, FRCPC
Staff Neonatologist, Sunnybrook Health
  Sciences Centre
Associate Professor, Paediatrics, University of
  Toronto
Toronto, Ont.

Robert J. Everett, MD, FRCPC, DABD
Clinical Assistant Professor, Department of
  Paediatrics
University of British Columbia
Vancouver, B.C.

Gail Fernandes, NNP, MN
Neonatal Nurse Practitioner
London Health Sciences Centre
London, Ont.

Shawn George, BSc, MD, FRCPC
Medical Director, B.C. Children's Hospital
  Chieng Family Medical Day Unit
Chair, Women's Infection Control Committee
Clinical Assistant Professor, Department of
  Paediatrics
University of British Columbia
Vancouver, B.C.

Beverley Harmston, RN
Clinical Nurse Educator, Interior Health
  Authority
Trail, B.C.

Lia Harris, MD, FRCPC
Paediatrician, North Okanagan Paediatric Clinic
Vernon, B.C.

Nancy Jackson, RN, BScN
Neonatal Intensive Care Unit and former
  Transport Clinician
Children's Hospital of Eastern Ontario
Ottawa, Ont.

Ann L. Jefferies, MD, MEd, FRCPC
Neonatologist, Mount Sinai Hospital
Professor, University of Toronto
Toronto, Ont.

Anne Marie Jekyll, MD, FRCPC
General Paediatrician, B.C. Women's Hospital
  and Health Centre
Consultant Paediatrician, Spinal Cord Clinic,
  B.C. Children's Hospital
Clinical Instructor, Faculty of Medicine,
University of British Columbia
Vancouver, B.C.

Sarah Jones, MD, PhD, FRCSC
Paediatric General Surgeon, London Health
  Sciences Centre
Associate Professor, Departments of Surgery and
  Paediatrics
Schulich School of Medicine and Dentistry,
Western University
London, Ont.

Majeeda Kamaluddeen, MD, MRCP (UK), FAAP
Neonatologist, Foothills Medical Centre
Clinical Associate Professor
University of Calgary
Calgary, Alta.

Eddie Kwan, RPh, BSc Pharm, PhD
NICU pharmacist, B.C. Women's Hospital and
 Health Centre,
B.C. Children's Hospital
Vancouver, B.C.

Pascal M. Lavoie, MDCM, PhD, FRCPC
Neonatologist, B.C. Women's Hospital and
 Health Centre
Associate Professor, Paediatrics
University of British Columbia
Vancouver, B.C.

Seth D. Marks, MD, MSc, FRCPC
Associate Professor, Department of Paediatrics
 and Child Health
Section Head, Paediatric Endocrinology and
 Metabolism
Medical Director, Diabetes Education Resource
 for Children and Adolescents (DER-CA)
Associate Head, Department of Paediatrics and
 Child Health
Max Rady College of Medicine Pediatrics and
 Child Health,
University of Manitoba
Winnipeg, Man.

Douglas D. McMillan, MD, FRCPC
Professor Emeritus,
University of Calgary
Calgary, Alta.
Professor Emeritus
Dalhousie University
Halifax, N.S.

Pradeep Merchant, MBBS, MD, FRCPC
Site Chief, Division of Neonatology
The Ottawa Hospital—Civic Campus
Assistant Professor, Department of Paediatrics
University of Ottawa, Faculty of Medicine
Ottawa, Ont.

Michael R. Narvey, MD, FRCPC, FAAP
Associate Professor, Department of Paediatrics
 and Child Health
Section Head, Neonatology and Medical
 Director, Child Health Transport Team
Max Rady College of Medicine, Pediatrics and
 Child Health
University of Manitoba
Winnipeg, Man.

Eugene Ng, MD, FRCPC, FAAP
Chief, Department of Newborn and
 Developmental Paediatrics
Sunnybrook Health Sciences Centre
Associate Professor, Paediatrics, University of
 Toronto
Toronto, Ont.

Shubhayan Sanatani, BSc, MD
Head, Division of Cardiology, B.C. Children's
 Hospital
Professor, Division of Cardiology, Department of
 Paediatrics
Faculty of Medicine, University of British
 Columbia
Vancouver, B.C.

Koravangattu Sankaran, BSc, FRCPC, MB, FCCM
Department of Paediatrics, Royal University
 Hospital
Professor Emeritus, Neonatology, College of
 Medicine
University of Saskatchewan
Saskatoon, Sask.

Michael Sgro, MD, FRCPC
Chief of Paediatrics, Women's and Children's
 Health Program
St. Michael's Hospital, Unity Health Toronto
Associate Professor, Faculty of Medicine,
 University of Toronto
Associate Scientist, Li Ka Shing Knowledge
 Institute, St. Michael's Hospital
Associate Faculty, Institute of Medical Sciences,
 University of Toronto
Toronto, Ont.

Katharine L. Smart, MD, FRCPC
Community Paediatrics, Clinical Assistant
  Professor, Department of Paediatrics
University of British Columbia
Whitehorse, YT

Paul Thiessen, MD, FRCPC
Clinical Professor, Paediatrics, University of
  British Columbia
Vancouver, B.C.

**Joseph Ting, MPH, MBBS, MRCPCH,
  FRCPC, DRCOG**
Neonatologist, B.C. Women's Hospital and
  Health Centre
Clinical Associate Professor, Neonatology
University of British Columbia
Vancouver, B.C.

Mónica Villa Guillèn, MD
Medical Director, Hospital Infantil de México
  Federico Gómez
Mexico City, Mexico

Bonnie Wilkie, BPE, RN
Nurse Educator, Kelowna General Hospital
Kelowna, B.C.

***For providing radiographs,
medical photographs, and other
special elements, we are most
grateful to:***

Dr. Anna Smyth
Paediatric Radiology Fellow, B.C. Children's
  Hospital
Vancouver, B.C.

Dr. Jacob Langer
Staff Surgeon, The Hospital for
  Sick Children
Professor, Surgery, University of Toronto
Toronto, Ont.

Dr. Peter J. Murphy
Consultant in Paediatric Anesthesia
Bristol Royal Hospital for Children
Bristol, U.K.

Dr. Joseph J Tepas
Emeritus Professor of Surgery and Paediatrics
University of Florida College of Medicine
Jacksonville, Fla.

Contributors to the French edition
Geneviève H. Piuze, MD, FRCPC
Chief of Staff, Neonatology, CHU de Québec
Neonatologist, CHU de Québec Université Laval
Chair, ACoRN French language working group
Quebec City, Que.

Ahmed Moussa, MD, FRCPC
Neonatologist, CHU Sainte-Justine
President, Neonatal Resuscitation Committee
Associate Professor, Department of Paediatrics
University of Montreal
Montreal, Que.

***Participants in the 2015 ACoRN
text review***

In 2015, this book underwent a content review.
The following experts lay the groundwork for the
current edition, and we thank them for pointing
the way.

Steve Arnold, MD, FRCPC

Debbie Aylward, RN, BScN, MScN

Kirsten A. Blaine, MD

Nancy Couto, NP-Paediatrics

Marion DeLand, RNC-NIC, MN

Gail Fernandes, NNP, MN

Charlotte Foulston, MD

Lia Harris, MD, FRCPC

Adele Harrison, MD

Nancy Jackson, RN, BScN

**Majeeda Kamaluddeen, MD,
  MRCP(UK), FAAP**

Al McDougal, MD

David Price, MD

Joseph Ting, MPH, MBBS, MRCPCH, FRCPC, DRCOG

Mónica Villa Guillèn, MD

Vicky Ward, RN

Text Development and Production

Project Manager: Jackie Millette, Director, Education and Guideline Development, Canadian Paediatric Society

Coordination and editing: Jennifer Strickland, Senior Editor, Canadian Paediatric Society

Cover and special elements: John Atkinson, Fairmont House Design

Translation and review: Dominque Paré (Le bout de la langue)

Special Elements

(Tables, figures, radiographs, and text boxes)

Tables

Figures

Radiographs and ECG tracings

Chapter 3: Respiratory

Chapter 4: Cardiovascular

Chapter 6: Surgical Conditions

Transition

Educational objectives

Upon completion of this chapter, you will be able to:

- Describe normal physiological transition from fetal to neonatal life.
- Explain how disruptions during transition impact the newborn.
- Explain how transition relates to resuscitation and stabilization processes in the at-risk or unwell newborn.
- Recognize infants who are at increased risk for problems during transition.
- Apply an appropriate surveillance plan for newborns during transition.
- Identify signs and symptoms of common problems during transition.
- Anticipate possible clinical trajectories of infants during transition.

Key concepts

1. Progression through transition is influenced by gestational age (GA), intrauterine environment, absence, or progress of labour, mode of birth, and the need for resuscitation.
2. Abnormal transition is a common pathway in many at-risk or unwell infants.
3. Some aspects of transition take place at birth, such as the separation of the placenta, onset of breathing, and the switch from fetal to neonatal circulation.
4. Cardiorespiratory, neurologic, glycemic, and thermal adaptations occur over several minutes, as extrauterine life begins.
5. Endocrine, metabolic, and immunological adaptations unfold over several hours and days.
6. Delayed cord clamping helps cardiovascular stabilization by increasing the newborn's blood volume by up to 30%, with most of this volume gained in the first minute post-birth. Cord clamping before the spontaneous onset of breathing interferes with placental transfusion.
7. Early skin-to-skin care and maternal touch reduce infant stress, facilitating successful transition to extrauterine life.

'Transition' is the process of change from fetal physiology to neonatal physiology and is the single most complex and extensive process of adaptation in the human life cycle. To transition successfully, the fetus undergoes a series of adaptations as GA progresses and the time of birth approaches. When the fetus separates from the mother and takes full charge of vital functions, every organ and system is involved.

Some aspects of transition take place immediately at birth, such as the separation of the placenta, the onset of breathing, and the switch from fetal to neonatal circulation. Others occur over minutes, including the cardiorespiratory, neurologic, glycemic, and thermal adaptations upon which extrauterine life depends. Yet others unfold over several hours and days. These include endocrine, metabolic, and immunological adaptations.

Observation and support of transition is important in all births and, for most, will be minimally invasive. For other births, however, close surveillance and focused support are needed, and, for a few births, intensive care is required.

Understanding transition is essential to understanding the ACoRN approach to newborn stabilization. This chapter discusses transition from the perspective of wellness and explains how altered transition can affect at-risk or unwell newborns.

Respiratory transition

In utero, the lung is an organ without a respiratory role but is open and stable because it is fluid-filled. This fluid is produced in the lung and is distinct from the amniotic fluid. Fetal lung fluid slowly drains into the amniotic fluid as both are at a similar hydrostatic pressure.

The first stage of lung development leads to formation of the conducting airways and is completed by 16 weeks. After this time, airways elongate and widen, and the gas-exchanging portion of the lung is gradually formed and vascularized (the canalicular phase). By 20 weeks, very thin, membrane-like cells appear in the terminal airways across which gas exchange will occur after birth. These cells are called type 1 pneumocytes. At the same time, type 2 pneumocytes appear, whose role will be to produce, store, release, and recycle surfactant. The canalicular phase is critically dependent on the developing lung being fluid-filled and cyclically stretched by intermittent fetal breathing.

> Failure of the progression described here can cause **pulmonary hypoplasia**. This condition occurs when, at an early developmental stage, the fetal lung is insufficiently fluid-filled, such as in severe early oligohydramnios, or insufficiently stretched, such as in severe congenital neuromuscular disorders, or exposed to a large space-occupying mass, such as a congenital diaphragmatic hernia.

After 24 weeks, there is a gradual decrease in the interstitium that separates the air spaces, a thinning of air space walls, and a proliferation of distal saccules to support gas exchange between the lung and the circulation. At the same time, the vascular bed that will support gas exchange expands and becomes intimately integrated with the developing respiratory surface (Figure 1.1).

The distal saccules are called respiratory bronchioles and alveolar ducts. These saccules continue to mature into alveoli following birth (the alveolar phase) and achieve their 'adult' configuration at approximately 5 weeks post-birth. Alveoli provide an increased surface area for gas exchange. Lung growth continues after birth as respiratory bronchioles and alveoli proliferate.

The immature lung has fewer and less developed air sacs, has a thicker interstitial layer, and is poorly vascularized. The area for gas exchange is smaller and the blood–gas barrier is greater than in the mature lung, which has more air spaces, has a thinner interstitium, and is more vascularized. Tissues in the immature lung are less elastic and more fragile. Hyperoxia is a powerful proinflammatory stimulus in the immature lung that can impede alveolar development.

For the lung to become a respiratory organ at birth, fetal lung fluid production must stop, and existing fluid must be rapidly reabsorbed. Fetal stress and labour stimulate this process. Starting before onset of labour, endocrine adaptations involving cortisol, thyroid hormones, and catecholamines promote fetal lung fluid clearance. Labour and vaginal birth further decrease lung fluid volume. At birth, any remaining lung fluid is absorbed first into the interstitium and then into the pulmonary circulation, enhancing the circulating volume.

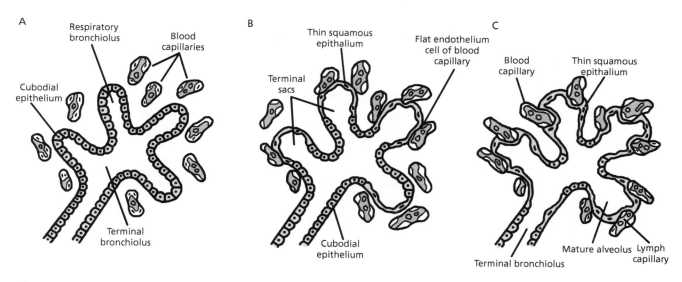

Figure 1.1. Lung development. A: In the canalicular stage (16 to 25 weeks), the cells lining the terminal airways are cuboidal and the capillary network is not in contact. B: In the saccular stage (25 to 40 weeks), cuboidal cells become very thin and closely associated with the capillary network. C: In the alveolar stage, capillaries make full contact with the alveolar membrane.

Water continues to be necessary to humidify and keep the linings of air-filled lungs healthy and functional. The natural attraction of water molecules for one another manifests as surface tension. Surface tension is the force that causes water to form droplets. In the lung, surface tension can be strong enough to cause the small respiratory airways, saccules, and alveoli to collapse. Surfactant decreases surface tension by separating water molecules. Surfactant-like activity occurs, for example, when soap stabilizes bubbles that do not form naturally in water. The air-filled lung requires surfactant production, release, and recycling to remain open and stable.

Surfactant production, release, and recycling are happening as early as 23 to 24 weeks gestation but may not be sustainable. Also, these processes may be impaired by inflammation, infection, or disruption of the respiratory lining by ventilation at any GA. In extremely premature infants, even the stretch of spontaneous breathing can impact the delicate respiratory lining of the lung.

The clinical consequence of delayed reabsorption of fetal lung fluid is called 'wet lung' or **transient tachypnea of the newborn (TTN)**.

The clinical consequence of insufficient surfactant production, release, and recycling is called **respiratory distress syndrome (RDS)**.

Surfactant production, release, and recycling can be improved by administering antenatal steroids to mothers who are likely to deliver a preterm infant within 48 h.

Surfactant production, release, and recycling may not be sustainable in prematurity or in the presence of inflammatory or infectious processes.

Meconium or amniotic fluid aspiration, or disruption of the alveolar lining caused by spontaneous breathing or mechanical ventilation, can also interfere with surfactant function.

In infants with TTN, there may be a degree of surfactant deficiency, albeit less than with RDS. This can cause an initial TTN presentation to evolve into a clinical and radiological picture consistent with RDS.

For respiratory transition to be successful at birth, the most important events are:

- Aeration—the establishment of a stable, air-filled lung,
- The establishment of ventilation of air spaces,
- The opening of the pulmonary vascular bed, and
- The matching of air space ventilation and vascular perfusion at the alveolar level.

Aeration allows the lung to stay open throughout the respiratory cycle. The volume of air present in the lung at the end of expiration is called the 'functional residual capacity' (FRC). Having air present in the air spaces at the end of expiration allows gas exchange with the pulmonary circulation to continue during expiration.

The establishment of ventilation allows for renewal of the gas in air spaces. 'Compliance' is the term that expresses the volume of air that can be mobilized with each breath for a given unit of change in pressure generated by the respiratory muscles or by supported ventilation.

Increasing respiratory rate is the infant's attempt to mobilize more volume every minute while saving the energy that would be needed to increase pressure with each breath.

Respiratory distress is observed when the respiratory muscles have to generate increased pressure while trying to mobilize the volume of air needed to maintain circulatory carbon dioxide (CO_2) within the normal range.

The opening of the pulmonary vascular bed allows the gas in air spaces to be exchanged with gases brought into the lung by circulating blood (Figure 1.2). Gas exchange is optimal when ventilation and perfusion are matched in each gas exchange unit.

When lung units are poorly expanded or ventilated, oxygen is not replenished fast enough for hemoglobin in the blood perfusing those areas to become fully saturated (Figure 1.3). Oxygenation can be normalized in this situation by improving the aeration of lung units and increasing the oxygen concentration in respiratory gases ventilating the lung.

The passage of blood through parts of the lung that are not ventilated is called 'intrapulmonary shunting' (Figure 1.4). Intrapulmonary shunting lowers the oxygen tension and oxygen saturation in the pulmonary

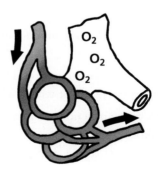

Figure 1.2. Opening of the lung and pulmonary vascular bed. In the healthy lung, alveoli are well inflated and ventilated, and the capillaries in contact with the alveoli are well perfused.
De-oxygenated blood (blue) entering to the alveolar capillary network becomes oxygenated (red) by air inside the alveolus.

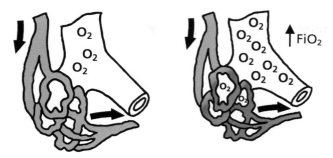

Figure 1.3. The poorly ventilated lung. With respiratory distress or respiratory failure, de-oxygenated blood (blue) entering the alveolar capillary network cannot be fully oxygenated by poorly ventilated air in the alveolus (left). Ventilation and administered oxygen can improve gas exchange as more oxygen is added to air inside the alveolus (right).

veins by mixing deoxygenated blood returning from shunted areas with oxygenated blood from matched areas. The decrease in oxygen tension and oxygen saturation in the pulmonary veins is proportional to the degree of intrapulmonary shunting. Intrapulmonary shunting can also occur when normally aerated lungs are diseased or filled with fluid (meconium, blood, or serous fluid as in pulmonary edema).

> The desaturating effect of pulmonary shunting is not influenced by administered oxygen because shunting occurs in areas where gas exchange does not occur.

Anatomically, an infant's airways and lungs are capable of sustaining life from 22 to 23 weeks GA onward, but transition is significantly impaired this early in development. Structural anomalies of the airway, neck, and chest are especially challenging because the need to breathe after birth is urgent. Congenital obstructions of the airway include rare conditions such as narrowing of the nasal passages (choanal atresia), midline cleft palate (Pierre-Robin sequence), and laryngeal and tracheal anomalies. Problems may arise in the chest, including diaphragmatic hernia, pulmonary hypoplasia, and skeletal anomalies of the chest wall. Many congenital conditions are detected antenatally, which facilitates anticipatory expert consultation before birth. A resuscitation team should be prepared for these situations.

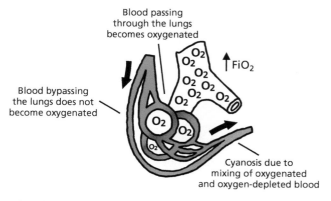

Figure 1.4. Shunting. This diagram shows blood bypassing the ventilated alveoli or the lungs altogether. Blood shunted away from ventilated alveoli cannot be oxygenated by administered oxygen. This blood mixes downstream with oxygenated blood, and downstream SpO2 depends on proportions of oxygenated versus deoxygenated blood in the mixture.

Some newborns with early respiratory difficulty may be transitioning with congenital anomalies of the head, neck, and thorax. If not diagnosed antenatally, these conditions may be unexpected causes of abnormal transition.

Abnormalities of respiratory transition are the most common destabilizing conditions in newborns. Respiratory illnesses are discussed in detail in Chapter 3, Respiratory.

Cardiovascular transition

Profound changes in the cardiovascular system occur during transition (Figure 1.5). The placenta's role as the source of fetal gas exchange and nutrition ends, the pulmonary vascular bed opens, and the

(A)

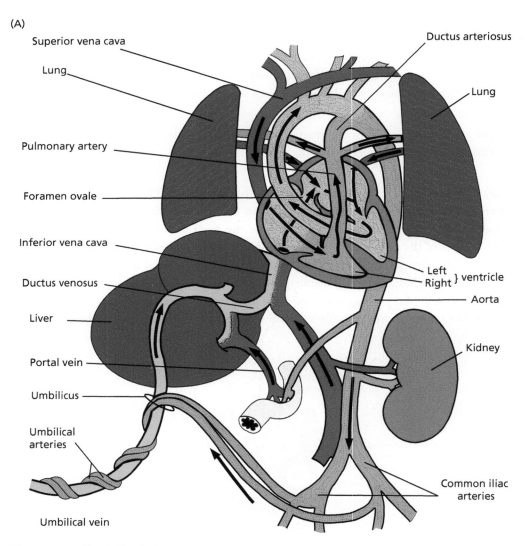

Figure 1.5. Fetal circulation.

Reprinted from Education in Anaesthesia, Critical Care and Pain 5. Peter J Murphy. The fetal circulation:107–12, 2005. With permission.

circulation converts from in-parallel to in-series. The total cardiac output nearly doubles during this process, increasing blood flow to the lungs, heart, kidneys, and gastrointestinal tract to meet higher basal metabolism, the work of breathing, and thermogenesis.

In the fetus, there is high vascular pressure within the nondistended lungs and low vascular pressure systemically, due to the large, compliant vascular bed of the placenta. This pressure difference causes blood in the fetus to be preferentially shunted away from the lungs.

The placenta is the organ of gas exchange in the fetus, which is why blood in the umbilical vein has the highest oxygen saturation in the fetus. Relatively well-oxygenated blood from the placenta flows through the umbilical cord and ductus venosus to the right atrium via the inferior vena cava. This oxygenated blood flow is under higher pressure than the fetal systemic return and streams into the right atrium separately from desaturated systemic venous blood. At least 25% of this oxygenated blood crosses the foramen ovale into the left atrium, where it mixes with the small

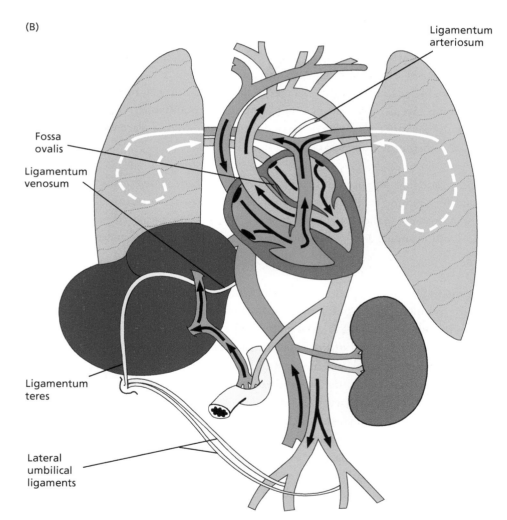

Figure 1.5. Neonatal circulation.

Reprinted from Education in Anaesthesia, Critical Care and Pain 5. Peter J Murphy. The fetal circulation:107–12, 2005. With permission

amount of blood returning from the fetal lungs. The normal oxygen saturation (SpO2) of blood in the fetal left atrium is about 65%. Of the blood ejected from the left ventricle, 60% reaches the coronaries and the brain.

The other 75% of placental blood that does not stream into the left atrium mixes with fetal venous return in the right atrium, flows to the right ventricle and then into the pulmonary artery. Most of this blood bypasses the lungs by exiting through the ductus arteriosus; it then mixes with blood from the left ventricle to reach the lower body and return to the placenta. The ductus arteriosus is kept open in the fetus by low oxygen tension and high levels of circulating prostaglandins, primarily produced by the placenta. Thus, both ventricles contribute to the systemic blood flow during fetal life, with the right ventricle contributing 60% of the combined cardiac output. The fetus's circulation depends on connections between the systemic and pulmonary circuits via the foramen ovale and ductus arteriosus. The right ventricle predominates in the fetus, with most of its output entering the descending aorta via the ductus arteriosus.

How much oxygen reaches the tissues is determined by cardiac output, hemoglobin concentration, and hemoglobin saturation. Because hemoglobin saturation is low in the fetus, high cardiac output and hemoglobin concentrations are needed to meet oxygen requirements. Also, fetal hemoglobin is able to carry more oxygen at lower tension than adult hemoglobin. During labour, the human fetus tolerates oxygen saturations as low as 30% without developing acidosis.

After birth, two major factors trigger changes in the circulation. The first is initiation of breathing, with lung expansion, alveolar gas exchange, and opening of the pulmonary vascular bed, which causes pulmonary vascular resistance to drop. The second factor is removal of placental circulation, caused by cessation of flow through the umbilical cord.

Delayed cord clamping supports cardiovascular stabilization by allowing the transfusion of placental blood to continue while pulmonary circulation capacity increases. Placental transfusion increases blood volume in the newly born by up to 30%, with the greatest gains in the first minute after birth. Cord clamping before the spontaneous onset of breathing interferes with placental transfusion.

Clamping the umbilical cord drastically reduces blood return to the right atrium as placental flow ceases. Capacity and filling of the pulmonary circulation increase with the onset of breathing, as does blood return to the left atrium and left atrial pressure. The latter, coupled with increasing systemic (left-sided) pressure caused by removal of the low-resistance placental vascular bed, forces the flap of the foramen ovale up against the atrial wall, functionally closing it. The foramen ovale can reopen, however, in clinical conditions where right atrial pressure exceeds left atrial pressure.

These same changes to pulmonary and systemic pressure immediately after birth also reduce flow from the pulmonary artery through the ductus arteriosus to the descending aorta. At the same time, the ductus arteriosus constricts and functionally closes due to increasing oxygen tension with onset of breathing and elimination of the placenta as the primary source of prostaglandin, which maintained ductal patency during fetal life. This process is followed by full anatomic closure, which converts the ductus arteriosus into a fibrous ligament (the ligamentum arteriosus) over the next several days or weeks.

Initiation of breathing and lung expansion at birth gradually increases pre-ductal saturation in term infants, from an in utero value of about 65% to about 90% by 5 to 10 min of age (see Figure 1.6).

Pre-ductal saturation, measured by pulse oximetry in the newborn's right hand or wrist, reflects the SpO2 of blood coming from the lungs plus any residual right-to-left shunting still occurring through the foramen ovale.

The left subclavian artery rises from the area of the aortic arch where the ductus arteriosus inserts. That is why the left hand or wrist SpO2 can reflect the pre-ductal, post-ductal, or mixed blood.

A rapid rise in pre-ductal SpO2 indicates that ventilation, lung stability, pulmonary circulation, and increased pulmonary flow are being established at the right pace in the healthy lung. Rapid rise also indicates that, as pulmonary venous return has increased, right-to-left flow through the foramen ovale has become minimal.

Post-ductal saturation, best measured in the feet, reflects the SpO2 of blood in the descending aorta plus residual right-to-left shunting still occurring at ductal level.

The mixing of deoxygenated blood from a right-to-left shunt through the open ductus arteriosus in early transition is reflected in a post-ductal SpO2 that is lower than the pre-ductal SpO2. Thus, it is normal for the rise in post-ductal SpO2 to lag behind the rise in pre-ductal SpO2 during the first 20 to 30 min post-delivery (Figure 1.6). When the post-ductal SpO2 continues to be lower than the pre-ductal SpO2, this may indicate persistently high pulmonary artery pressures.

Abnormal cardiovascular transition may indicate the presence of a congenital cardiovascular abnormality. Such conditions are discussed in detail in Chapter 4, Cardiovascular.

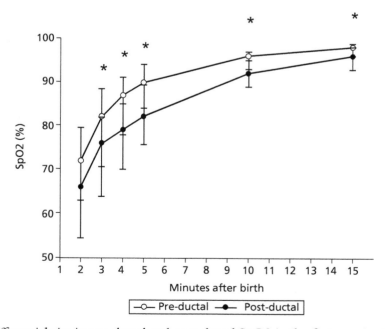

Figure 1.6. Differential rise in pre-ductal and post-ductal SpO2 in the first 15 minutes post-birth.

Source: Mariani G, Dik PB, Ezquer A, et al. Pre-ductal and post-ductal O2 saturation in healthy term neonates after birth. J Pediatr 2007;150(4):418–21. With permission.

Neurobehavioural transition

The most immediate and critical neurobehavioural transition in newborns is the establishment of regular breathing. Breathing requires coordinated respiratory activity in response to mechanical and chemical receptors. A healthy brain and respiratory system maintain tight control on both blood pH and carbon dioxide levels through normal breathing activity.

Failure to initiate breathing, either spontaneously or despite stimulation, occurs when the central nervous system (CNS) is depressed at birth. This is the most common reason for neonatal resuscitation at birth.

Respiratory drive is usually strong at the time of birth. Conditions that affect respiratory drive, such as prematurity, maternal medications, or fetal illness, may impede this critical neurobehavioural transition.

To ensure a normal neurobehavioural transition, healthy newborns should be skin-to-skin with their mothers for at least 1 h following birth. Routine medical and nursing interventions, such as weighing and vitamin K therapy, should be deferred.

During transition, infants are increasingly able to integrate and modulate neurobehaviours in a process referred to as 'self-regulation'. Self-regulation develops in the womb and throughout the birth process but is especially challenged in the first hours and days after birth. Balanced regulation of motor activity and state control appear to depend more on environmental stimuli than on specific cardiac and respiratory adjustments, and both domains are highly sensitive to maternal facilitation.

Well newborns have normal sleep–wake states and respond appropriately to the environment and handling. They show normal tone and activity, with no abnormal movements. When they are wakened, disturbed, or cry, they settle with comfort or feeding. Skin-to-skin care and parental voice and touch reduce infant stress. Signs of normal regulation include smooth, flexed movements, increasing quiet (versus active) sleep, less extensor movement, improving synchronization of motor and state subsystems, and lower cortisol levels.

Newborns showing suboptimal regulation may be hypo- or hyper-responsive to stimulation, lethargic, irritable, or have high or low tone or abnormal movements. These infants need careful observation and formal assessment.

Two-thirds of healthy newborns have fine tremors during periods of alertness and when startled, crying, or upset. Most tremors are benign and disappear by day 3. Tremors can also be caused by CNS disorders or metabolic conditions, especially when they are frequent or pronounced. Tremors and other abnormal movements are discussed in Chapter 5, Neurology.

Feeding transition

In utero, the healthy fetus swallows significant quantities of amniotic fluid, which is digested and absorbed by the gut. Healthy newborns have coordinated suck-swallow-breathe mechanisms from birth and are neurobehaviourally ready for breastfeeding during the first hour of skin-to-skin care.

During initial feeding, the breast produces colostrum, a protein-rich nutrient that promotes healthy gut and immune function. Regular breastfeeding happens on cue with increasing frequency over the first few days post-birth, with the production of breast milk after 2 to 3 days. Healthy infants do not require supplementation.

Breastfeeding promotes gut motility, and the first stool, consisting of dark green or black meconium, is produced by 24 to 36 h. As the infant ingests colostrum, then breast milk, stool colour lightens, and consistency normalizes. Failure to pass meconium by 48 h of age requires evaluation.

A number of conditions requiring surgery can interfere with normal feeding transition and will be discussed in Chapter 6, Surgical Conditions.

Glycemic transition

For most of gestation, fetal glucose concentrations are about two-thirds of maternal glucose levels, with a lower limit of approximately 3 mmol/L. Although the fetal liver is capable of gluconeogenesis from early gestation, the fetus does not produce glucose during normal homeostasis. Rather, fetal energy needs are supported primarily by the transplacental transfer of glucose, amino acids, free fatty acids, ketones, and glycerol. As term gestation approaches, glucose and other substrates are stored increasingly as glycogen and fat, in response to high insulin-like factors and low glucagon levels in the fetus.

When flow in the umbilical cord ceases, so does the newborn's glucose supply from the mother, causing a physiological dip in glucose levels. This glucose 'trough' is normal in healthy infants but can be of concern in those who are born unwell or at risk. In healthy newborns, the glucose trough triggers counter-regulation and a subsequent rise in glucose levels. This return to normal glucose levels is essential for healthy brain function and development.

Counter-regulation also includes the following metabolic processes:

- Making new glucose from internal sources (glycogenolysis and gluconeogenesis)
- Using alternative fuels as substrate for brain metabolism (lactate, ketones, amino acids, and fatty acids)
- Lowering the utilization of glucose by the body in response to limited availability

Healthy newborns with no risk factors do not need glucose monitoring.

Counter-regulation raises a newborn's glucose level in the first few hours after birth and ensures successful transition. In healthy term infants, the lowest point in blood glucose (BG) levels occurs at 1 to 2 h of age. By 2 to 4 h of age, BG recovers to late gestation levels. Glucose values achieve adult levels by 72 h of age (Figure 1.7).

Hepatic glycogen stores are a rapid, ready source of glucose for the newborn's first hours of extrauterine life. However, evidence suggests that even in well term infants, this source provides sufficient glucose for only the first 10 h post-delivery. The next pathway for maintaining glucose homeostasis involves gluconeogenesis (making glucose using fatty acids, glycerol, amino acids, and lactate) and ketogenesis (making ketones from fatty acids). Gluconeogenesis is supported by glucagon and counter-regulatory hormones, growth hormone, and cortisol and is established by 4 to 6 h of age.

Counter-regulation is a critical adaptation that almost never fails in healthy newborns. However, at-risk, unwell, or premature newborns may not be able to mobilize these systems effectively or in as sustained a manner and are at greater risk for disrupted glucose homeostasis and hypoglycemia. Newborns of diabetic mothers who had trouble controlling their glucose during pregnancy are at risk for high insulin levels, stimulated by elevated circulating BG in utero. After birth, these high insulin levels may persist and are associated with hypoglycemia. Preterm and small for GA infants may have minimal glycogen and fat stores, such that energy substrates during transition can be

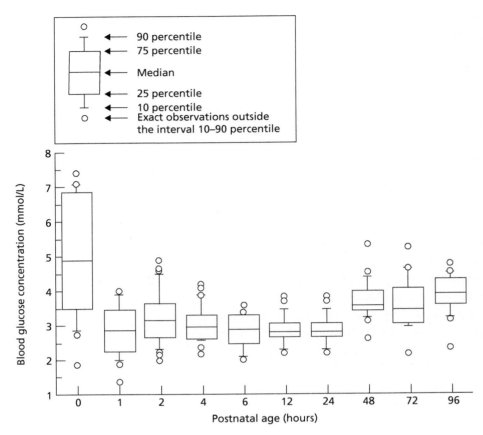

Figure 1.7. Blood glucose concentration in the first 96 h post-birth.

Source: Hoseth E, Joergensen A, Ebbeson F, Moeller M. Blood glucose levels in a population of healthy, breastfed, term infants of appropriate size for gestational age. Arch Dis Child Fetal Neonatal Ed 2000;83(2):F117–9. Reprinted with permission.

severely challenged. They may need an intravenous (IV) infusion of glucose to prevent or treat hypoglycemia.

> Hypoglycemia must be anticipated in at-risk infants, but not all will develop low BG. Nor will all newborns with transient hypoglycemia need IV fluids or transfer to intensive care. However, infants with hypoglycemia who do not respond to initial care must be recognized early and managed effectively in a specialized nursery. A stepwise approach to stabilization and care is described in Chapter 7, Fluid and Glucose.

Renal transition

Human kidney development starts at 5 weeks of gestation. Primitive glomeruli appear at approximately 9 weeks, and nephrogenesis is complete by 32 to 35 weeks. The number of nephrons does not increase following birth.

During pregnancy, fetal fluid homeostasis is maintained by the bidirectional exchange between mother and fetus, through the placenta. Urine production begins between the 10th and 12th week and increases throughout gestation, reaching 10 mL/h to 20 mL/h at term. Because water is exchanged freely with the mother, there is no need for renal concentrative function in the fetus.

An important role of fetal renal excretory function is its contribution to amniotic fluid production, of which fetal urine is the main component. Surrounding amniotic fluid allows the fetus to move as muscle and bone develop, and aids lung development by slowing drainage of fetal lung fluid and making room for fetal breathing.

While premature rupture of membranes is the most common cause of severe oligohydramnios (insufficient amniotic fluid), other causes include renal dysplasia or agenesis, polycystic kidneys, urinary tract obstruction, and fetal renal compromise secondary to maternal medication exposure. Early, severe oligohydramnios may lead to fetal demise, musculoskeletal abnormalities (e.g., facial distortion, club foot), pulmonary hypoplasia, and intrauterine growth restriction. Later complications include umbilical cord compression.

Common causes of polyhydramnios (excessive amniotic fluid) are maternal diabetes leading to fetal hyperglycemia and polyuria, fetal gastrointestinal obstruction, CNS or neuromuscular diseases that impede swallowing of amniotic fluid, or conditions leading to hydrops fetalis. In twin-to-twin transfusion syndrome, the amniotic fluid volume may be higher in the recipient twin and lower in the donor.

At term birth, total body water is mostly extracellular fluid and comprises 75% of the newborn's weight. Because of the free passage of small chemical particles across the placenta, electrolyte and creatinine levels at time of birth reflect maternal values. In the immediate postnatal period, normal urine output is about 1 mL/kg/h, but infants may not void until 12 to 24 h of age. By day 3, diuresis is common, with output reaching 5 mL/kg/h to 7 mL/kg/h. Urine output then decreases to reflect fluid intake. Total body water decreases in the first days post-birth, due to minimal fluid intake and a rising glomerular filtration rate. This process results in a physiologically normal weight loss of 5% to 10% in term newborns and, typically, somewhat more in premature newborns.

While glomerular and tubular function in newborns is low compared with older children and adults, a term infant's kidneys are well equipped to manage homeostasis and sustain normal development and maturation from the moment of birth. Specifically, the concentrating capacity of the kidneys increases as the renal gradient of osmolarity becomes established in the first days post-birth.

The newborn kidney's ability to adapt to hypovolemia, hypotension, or fluid overload is limited. Similarly, it is difficult for newborn kidneys to adapt to hypoxemia or exposure to nephrotoxic medications, such as aminoglycosides, especially before 32 to 35 weeks gestation, when nephrogenesis is still incomplete.

Healthy renal transition is facilitated by exclusive breastfeeding, which provides the optimal balance of water, sodium, potassium, phosphorus, and other nutrients. In unwell infants, fluid and nutrient intake needs careful monitoring.

The kidneys also manage acid-base balance in well newborns. Healthy term infants have bicarbonate levels of 20 mEq/L to 24 mEq/L. These levels can fall as low as 14 mEq/L in premature infants. All newborns have limited ability to tolerate metabolic stress, and they can easily develop metabolic acidosis when unwell.

Disease states, fluid administration, and drug therapy can impact acid-base balance significantly, leading to acidosis or alkalosis.

Hepatic transition

Bilirubin is a naturally occurring, orange-yellow pigment made during the breakdown of hemoglobin, a process that starts in the spleen as red blood cells are broken down by macrophages. Unconjugated bilirubin is the initial fraction of bilirubin, and it circulates, bound to albumin, in blood. In the fetus, the placenta is the main excretory pathway for unconjugated bilirubin.

After birth, the infant's liver must deal with circulating unconjugated bilirubin (Figure 1.8). The newborn has a naturally high bilirubin load because of overproduction, due to a large red cell mass and a reduced red cell lifespan. In some newborns, hemolytic conditions may accelerate red cell breakdown and turnover. Bilirubin is conjugated in the liver, such that it can be added

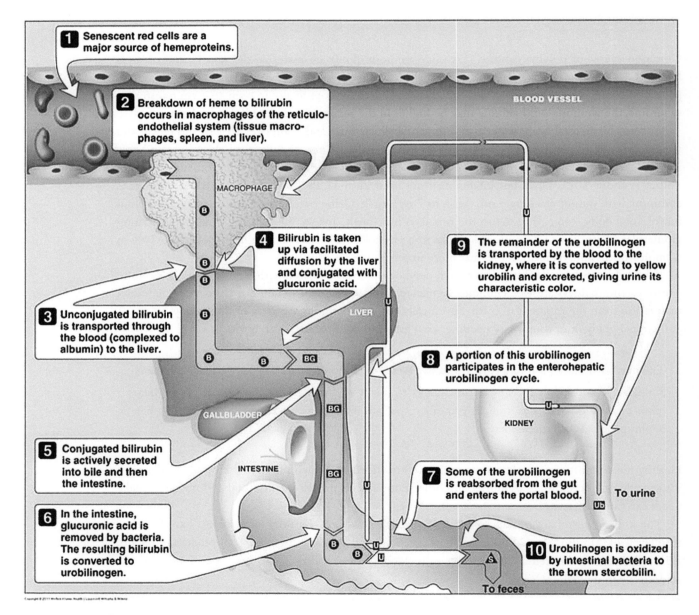

Figure 1.8. Bilirubin excretion pathway.

Source: Ferrier D (ed.). Lippincott Illustrated Reviews: Biochemistry, 5th edition. Used with permission.

to bile and excreted into the small bowel. 'Enterohepatic' circulation of bilirubin allows it to be reabsorbed and excreted again in different chemical forms. In well infants, this process facilitates excretion and gives stool its natural colour. However, infants who have difficulty feeding are at risk for high bilirubin levels, and very pale stools may indicate liver disease. Preterm infants are especially vulnerable to high levels of bilirubin because enzyme activity in their livers cannot conjugate bilirubin efficiently.

In excess concentrations, unconjugated bilirubin is neurotoxic. Certain drugs, such as sulphonamides and salicylates, will displace bilirubin from albumin, increasing risk for toxicity. Illnesses that threaten the blood–brain barrier, such as sepsis or acidosis, may further increase risk for toxicity. Acute bilirubin encephalopathy (ABE) is the acute neurologic manifestation of bilirubin toxicity. Kernicterus, the chronic sequela of ABE, is a serious condition associated with permanent neurological damage. Factors that increase risk for kernicterus are discussed in Chapter 8, Jaundice. The clinical manifestation of raised bilirubin levels (hyperbilirubinemia) is 'jaundice'. Jaundice is present in up to two-thirds of healthy newborns, making detection of pathological jaundice a continual challenge.

> Difficulty feeding and dehydration, often associated with a greater than 10% to 15% weight loss, may contribute to toxic bilirubin levels. This relationship is clinically important and is discussed in Chapter 8, Jaundice.

Much less commonly, the conjugated fraction of bilirubin becomes elevated post-birth. This is called 'cholestatic jaundice'. Cholestatic jaundice may be seen when there is excessive bilirubin load, such as in hemolytic diseases (e.g., erythroblastosis fetalis), or in hepatocellular injury from toxic, infectious, or metabolic causes, or in bile flow obstruction (e.g., biliary atresia). Conjugated bilirubin concentrations greater than 18 μmol/L, or 20% of the total serum bilirubin concentration, warrant further investigation. Infants with stool that is pale yellow, chalky white, or clay-coloured need investigation. These are warning signs of biliary atresia, a life-threatening liver disease presenting in the first month of life. Early intervention is critical for infants with this diagnosis.

> Counsel parents to be alert to their infant's stool colour during the first month post-birth. If stools are pale or clay-coloured, or a parent is concerned about stool colour, the infant should be assessed by a physician.

Thermal transition

Fetal body temperature is about 0.5°C above maternal temperature. Although the fetus produces heat from metabolism, this heat disperses across the placenta and fetal membranes. The thermogenic response potential develops during late gestation, with increasing brown adipose tissue around the kidneys and interscapular areas of the back. Brown adipose tissue comprises about 1% of fetal weight at term.

At birth, cardiorespiratory changes and cold stimulus to the skin activate thermogenesis in brown adipose tissue. Brown adipose tissue generates heat by uncoupling oxidative metabolism from adenosine triphosphate synthesis in the mitochondria, with the release of heat. This process is modulated by the same hormones that modulate the fetal preparation for birth and the transition period. Infants born preterm may not have developed enough brown adipose tissue to protect against cold stress. Term infants can generate some additional heat by shivering thermogenesis, a mechanism which increases skeletal muscle activity but is of secondary importance as a heat source in newborns.

Four basic concurrent mechanisms cause heat loss (or gain) in newborns through environmental transfer (Figure 1.9):

- Conduction: Through direct contact with cold (or warm) surfaces
- Convection: As air currents draw heat from the body
- Evaporation: As skin loses heat when water molecules change from liquid to a gaseous state
- Radiation: Through thermal waves to a colder surface (e.g., a wall or window) or from a heat source (e.g., a radiant warmer)

Preterm newborns are more susceptible to heat loss through evaporation. Transepidermal water loss through evaporation correlates inversely with GA. For example, infants born at 25 weeks lose 15 times more water than term infants, because their skin is thinner than a term newborn's skin. In low birth weight and preterm infants, evaporative heat loss is the main form of heat loss during the first week of life.

> When infant condition allows, skin-to-skin care minimizes cold stress and facilitates thermal transition.

All at-risk or unwell infants are vulnerable to thermal stress and require close monitoring and care, as described in Chapter 9, Thermoregulation.

(A) (B)

(C) (D)

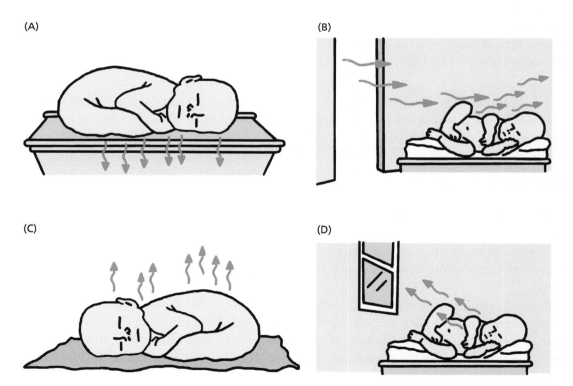

Figure 1.9. Mechanisms of heat loss. (A) Conduction; (B) Convection; (C) Evaporation; (D) Radiation.

Immunological transition

The immune system includes innate and adaptive immune components. Innate immunity refers to non-specific defence mechanisms, including physical barriers (such as skin), certain chemicals in the blood, and immune system cells that can recognize and attack pathogenic micro-organisms.

The fetal and neonatal immune systems function to:

- Protect against infection,
- Mediate the transition between the relatively sterile intrauterine environment and the foreign, antigen-rich environment of the outside world, and
- Avoid potentially harmful reactions against maternal (alloimmune) and fetal (autoimmune) factors, a process known as 'immunological tolerance'.

The fetal innate immune system is biased toward anti-inflammatory or tolerogenic responses. After birth, however, there is an age-dependent maturation of the immune response as the neonatal skin and gut are rapidly colonized with microbial flora. Newborns are exposed to environmental and commensal bacteria in natural settings:

- By exposure to vaginal bacteria in labour,
- By passage through the birth canal,
- By skin-to-skin contact with parents, and
- By breastfeeding and consuming colostrum.

Breast milk contains diverse immunological factors that modulate the inflammatory response and help to establish beneficial intestinal flora. There is increasing evidence that the overall load and type of bacteria in a newborn's gut influence health in later life, including risk of early-onset infections, abnormal gut function, and allergic status. Breast milk is associated with a diminished risk of subsequent atopy.

Immunological challenges during transition include:

- Maternal infections
- Antibiotic exposure before or after birth
- Delayed skin-to-skin contact
- Provision of oxygen or mechanical ventilation
- Medical and nursing interventions that risk colonization with pathogens or break the skin (e.g., blood tests or IV cannulae)
- Artificial nutrition and nutritional supplements
- Neonatal infections

In the first days post-birth, about one-half of newborns develop a prominent but transitory rash, characterized by small erythematous papules, often surrounded by a diffuse erythematous halo, known as 'erythema toxicum neonatorum'. Emerging evidence indicates that this rash is caused by reaction of neonatal skin to commensal flora, in particular Gram-positive staphylococci that colonize the skin and often penetrate into hair follicles. At rash sites, neonatal macrophages produce an acute-phase response triggering hepatocyte production of plasma proteins, such as C-reactive protein, which have roles in the clearance and detoxification of microbes and microbial toxins.

Neonatal intestinal function and immunity is altered by the use of non-human milk formula, especially in the premature infant. And while processing human breast milk (e.g., by freezing or pasteurization) is sometimes necessary to avoid the transmission of infection, it can alter its immunological properties significantly.

The transition in the human life cycle from dependent fetus to independent newborn is complex and involves all body systems. This chapter highlighted the most important changes. Knowledge of transition is crucial to assessing and, if necessary, resuscitating and stabilizing the neonate. It is the foundation on which ACoRN is based.

Transition: Review

1. **Delayed cord clamping:**
   - ☐ Interferes with cardiovascular stabilization, because it may drain the infant's blood into the placenta.
   - ☐ Should be delayed for at least 5 min to facilitate transition.
   - ☐ Should precede the onset of breathing.
   - ☐ May overload the pulmonary circulation, especially as the infant is transitioning from intrauterine life.
   - ☐ Increases blood volume in the newly born by up to 30%, due to placental transfusion.

2. **A pre-ductal saturation (SpO2) is measured by pulse oximetry on the infant's:**
   - ☐ Right hand or wrist.
   - ☐ Right foot.
   - ☐ Left hand or wrist.
   - ☐ Left foot.

3. **A normal rise in pre-ductal SpO2 indicates that the following are being established at the right pace in the healthy lung. Tick all that apply.**
   - ☐ Ventilation.
   - ☐ Splanchnic circulation.
   - ☐ Increased pulmonary blood flow.
   - ☐ Increased cerebral blood flow.

4. **Which statements relating to neurobehavioural transition are correct? Tick all that apply.**
   - ☐ The most immediate and critical neurobehavioural transition in newborns is the establishment of regular breathing.
   - ☐ Failure to initiate breathing is not a common reason for neonatal resuscitation at birth.
   - ☐ Early skin-to-skin care and maternal touch reduce infant stress.
   - ☐ Healthy newborns often exhibit fine tremors during periods of alertness and when startled, crying, or upset.

5. **An infant born vaginally, at term, in the presence of meconium, is grunting at 20 min of age. He has good tone and is only crying intermittently. He is being cuddled skin-to-skin by his mother, under a dry towel, in a low-lit room. Tick the next appropriate care steps.**
   - ☐ Administer oxygen to improve saturations.
   - ☐ Administer CPAP to facilitate lung aeration and maintain adequate end-expiratory volume.
   - ☐ Take the infant to the radiant warmer to facilitate observation.
   - ☐ Initiate breastfeeding, to settle him.
   - ☐ Perform pre-ductal oximetry to obtain saturations.

6. **When cord clamping removes the maternal glucose supply, maintaining an adequate blood glucose concentration is essential. Neurological compromise can occur if the brain is deprived of glucose. Tick all statements that apply.**
   - ☐ Adequate BG levels are achieved by a process known as 'counter-regulation'.
   - ☐ New glucose is made from internal sources through glycogenolysis and gluconeogenesis.
   - ☐ Alternative fuels used as substrate for brain metabolism include lactate, ketones, amino acids, and fatty acids.
   - ☐ Insulin is the main hormone supporting a gradual rise in serum BG in the first few hours post-birth.
   - ☐ Glucagon is a catabolic hormone, and its rise at birth can have negative consequences for the newborn.

7. **Conjugated bilirubin is produced by the liver and excreted in bile. Tick all statements that apply.**
   - ☐ Elevated serum conjugated bilirubin is common in infants.
   - ☐ Parents should be alert to their infant's stool colour during the first month.
   - ☐ Early assessment by a physician is urgent for babies whose stool is an abnormal colour.
   - ☐ Biliary atresia is a life-threatening liver disease that presents in the first month of age and is the most common cause of liver transplantation in childhood.

8. **All infants are at risk for developing cold stress. Four mechanisms cause heat loss (or gain) in newborns through environmental transfer. Match each mechanism with its correct definition.**

   a. Conduction   ____ Heat transfer through thermal waves to a colder surface, such as a wall or window, or from a warm source, such as a radiant warmer.

   b. Convection   ____ Transfer of heat to water molecules during transition from liquid to gas.

   c. Evaporation   ____ Transfer of heat to air currents.

   d. Radiation   ____ Direct transfer of heat to a cold (or from a warm) surface.

9. **Challenges to the neonatal immune system during transition include: (Tick all that apply.)**
   ☐ Maternal infections
   ☐ Antibiotic exposure before or after birth
   ☐ Delayed skin-to-skin contact
   ☐ Provision of oxygen or mechanical ventilation
   ☐ Interventions that can introduce pathogens or break the skin (e.g., blood tests or intravenous cannulae)
   ☐ Artificial nutrition and nutritional supplements
   ☐ Invasive neonatal infections

Bibliography

Alvaro R, Rigatt H. Breathing in fetal life and onset and control of breathing in the neonate. In: Polin RA, Abman SH, Rowitch DH, Benitz WE, Fox WW, eds. Fetal and Neonatal Physiology, 5th ed. Philadelphia, PA: Elsevier; 2017.

Baldwin HS, Dees E. Embryology and physiology of the cardiovascular system. In: Gleason CA, Devaskar SU. Avery's Diseases of the Newborn, 9th ed. Philadelphia, PA: Elsevier/Saunders; 2012.

Bhatt S, Alison BJ, Wallace EM, et al. Delaying cord clamping until ventilation onset improves cardiovascular function at birth in preterm lambs. J Physiol 2013;591(8):2113–26.

Botwinski CA, Falco GA. Transition to postnatal renal function. J Perinat Neonatal Nurs 2014;28(2):150–4.

DiFiore JW, Wilson JM. Lung development. Semin Pediatr Surg 1994;3(4):221–32.

Gregory GA, Kitterman JA, Phibbs RH, Tooley WH, Hamilton WK. Treatment of the idiopathic respiratory-distress syndrome with continuous positive airway pressure. N Engl J Med 1971;284(24):1333–40.

Harding R, Hooper SB. Regulation of lung expansion and lung growth before birth. J Appl Physiol (1985) 1996;81(1):209–24.

Hillman NH, Kallapur SG, Jobe AH. Physiology of transition from intrauterine to extrauterine life. Clin Perinatol 2012;39(4):769–83.

Hoseth E, Joergensen A, Ebbeson F, Moeller M. Blood glucose levels in a population of healthy, breastfed, term infants of appropriate size for gestational age. Arch Dis Child Fetal Neonatal Ed 2000;83(2):F117–9.

Kiserud T, Haugen G. Umbilical circulation. In: Polin RA, Abman SH, Rowitch DH, Benitz WE, Fox WW, eds. Fetal and Neonatal Physiology, 5th ed. Philadelphia, PA: Elsevier; 2017.

Kumar S. Fetal and placental physiology. In: Bennett P, Williamson C, eds. Basic Science in Obstetrics and Gynaecology, 4th ed. Edinburgh, UK: Churchill Livingstone/Elsevier; 2010.

Lindower JB. Water balance in the fetus and neonate. Semin Fetal Neonatal Med 2017;22(2):71–5.

Lumb AB. Applied physiology: Pregnancy, neonates and children. In: Lumb AB. Nunn's Applied Respiratory Physiology, 8th ed. Edinburgh, UK: Elsevier; 2017.

Mariani G, Dik PB, Ezquer A, et al. Pre-ductal and post-ductal O2 saturation in healthy term neonates after birth. J Pediatr 2007;150(4):418–21.

McDonald SJ, Middleton P, Dowswell T, Morris PS. Effect of timing of umbilical cord clamping of term infants on maternal and neonatal outcomes. Cochrane Database Syst Rev 2013(7):CD004074.

Merklin RJ. Growth and distribution of human fetal brown fat. Anat Rec 1974;178(3):637–45.

Murphy PJ. The fetal circulation. Continuing Education in Anaesthesia, Critical Care and Pain 2005;5(4):107–12.

Polglase GR, Dawson JA, Kluckow M, et al. Ventilation onset prior to umbilical cord clamping (physiological-based cord clamping) improves systemic and cerebral oxygenation in preterm lambs. PLoS One 2015;10(2):e0117504.

Power G, Blood A. Thermoregulation. In: Polin R, Fox W, Abman S, eds. Fetal and Neonatal Physiology, 4th ed. Philadelphia, PA: Saunders/Elsevier; 2011.

Noori S, Seri I, Stavroudis TA. Principles of developmental cardiovascular physiology and pathophysiology. In: Kleinman CS, Seri I, eds. Hemodynamics and Cardiology: Neonatology Questions and Controversies, 2nd ed. Philadelphia, PA: Saunders/Elsevier; 2012.

Segar JL. Renal adaptive changes and sodium handling in the fetal-to-newborn transition. Semin Fetal Neonatal Med 2017;22(2):76–82.

Schoenwolf GC, Bleyl SB, Brauer PR, Francis-West PH. Human Embryology, 5th ed. Philadelphia, PA: Churchill Livingstone/Elsevier; 2015.

Sulemanji M, Vakili K. Neonatal renal physiology. Semin Pediatr Surg 2013;22(4):195–8.

Tourneur E, Chassin C. Neonatal immune adaptation of the gut and its role during infections. Clin Dev Immunol 2013;270301.

Ward Platt M, Deshpande S. Metabolic adaptation at birth. Semin Fetal Neonatal Med 2005;10(4):341–50.

What-when-how: In-depth tutorials and information. Care of the Normal Newborn (Maternal and Newborn Nursing) Part 1: http://what-when-how.com/nursing/care-of-the-normal-newborn-maternal-and-newborn-nursing-part-1/ (Accessed March 5, 2019).

Whitsett JA, Weaver TE. Hydrophobic surfactant proteins in lung function and disease. N Engl J Med 2002;347(26):2141–8.

Answer key: Transition

1. **Delayed cord clamping:**
   - ☐ Interferes with cardiovascular stabilization, because it may drain the infant's blood into the placenta.
   - ☐ Should be delayed for at least 5 min to facilitate transition.
   - ☐ Should precede the onset of breathing.
   - ☐ May overload the pulmonary circulation, especially as the infant is transitioning from intrauterine life.
   - ✓ Increases blood volume in the newly born by up to 30%, due to placental transfusion.

2. **A pre-ductal saturation (SpO2) is measured by pulse oximetry on the infant's:**
   - ✓ Right hand or wrist.
   - ☐ Right foot.
   - ☐ Left hand or wrist.
   - ☐ Left foot.

3. **A normal rise in pre-ductal SpO2 indicates that the following are being established at the right pace in the healthy lung.**
   - ✓ Ventilation
   - ☐ Splanchnic circulation
   - ✓ Increased pulmonary blood flow
   - ☐ Increased cerebral blood flow

4. **Which statements relating to neurobehavioural transition are correct?**
   ✓ The most immediate and critical neurobehavioural transition in newborns is the establishment of regular breathing.
   ☐ Failure to initiate breathing is not a common reason for neonatal resuscitation at birth.
   ✓ Early skin-to-skin care and maternal touch reduce infant stress.
   ✓ Healthy newborns often exhibit fine tremors during periods of alertness, and when startled, crying, or upset.

5. **An infant born vaginally, at term, in the presence of meconium, is grunting at 20 min of age. He has good tone and is only crying intermittently. He is being cuddled skin-to-skin by his mother, under a dry towel, in a low-lit room. Tick the next appropriate care steps.**
   ☐ Administer oxygen to improve saturations.
   ☐ Administer CPAP to facilitate lung aeration and maintain adequate end-expiratory volume.
   ✓ Take the infant to the radiant warmer to facilitate observation.
   ☐ Initiate breastfeeding, to settle him.
   ✓ Perform pre-ductal oximetry to obtain saturations.

6. **When cord clamping removes the maternal glucose supply, maintaining an adequate blood glucose concentration is essential. Neurological compromise can occur if the brain is deprived of glucose. Tick all statements that apply.**
   ✓ Adequate BG levels are achieved by a process known as 'counter-regulation'.
   ✓ New glucose is made from internal sources through glycogenolysis and gluconeogenesis.
   ✓ Alternative fuels used as substrate for brain metabolism include lactate, ketones, amino acids, and fatty acids.
   ☐ Insulin is the main hormone supporting a gradual rise in serum BG in the first few hours post-birth.
   ☐ Glucagon is a catabolic hormone, and its rise at birth can have negative consequences for the newborn.

7. **Conjugated bilirubin is produced by the liver and excreted in bile. Tick all statements that apply.**
   ☐ Elevated serum conjugated bilirubin is common in infants.
   ✓ Parents should be alert to their infant's stool colour during the first month.
   ✓ Early assessment by a physician is urgent for babies whose stool is an abnormal colour.
   ✓ Biliary atresia is a life-threatening liver disease that presents in the first month of age and is the most common cause of liver transplantation in childhood.

8. **All infants are at risk for developing cold stress. Four mechanisms cause heat loss (or gain) in newborns through environmental transfer. Match each mechanism with its correct definition.**

a. Conduction	_d_ Heat transfer through thermal waves to a colder surface, such as a wall or window, or from a warm source, such as a radiant warmer.
b. Convection	_c_ Transfer of heat to water molecules during transition from liquid to gas.
c. Evaporation	_b_ Transfer of heat to air currents.
d. Radiation	_a_ Direct transfer of heat to a cold (or from a warm) surface.

9. **Challenges to the neonatal immune system during transition include:**
   ✓ Maternal infections
   ✓ Antibiotic exposure before or after birth
   ✓ Delayed skin-to-skin contact
   ✓ Provision of oxygen or mechanical ventilation
   ✓ Interventions that can introduce pathogens or break the skin (e.g., blood tests or intravenous cannulae)
   ✓ Artificial nutrition and nutritional supplements
   ✓ Invasive neonatal infections

The ACoRN Process

2

Educational objectives

Upon completion of this chapter, you will be able to:

- Identify the unwell or at-risk infant who will benefit from the Acute Care of at-Risk Newborns (ACoRN) Process.
- Determine whether an infant needs immediate resuscitation or stabilization.
- Use the **ACoRN Primary Survey** to conduct systematic evaluations of infants.
- Apply the **Consolidated Core Steps** while performing the Primary Survey, to facilitate earlier stabilization.
- Generate a prioritized **Problem List**.
- Describe the basic structure and navigation of the **ACoRN Sequences**.
- Identify essential ACoRN tools in specific sequences that help to organize care.
- Assess an infant's **Level of Risk** (green, yellow, or red), depending on acuity, specific care needs, and the current care setting.
- Describe types of support that may be needed by the infant, the family, and the health care team.
- Evaluate available resources for newborn care in local and referral facilities and prepare infants for transport when required.

Key concepts

1. ACoRN is a post-resuscitation stabilization program.
2. Infants who are unwell, at-risk, or post-resuscitation require close observation for early detection, intervention, treatment, and (ideally) prevention of problems.
3. The **Primary Survey** is a rapid, thorough, systematic, and sequential assessment of eight areas of potential concern that is completed with minimal disturbance to the infant.
4. The **Consolidated Core Steps** are a rapid series of supportive actions performed at the same time as the Primary Survey.
5. **Alerting Signs** are used to identify infants with system-specific risks or problems who will benefit from the ACoRN Process.
6. The **Problem List**, which is generated after completing the Primary Survey, ensures that all the appropriate sequences are addressed in a standardized and prioritized order.
7. **ACoRN Sequences** are algorithms that systematically guide care in each area of concern identified in the Problem List.
8. **Level of Risk** is designated based on an infant's presentation, anticipated clinical course, and the site's capacity to deliver the care required.

9. **Support**, an integral component of the ACoRN Process, begins at the time of the first contact with the infant and family, and is an important determinant of neonatal outcomes.

10. The ACoRN Process helps the provider to complete necessary assessments and tasks within one hour of the initial encounter—the 'Golden Hour'.

11. Consultation and preparation for transport are essential elements of stabilization and should be considered early in the infant's course.

Like neonatal resuscitation, stabilization is most effective when performed by a well-coordinated team. The ACoRN program uses educational techniques to promote and support team learning and practice. This chapter focuses on practical essentials: the knowledge and tools you need to understand and navigate the ACoRN Process. However, successful use of ACoRN in clinical practice requires a thorough understanding and familiarity with the ACoRN materials. This knowledge and skill acquisition can be facilitated by using the ACoRN Process to work through clinical cases and simulations as well as in the clinical setting.

ACoRN uses Alerting Signs, which are clinical observations, assessments, or laboratory values that identify infants who are at-risk or unwell, to guide entry into different care pathways. Alerting Signs are different for each of the eight system-based areas of potential concern. Any infant with ACoRN Alerting Signs requires ongoing observation, and may need intervention and management, to achieve or maintain stability.

The objective of ACoRN is to optimize care and outcomes for at-risk or unwell newborns in any clinical setting, using this textbook and related tools and resources at www.cps.ca/en/acorn.

The 'Golden Hour'

In ACoRN, the 'Golden Hour' refers to the first, crucial care window following initial patient contact, when a health care team must ensure that an infant is properly monitored, and that all organ systems have been evaluated and appropriately stabilized using a prioritized, systematic, evidence-based approach. This is achieved using the ACoRN Process. The concept of the Golden Hour was born in field medicine and has been imported into neonatal care via trauma and emergent care over the last two decades. Its focus on deploying resources efficiently, minimizing complications, and achieving rapid stabilization, consultation, and transfer, have particular relevance for early newborn care. Optimizing care during this first hour has immediate and long-term benefits.

Resuscitation and stabilization are critical processes that require effective team dynamics and timed outputs. During the first hour of patient contact, the neonatal team focuses on initial stabilization, orders diagnostic tests (e.g., radiographs and blood gases) to support decision-making, and identifies the need for consultation or transport.

The Golden Hour ends when all individualized ACoRN assessments and tasks are completed, including an evaluation of the infant's Level of Risk. The clinical course is anticipated, interventions to prevent deterioration have been implemented, and the decisions whether to consult with a specialist or arrange for transport have been reached.

The ACoRN Process

ACoRN provides a logical, system-based approach to gathering and organizing clinical information, establishing priorities, and intervening appropriately for infants who are unwell, or at risk for becoming unwell, in the first few hours or days post-birth. ACoRN is designed to be useful regardless of the complexity of an infant's condition or the frequency with which a practitioner is called upon to manage it.

The ACoRN Process (Figure 2.1) has nine key steps:

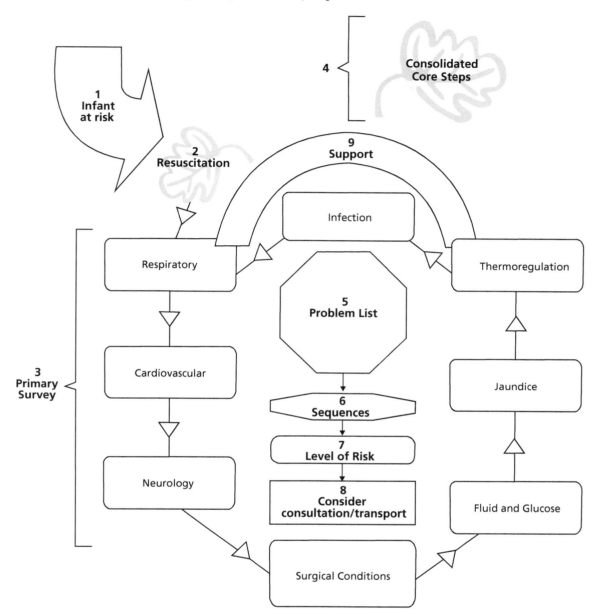

Figure 2.1. The ACoRN Process.

1. Identify the **at-risk infant** who will benefit from the ACoRN Process:
   The infant at risk is unwell or at risk for becoming unwell, based either on identified risk factors or is post-resuscitation and requires stabilization.

2. Determine whether **Resuscitation** is required:
   ACoRN is not a neonatal resuscitation program, but it recognizes that some unwell infants may require resuscitation before, or possibly during, stabilization. ACoRN links the resuscitation and stabilization processes in each sequence by prioritizing a return to resuscitation care, or post-resuscitation care, when necessary.

3. Perform a systematic assessment of the infant, using the **ACoRN Primary Survey**:

   The ACoRN Primary Survey identifies the presence or absence of Alerting Signs in eight system–based areas of potential concern:

1. Respiratory	5. Fluid and Glucose
2. Cardiovascular	6. Jaundice
3. Neurology	7. Thermoregulation
4. Surgical Conditions	8. Infection

4. Perform the **Consolidated Core Steps**:

   These actions and assessments are performed at the same time as the Primary Survey, to support the infant, obtain needed information, and establish monitoring.

5. Identify the prioritized **Problem List**:

   When an Alerting Sign is present, the appropriate care sequence is identified on the Problem List, in order of priority:

1. Respiratory	5. Fluid and Glucose
2. Cardiovascular	6. Jaundice
3. Neurology	7. Thermoregulation
4. Surgical Conditions	8. Infection

6. Work through each **ACoRN Sequence** in priority order.

   All care sequences are constructed following the **ACoRNs mnemonic** (Figure 2.2):

A . . . Alerting Signs	Specific indicators of a problem within each system
C . . . Core Steps	Essential tasks to assist decision–making and organize care
O . . . Organization of Care	A prioritized approach to meeting the infant's stabilization requirements
R . . . Response	Immediate, necessary steps to stabilize the infant
N . . . Next Steps	Tasks (including a focused history and physical exam) that provide information to formulate a specific diagnosis and management plan
S . . . Specific Diagnosis and Management	Identifying cause, treatment, and the need for specialized consultation and management

7. Identify the infant's **Level of Risk**:

   This assessment considers the ongoing needs of the infant, the expected clinical trajectory of the illness, and the capacity of the site providing care. This tool helps identify the need for early consultation and/or transport.

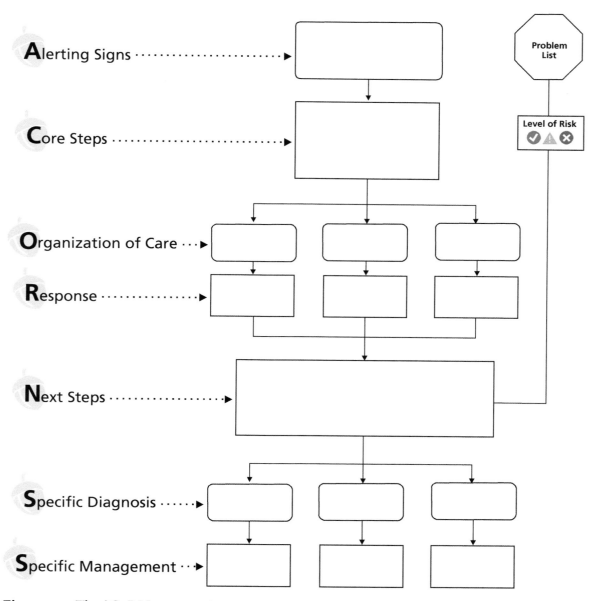

Figure 2.2. The ACoRNs mnemonic.

8. Consider **consultation/transport:**
   Early consultation with an on-site specialist or a regional referral centre optimizes care but does not always entail need for transport.
9. Provide **Support** to infants, families, and health care providers, using appropriate strategies and principles:
   Support is an overarching component of the ACoRN Process and begins at the point of first contact with infants and families. Supportive care is an important determinant of neonatal outcomes and should always be attended to as medical problems are addressed.

The ACoRN Primary Survey

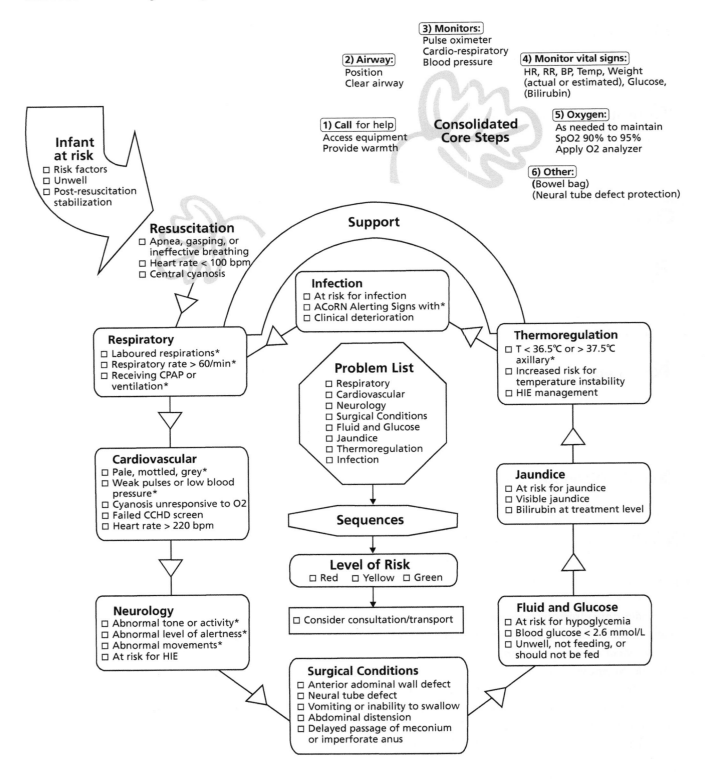

3) Monitors:
Pulse oximeter
Cardio-respiratory
Blood pressure

2) Airway:
Position
Clear airway

4) Monitor vital signs:
HR, RR, BP, Temp, Weight
(actual or estimated), Glucose,
(Bilirubin)

1) Call for help
Access equipment
Provide warmth

Consolidated Core Steps

5) Oxygen:
As needed to maintain
SpO2 90% to 95%
Apply O2 analyzer

6) Other:
(Bowel bag)
(Neural tube defect protection)

Infant at risk
□ Risk factors
□ Unwell
□ Post-resuscitation stabilization

Resuscitation
□ Apnea, gasping, or ineffective breathing
□ Heart rate < 100 bpm
□ Central cyanosis

Support

Infection
□ At risk for infection
□ ACoRN Alerting Signs with*
□ Clinical deterioration

Respiratory
□ Laboured respirations*
□ Respiratory rate > 60/min*
□ Receiving CPAP or ventilation*

Thermoregulation
□ T < 36.5°C or > 37.5°C axillary*
□ Increased risk for temperature instability
□ HIE management

Problem List
□ Respiratory
□ Cardiovascular
□ Neurology
□ Surgical Conditions
□ Fluid and Glucose
□ Jaundice
□ Thermoregulation
□ Infection

Cardiovascular
□ Pale, mottled, grey*
□ Weak pulses or low blood pressure*
□ Cyanosis unresponsive to O2
□ Failed CCHD screen
□ Heart rate > 220 bpm

Jaundice
□ At risk for jaundice
□ Visible jaundice
□ Bilirubin at treatment level

Sequences

Level of Risk
□ Red   □ Yellow   □ Green

Neurology
□ Abnormal tone or activity*
□ Abnormal level of alertness*
□ Abnormal movements*
□ At risk for HIE

□ Consider consultation/transport

Fluid and Glucose
□ At risk for hypoglycemia
□ Blood glucose < 2.6 mmol/L
□ Unwell, not feeding, or should not be fed

Surgical Conditions
□ Anterior adominal wall defect
□ Neural tube defect
□ Vomiting or inability to swallow
□ Abdominal distension
□ Delayed passage of meconium or imperforate anus

Identifying the infant at risk

The ACoRN Process begins with distinguishing the infant who seems well from the infant who does not. The well infant has normal vital signs, colour, activity, feeding patterns, and has passed meconium and urine within the first 24 h post-birth.

The unwell infant

Indications that an infant is unwell may be as subtle as a weak sucking reflex or as obvious as cyanosis unresponsive to oxygen. Close observation and a timely review of maternal and birth histories and findings on physical examination are warranted. An intuitive sense that something is 'just not right' with an infant is as valid as more overt signs. Both should trigger the provider to start the ACoRN Process.

The at-risk infant

Of the infants who appear well initially, some are at greater risk of becoming unwell than the general newborn population. These 'at-risk' infants are broadly identified on the basis of their gestational age, weight, and the presence of risk factors in the antepartum, intrapartum, and/or neonatal histories. Examples include:

- Infants who are preterm, including late preterm (34 to 36 weeks) or small for gestational age
- Infants of diabetic mothers
- Infants born exposed to licit or illicit drugs
- Infants born following prolonged rupture of membranes
- Infants who have been exposed to abnormally warm or cold environments

Managing at-risk infants using the ACoRN Process ensures close observation, early detection of problems, timely interventions, appropriate treatment, and prevents problems or conditions from developing or deteriorating. Specific neonatal risk factors are discussed in each system-based chapter of this text.

Post-resuscitation requiring stabilization

The ACoRN Process is also used to stabilize infants who required resuscitated at birth.

Resuscitation

The first priority in caring for an unwell or at-risk infant is to determine whether immediate resuscitation is needed to establish adequate cardiorespiratory function. That is why, in the ACoRN Process, the Resuscitation Sequence is positioned before entry into the Primary Survey. The need for immediate resuscitation takes precedence over all other concerns. The most common cause of cardiorespiratory instability in the newborn is hypoxemia (decreased oxygen content in the blood), and the most common cause of poor response to resuscitation is failure to correct this condition. Therefore, interventions in the Resuscitation Sequence aim to establish effective ventilation, improve oxygenation, and stabilize cardiac output.

The Resuscitation Sequence (Figure 2.3) links ACoRN with the resuscitation algorithm published by the International Liaison Committee on Resuscitation. The algorithm was adapted by the American Academy of Pediatrics in their *Textbook of Neonatal Resuscitation*. The concepts, sequences, and skills related to infant resuscitation are taught in the Neonatal Resuscitation Program (NRP).

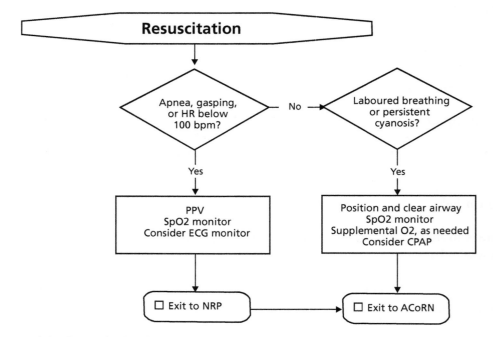

Resuscitation
- ☐ Apnea, gasping, or ineffective breathing
- ☐ Heart rate < 100 bpm
- ☐ Central cyanosis

Figure 2.3. The Resuscitation Sequence.

Any infant who shows one or more of the three **Resuscitation Alerting Signs** enters the Resuscitation Sequence.

Apnea, gasping, or ineffective breathing

Infants who are apneic or gasping cannot generate sufficient air movement to oxygenate or ventilate their lungs effectively. Infants with ineffective breathing may not be able to maintain consistent gas exchange and may have an airway obstruction caused by poor positioning, secretions, aspiration, or anatomic abnormality.

Heart rate less than 100 beats / min

A heart rate less than 100 bpm in an unwell infant often indicates ineffective breathing and hypoxemia. Some healthy term infants have a slow resting heart rate, in the range of 80 to 100 bpm. These infants look well, and their cardiac rhythm is sinus. A slow heart rate caused by congenital heart block is rare, and usually presents with a fixed heart rate less than 80 bpm. These infants are usually identified during the antepartum or intrapartum period, and they do not enter the Resuscitation Sequence.

Central cyanosis

Central cyanosis typically presents as a bluish discolouration (duskiness) of the body, lips, and mucous membranes. However, cyanosis should always be suspected when an infant's colour is not obviously 'pink' or healthy looking. Factors that can influence an infant's colour include degree of oxygenation, skin thickness, natural skin colour, perfusion, hemoglobin concentration, and ambient light level. Pulse oximetry has an essential role in the assessment of cyanosis.

Central cyanosis is always abnormal and indicates hypoxemia, which is often caused by ineffective ventilation and lung disease, accompanied by respiratory distress. Central cyanosis may also occur in conditions where venous and arterial blood mix, such as persistent pulmonary hypertension of the newborn (PPHN, previously known as persistent fetal circulation), and congenital cardiac anomalies. Mixing of venous with arterial blood reduces oxygen content in the arterial blood.

A bluish discolouration of the hands and feet with a pink body and mucous membranes is called peripheral cyanosis (or acrocyanosis). This effect is commonly seen in the first hours post-birth and may indicate cold stress. Peripheral cyanosis is caused by peripheral vasoconstriction, not hypoxemia, and does not require oxygen therapy.

Organization of Care depends on whether the infant

- Is apneic, gasping, or has a heart rate less than 100 bpm, or
- Has laboured breathing and/or persistent cyanosis, despite supplemental oxygen.

Response for the infant who is gasping, apneic, or has a heart rate less than 100 bpm is to exit ACoRN and provide resuscitation as per the NRP until the infant's heart rate is 100 bpm or greater.

The infant whose heart rate is 100 bpm or greater and has laboured breathing and/or persistent cyanosis despite supplemental oxygen exits to the ACoRN Primary Survey.

Every infant who has entered the Resuscitation Sequence is considered unwell and, upon successful completion of resuscitation, should be immediately assessed using the ACoRN Primary Survey. When proceeding though the ACoRN Process, a return to the Resuscitation Sequence may be needed at any point should the infant's condition deteriorate or any of the Resuscitation Alerting Signs become evident.

The Primary Survey

The ACoRN Primary Survey is a rapid, thorough, systematic, and sequential assessment of eight areas of potential concern in the unwell or at-risk infant. It relies heavily on observation and is completed with minimal disturbance to the infant. The eight areas are:

1. Respiratory
2. Cardiovascular
3. Neurology
4. Surgical conditions
5. Fluid and glucose
6. Jaundice
7. Thermoregulation
8. Infection

Alerting Signs

Each area has its own specific Alerting Signs, to indicate whether the infant is having a problem in that system.

For example:

> **Respiratory**
> ☐ Laboured respirations*
> ☐ Respiratory rate > 60/min*
> ☐ Receiving CPAP or ventilation*

Each Alerting Sign is assessed as follows:

☑ Check when sign is present.

☐ Leave box blank when sign is absent.

❓ Put a question mark if an evaluation is pending (e.g., when you are waiting for results from a blood pressure or blood glucose test).

Alerting Signs for Infection emerge as the Primary Survey is being completed.

> Any ACoRN Alerting Sign marked with an asterisk (*) in the Primary Survey suggests that infection may also be present.

Infection is also suspected in infants with a risk factor for infection identified on the focused history or physical exam completed in any ACoRN Sequence and/or when clinical deterioration occurs. Early recognition and prompt treatment with antibiotics will improve outcome in infants with bacterial infections.

The Consolidated Core Steps

Consolidated Core Steps are a rapid series of supportive actions performed at the same time as the ACoRN Primary Survey. They, too, are prioritized:

1. Call:
   - Call for help refers to the immediate need for additional staff. A specialist consult within your own care setting or a timely call to a regional referral centre can significantly impact course of treatment and infant outcome. Be mindful that the more information you can obtain by reviewing the Primary Survey or Sequences before calling for help, the better a specialist's guidance is likely to be.
   - Access equipment needed for clinical support.
   - Provide warmth to minimize stress.

2. Airway:
   - Position the infant's head in a neutral position to open the airway.
   - Clear airway of secretions. Suction the oropharynx and nose if needed.
   - Contain the infant to provide comfort. Nest the infant whenever possible.

3. Monitors:
   - Apply pulse oximeter to the infant's right hand or wrist and ensure upper and lower limits have been set.
   - Attach cardiopulmonary leads and ensure upper and lower limits have been set.
   - Use a blood pressure monitor and a cuff of the correct size.

4. Monitor vital signs:
   - Obtain heart rate, respiratory rate, blood pressure, and axillary temperature.
   - Obtain point-of-care blood glucose when the infant is unwell.

- Weigh the infant (preferred) or estimate weight if the infant is too unstable.
- Obtain bilirubin (if applicable).

5. Oxygen:
   - Administer oxygen as needed to maintain SpO2 of 90% to 95%.
   - Measure oxygen continuously using a calibrated O2 analyzer if the infant is receiving oxygen in an oxygen hood or incubator without a built-in O2 analyzer.

6. Other:
   - Protect an infant's anterior abdominal wall defect with an appropriate clear cover or dressing.
   - Apply a sterile, moist cover to an open neural tube defect.

Infants entering the ACoRN Process because they are unwell or post-resuscitation are at risk for hypoglycemia and temperature instability. Timely blood glucose determination and thermal management are important parts of the Consolidated Core Steps.

Integration of the information obtained in the Consolidated Core Steps and Primary Survey is dependent on clear communication between the ACoRN team members performing these two functions.

The Problem List

The Problem List prioritizes the eight areas of concern in the Primary Survey.

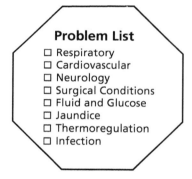

Problem List
- ☐ Respiratory
- ☐ Cardiovascular
- ☐ Neurology
- ☐ Surgical Conditions
- ☐ Fluid and Glucose
- ☐ Jaundice
- ☐ Thermoregulation
- ☐ Infection

If, for example, an infant has one or more of the Alerting Signs in the Cardiovascular Sequence, a corresponding check mark is added to Cardiovascular in the Problem List.

When test results to establish a particular Alerting Sign are pending (e.g., a blood glucose result is not yet available), the corresponding box in the Problem List (Fluid and Glucose in this case) should have a question mark to remind care providers to follow up as soon as possible, while other aspects of the ACoRN Process proceed.

Problem List
- ☐ Respiratory
- ✓ Cardiovascular
- ☐ Neurology
- ☐ Surgical Conditions
- ? Fluid and Glucose
- ☐ Jaundice
- ☐ Thermoregulation
- ☐ Infection

When the Primary Survey has been completed, the Problem List identifies the order that concerns should be addressed. Identified problems should be addressed in the specified order for optimal stabilization.

ACoRN Sequences

For each system of concern, there is a corresponding ACoRN Sequence that guides initial stabilization, helps the health care team to identify a working diagnosis, and culminates in a specific diagnosis and management plan.

The evaluation → decision → action cycle, familiar from NRP, is repeated throughout each ACoRN Sequence. The process of evaluation is represented by rounded boxes, decisions are depicted by arrows, and actions (including monitoring, interventions, and diagnostic tests) are indicated by rectangles. See an excerpt from the Respiratory Sequence, facing page.

The schematic structure of the sequences (Figure 2.2, page 29) is shown next.

A lerting Signs	The presence of the Alerting Signs identified in the Primary Survey is confirmed. If, upon entering a sequence, the Alerting Sign that prompted entry is no longer present, there is no need to proceed further within that sequence. The ACoRN provider can move to the next sequence in the Problem List.
C ore Steps	The Core Steps, which apply to all infants entering a given sequence, are performed. This step may require the use of a sequence-specific tool (e.g., the Respiratory Score) to aid decision-making and the Organization of Care.
O rganization of Care	The course of action is organized based on Alerting Signs, Core Steps, and specific, system-related physical findings, risks, or indicators, which are detailed in their respective chapters.
R esponse	The Response describes the interventions required to provide stabilization, based on the Organization of Care. Management options and results are reviewed.
N ext Steps	The focused history and physical examination are essential Next Steps in every sequence. Information-gathering toward a working diagnosis, reviewing the clinical course, and diagnostic testing to narrow differential diagnosis and support decision-making, are part of Next Steps. The ACoRN provider may also consider consultation or transport and return to the Problem List to address the next sequence of concern.
S pecific Diagnosis and Management	A specific diagnosis or diagnostic category is established based on the infant's condition, physical findings, and test results. The ongoing management specific to the diagnosis is provided while addressing any other areas of concern. Further management may include frequent monitoring, preventive care, and preparation for transport.

Different clinical information is acquired at each stage of the ACoRN Process, along with system-specific evaluations and actions to guide decision-making. The ACoRN provider inserts a check mark in each box that applies to an infant's condition, starting with the Core Steps. These check marks indicate that an observation has been made or an action has been taken.

The ACoRN provider navigates each sequence identified on the Problem List to the level of **Next Steps**. Progressing through the sequence allows the provider to collect information pertinent for a working diagnosis, provides guidance on actions or tasks to promote initial stabilization, and creates a list of other information or investigations for the ACoRN provider to collect on a 'to-do' list. The goal is to coordinate the recommended testing from all relevant sequences, minimize disruption to the infant, and promote timely return of information required to establish a specific diagnosis and management plan. At this stage, the ACoRN provider exits the sequence and moves on to the next one listed on the Problem List. As results come in, or the infant's condition changes, the provider can return to the sequence to continue management. See the following example.

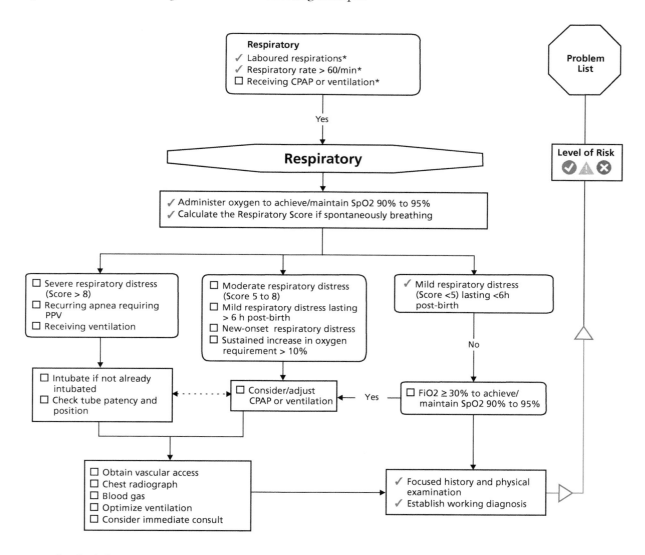

Level of Risk

Assessing an infant's Level of Risk considers the degree of ongoing attention the infant requires, the level of stability achieved, anticipated clinical course, and the need for early consultation and/or transport. Each sequence assigns a level of risk based on the working diagnosis, the type of support required, and on-site capacity to provide, and sustain the level of care an infant requires.

Level of Risk: The ACoRN Process	
In the ACoRN Primary Survey, level of risk is based on the highest level of risk assigned in any of the ACoRN sequences.	
	Green: • Infant is 35 weeks gestation or greater, clinically stable, and needs a low level of intervention and ongoing monitoring, **AND** • Ongoing requirements do not exceed site capability
	Yellow: • Infant is clinically stable but needs a higher level of observation or intervention, **OR** • Infant is clinically stable but a worsening clinical course is anticipated, **AND** • Site can provide appropriate management, investigations, and monitoring for the infant's condition **Infants at a Yellow Level of Risk require increased levels of attention and may require consultation. Transfer is required if needs exceed site capabilities.**
	Red: • Infant is unstable or unwell, needs a high level of observation or intervention, **OR** • Infant is anticipated to become unstable or unwell, **OR** • Infant requires care that is beyond the site's capacity to manage or monitor safely **Infants at a Red Level of Risk are considered unstable, and require level 3 care. Transfer is required if infant or care team needs exceed site capabilities.**

Even before infant condition is considered, the following risk factors should be top of mind:

- Infants with **Green Level of Risk** are those who are 35 weeks gestation or greater and medically stable.
- Infants with **Yellow Level of Risk** require a higher level of attention and may require consultation and/or transport, including well looking infants less than 35 weeks.
- Infants with unresolved **Red Level of Risk** issues are considered unstable, require close attention, and are likely to require consultation and transport.

Transfer is required if the infant's or care team's needs exceed site capacity.

Consult / Transport

When an infant's current condition or anticipated clinical course cannot be managed locally, the earlier the need for more specialized care is identified and the sooner the transport process is initiated, the better. The decision to consult on or transport an at-risk or unwell infant to another facility is based on discussions between the sending facility and the transport coordinating physician. Asking for a consult does not necessarily mean you want, or need to transport an infant to another facility. A number of factors are considered, including:

- The infant's current condition and anticipated clinical course
- Sending hospital resources (i.e., on-site personnel, expertise, equipment, and specialized services)
- Transport team availability
- Regional referral patterns
- Mode of transport
- Current or impending weather conditions

Each ACoRN sequence indicates when to consider obtaining a consultation or arrange for transport. Arrangements for transport should begin as soon as the need becomes apparent.

Support for the infant, family, and health care team

Support is an overarching component of ACoRN, permeating the whole program, and will be discussed in detail in Chapter 12, Support. The infant is the focus of everyone's attention, but the needs of the family and health care team are important and should not be overlooked. Support begins before the first contact with the infant and family and continues during the provision of care. Support is also about team performance and the recognition and management of stress.

Support includes controlling the environment, avoiding sensory overload, managing stress and pain, and promoting supportive approaches to the delivery of care.

The ACoRN Process: Case 1—Using ACoRN to initiate newborn stabilization

A mother presents in advanced preterm labour to your level 1 site. She is 32 years old, G2 P1 and 34 +2/7 weeks gestation. A 2100-g baby boy is born by vaginal delivery 2 hours later. At birth, the baby cries, heart rate is greater than 100, and his SpO2 is 68% and does not increase without supplemental oxygen. Apgars are 6 and 7. At 15 min of age, you note the baby has mild in-drawing and now requires 30% oxygen to maintain the SpO2 at 90%. The respiratory rate is 70.

1. **Which of the Alerting Signs for Infant at Risk would you check? Tick all that apply.**
   - ☐ Risk factors
   - ☐ Unwell
   - ☐ Post-resuscitation stabilization

2. **Are there current Alerting Signs for Resuscitation?**
   - ☐ Yes   ☐ No

You perform the ACoRN Primary Survey at the same time that a colleague performs the Consolidated Core Steps. As you do so, you make the following observations:

The baby has mild subcostal in-drawing, decreased breath sounds, grunting with handling, and his SpO2 is 92% on 30% oxygen delivered by T-piece. The heart rate is 160 bpm. The pulses are palpable, and his colour is pink. His tone and level of alertness are appropriate. There is no obvious surgical condition or visible jaundice. He is being cared for on an overbed warmer.

The **Primary Survey** prompts you to evaluate the eight areas of concern, using the **Alerting Signs** to ensure you have made observations pertinent to each area.

3. **Mark the Primary Survey on facing page based on the information you have so far. Check (✓) for what you know, and put a question mark (?) for any information still missing.**

Based on the Alerting Signs marked with a question mark, the Primary Survey prompts you to make additional observations. Some answers will be provided by your colleague completing the **Consolidated Core Steps**. Only when you have those observations can you develop a complete **Problem List**.

The Consolidated Core Steps add the following information: the infant's blood pressure is 58/32 mean of 41, blood glucose is 3.2 mmol/L, axillary temperature is 37°C.

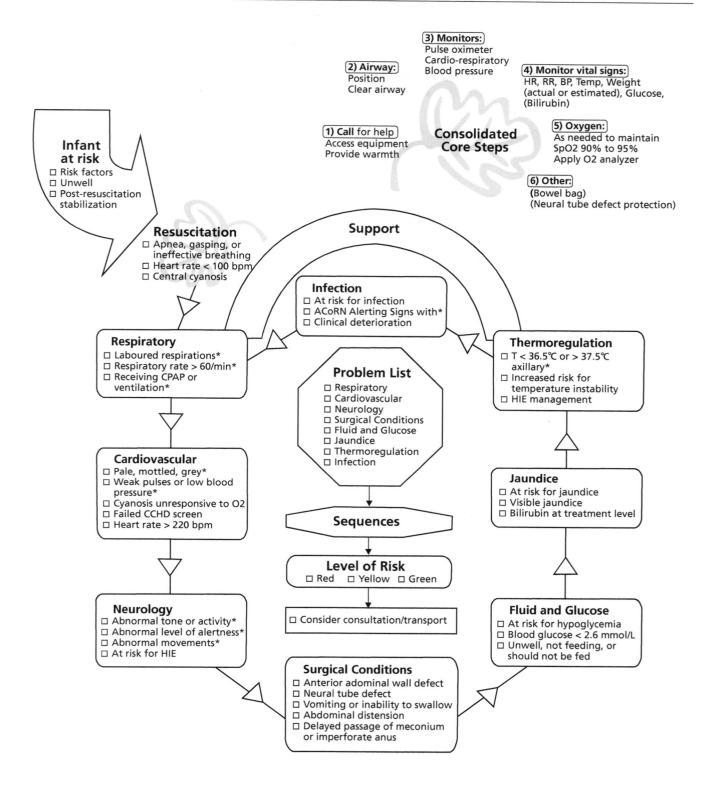

Infant at risk
- ☐ Risk factors
- ☐ Unwell
- ☐ Post-resuscitation stabilization

Resuscitation
- ☐ Apnea, gasping, or ineffective breathing
- ☐ Heart rate < 100 bpm
- ☐ Central cyanosis

Support

Consolidated Core Steps

1) Call for help
Access equipment
Provide warmth

2) Airway:
Position
Clear airway

3) Monitors:
Pulse oximeter
Cardio-respiratory
Blood pressure

4) Monitor vital signs:
HR, RR, BP, Temp, Weight (actual or estimated), Glucose, (Bilirubin)

5) Oxygen:
As needed to maintain SpO2 90% to 95%
Apply O2 analyzer

6) Other:
(Bowel bag)
(Neural tube defect protection)

Respiratory
- ☐ Laboured respirations*
- ☐ Respiratory rate > 60/min*
- ☐ Receiving CPAP or ventilation*

Infection
- ☐ At risk for infection
- ☐ ACoRN Alerting Signs with*
- ☐ Clinical deterioration

Thermoregulation
- ☐ T < 36.5°C or > 37.5°C axillary*
- ☐ Increased risk for temperature instability
- ☐ HIE management

Cardiovascular
- ☐ Pale, mottled, grey*
- ☐ Weak pulses or low blood pressure*
- ☐ Cyanosis unresponsive to O2
- ☐ Failed CCHD screen
- ☐ Heart rate > 220 bpm

Problem List
- ☐ Respiratory
- ☐ Cardiovascular
- ☐ Neurology
- ☐ Surgical Conditions
- ☐ Fluid and Glucose
- ☐ Jaundice
- ☐ Thermoregulation
- ☐ Infection

Jaundice
- ☐ At risk for jaundice
- ☐ Visible jaundice
- ☐ Bilirubin at treatment level

Sequences

Neurology
- ☐ Abnormal tone or activity*
- ☐ Abnormal level of alertness*
- ☐ Abnormal movements*
- ☐ At risk for HIE

Level of Risk
☐ Red   ☐ Yellow   ☐ Green

☐ Consider consultation/transport

Fluid and Glucose
- ☐ At risk for hypoglycemia
- ☐ Blood glucose < 2.6 mmol/L
- ☐ Unwell, not feeding, or should not be fed

Surgical Conditions
- ☐ Anterior adominal wall defect
- ☐ Neural tube defect
- ☐ Vomiting or inability to swallow
- ☐ Abdominal distension
- ☐ Delayed passage of meconium or imperforate anus

Within each of the sequences, as prioritized by the Problem List, you confirm the continued presence of the Alerting Signs and perform the Core Steps, using any sequence-specific tools to help you organize your care. The **Organization of Care** helps determine the initial **Response** required for immediate stabilization. You perform the **Next Steps**, including a focused history, physical examination, and putting any recommended investigations on your to-do list. You determine the working diagnosis and **Level of Risk** corresponding to each sequence and move to the next area of concern identified on the Problem List.

Specific tasks in each sequence may take time to complete and will be described in detail in their respective chapters.

In the Respiratory Sequence:
- You obtain a Respiratory Score and identify the degree of respiratory distress.
- You organize your care and work through the appropriate response according to the degree of respiratory distress.
- You determine the level of oxygen required by targeting SpO2 90% to 95%.
- You determine whether the infant requires respiratory support, such as CPAP or ventilation.
- You determine whether vascular access, a chest radiograph, and/or a blood gas are required.

In the Fluid and Glucose Sequence:
- You calculate fluid requirements based on age and condition.
- You organize your care on the basis of whether the infant can feed or not.
- You determine the initial glucose level and subsequent monitoring needs.
- You initiate intravenous dextrose at the hourly requirement for an infant who cannot feed or who is hypoglycemic after feeding support was attempted.
- You initiate a fluid balance sheet and calculate the glucose infusion rate needed to achieve target glucose levels.

In the Jaundice Sequence:
- You identify this is an infant at increased risk for jaundice due to prematurity. A screening bilirubin is recommended at 24 h.

In the Thermoregulation Sequence:
- You ensure the infant is in an environment where the temperature can be managed.
- You ensure his temperature is within the appropriate target range.

In the Infection Sequence:
- You identify additional risk factors for infection and complete the Infection Assessment Table.
- You organize your care based on the Infection Assessment Table recommendations.

Once all the sequences identified in your Problem List are completed, you can assess the infant's overall Level of Risk.

4. What is this infant's overall Level of Risk?
- ☐ The highest level of risk recorded
- ☐ The lowest level of risk recorded
- ☐ The average of all levels of risk recorded
- ☐ Green, yellow, and red
- ☐ Yellow

The last steps of stabilization in the ACoRN Process are to ensure that **Support** is being provided to the family and team and assess whether **Transport** to a facility that can provide a higher level of care is required.

As further information or investigations return, you re-enter each sequence to complete the **Specific Diagnosis and Management** steps of each sequence identified on your Problem List.

5. What will you communicate to the transport coordinating physician? Use the SBARR format.

Item	Verbalize	Description and example
S – situation	"This is my chief concern"	
B – background	"I want you to know"	
A – assessment	"This is the infant's condition"	
R – recommendation	"I need"	
R – readback/response	"Are there any questions?"	

While you are waiting for the transport team to arrive, the ACoRN Primary Survey is repeated at regular intervals *and* with any significant change in the infant's condition.

Answer key: The ACoRN Process Case 1—Using ACoRN to initiate newborn stabilization

1. **Which of the Alerting Signs for Infant at Risk would you check?**

   ✓ Risk factors

   ✓ Unwell

   ✓ Post-resuscitation stabilization

This baby satisfies all three Alerting Signs for entry into the ACoRN Process. He has risk factors (preterm birth), is unwell (laboured respirations and need for supplemental oxygen to maintain saturations within normal limits), and required resuscitation interventions at birth (provision of free flow oxygen to maintain saturations). Any one of these Alerting Signs on its own is sufficient to identify an infant that is in need of further observation and stabilization.

2. **Are there current Alerting Signs for Resuscitation?**

   ☐ Yes   ✓ No

None of the Alerting Signs for Resuscitation are present. The baby is breathing spontaneously, has a heart rate >100 bpm, and cyanosis has corrected with supplemental oxygen. If you are uncertain, enter the Resuscitation Sequence. Based on the absence of apnea or gasping and a heart rate above 100, you will navigate down the right-hand arm of the sequence and be directed to provide appropriate positioning, clear the airway, and deliver oxygen. CPAP can be considered. As you exit to ACoRN (stabilization) versus NRP (resuscitation), the Respiratory Sequence will provide additional guidance on the provision of CPAP and other respiratory supports for this infant.

3. **Mark the Primary Survey (facing page) based on the information you have so far. Check (✓) for what you know, and put a question mark (?) for any information still missing.**

This baby has obvious Respiratory Alerting Signs and it is the first prioritized sequence on your Problem List. The Consolidated Core Steps provided you with enough information to remove any ? marks from the Cardiovascular Alerting Signs. This baby's gestational age of 34 weeks puts him at risk for hypoglycemia despite the normal glucose obtained in the Consolidated Core Steps. At 34 weeks, he is not likely ready to take full oral volumes by mouth. Also, risk for aspiration increases when babies breathe at a rate of 70 breaths/min or greater. In a term or late preterm baby with mild respiratory distress, the decision whether the baby should be fed can be delayed for 1 to 2 h to see if the respiratory distress settles.

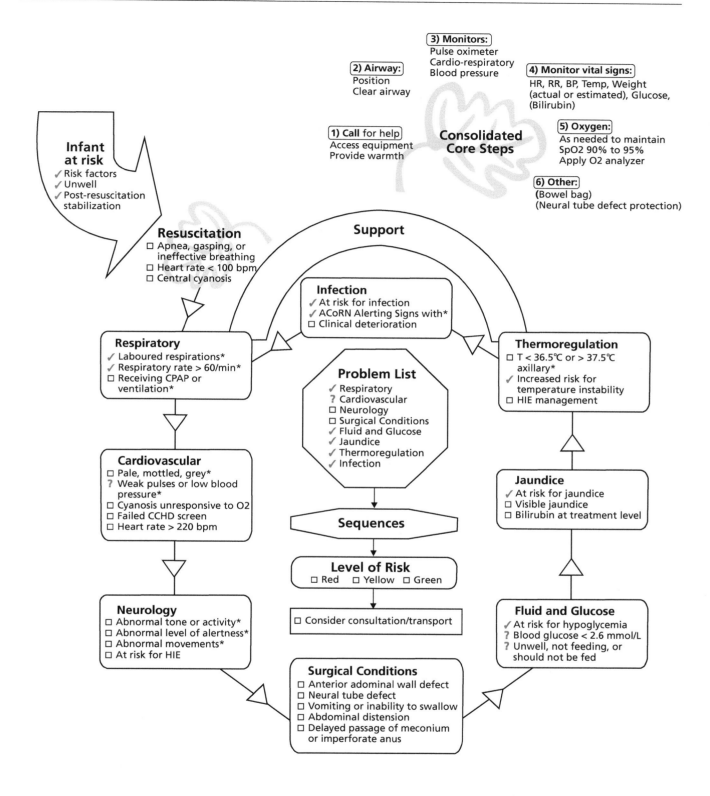

3) Monitors:
Pulse oximeter
Cardio-respiratory
Blood pressure

2) Airway:
Position
Clear airway

4) Monitor vital signs:
HR, RR, BP, Temp, Weight
(actual or estimated), Glucose,
(Bilirubin)

1) Call for help
Access equipment
Provide warmth

**Consolidated
Core Steps**

5) Oxygen:
As needed to maintain
SpO2 90% to 95%
Apply O2 analyzer

6) Other:
(Bowel bag)
(Neural tube defect protection)

**Infant
at risk**
✓ Risk factors
✓ Unwell
✓ Post-resuscitation
stabilization

Support

Resuscitation
☐ Apnea, gasping, or
ineffective breathing
☐ Heart rate < 100 bpm
☐ Central cyanosis

Infection
✓ At risk for infection
✓ ACoRN Alerting Signs with*
☐ Clinical deterioration

Respiratory
✓ Laboured respirations*
✓ Respiratory rate > 60/min*
☐ Receiving CPAP or
ventilation*

Thermoregulation
☐ T < 36.5℃ or > 37.5℃
axillary*
✓ Increased risk for
temperature instability
☐ HIE management

Problem List
✓ Respiratory
? Cardiovascular
☐ Neurology
☐ Surgical Conditions
✓ Fluid and Glucose
✓ Jaundice
✓ Thermoregulation
✓ Infection

Cardiovascular
☐ Pale, mottled, grey*
? Weak pulses or low blood
pressure*
☐ Cyanosis unresponsive to O2
☐ Failed CCHD screen
☐ Heart rate > 220 bpm

Jaundice
✓ At risk for jaundice
☐ Visible jaundice
☐ Bilirubin at treatment level

Sequences

Neurology
☐ Abnormal tone or activity*
☐ Abnormal level of alertness*
☐ Abnormal movements*
☐ At risk for HIE

Level of Risk
☐ Red   ☐ Yellow   ☐ Green

Fluid and Glucose
✓ At risk for hypoglycemia
? Blood glucose < 2.6 mmol/L
? Unwell, not feeding, or
should not be fed

☐ Consider consultation/transport

Surgical Conditions
☐ Anterior adominal wall defect
☐ Neural tube defect
☐ Vomiting or inability to swallow
☐ Abdominal distension
☐ Delayed passage of meconium
or imperforate anus

Entry into the Fluid and Glucose Sequence will help you determine the most appropriate method and rate of support for this infant. Preterm infants are at higher risk for delayed clearance of bilirubin and, therefore, jaundice. Routine screening at 24 h is recommended in the absence of additional Jaundice Alerting Signs.

Despite the fact that this baby's temperature is in the normal range at present, he is being cared for on an overbed warmer, away from skin-to-skin contact with parents, and is at increased risk for temperature instability as a result.

Lastly, this baby has ACoRN Alerting Signs with an *, so he meets the criteria for entry into the Infection Sequence. The spontaneous onset of preterm labour is also a known risk factor for infection. Additional risk factors may be identified on focused history or physical examination.

4. What is this infant's overall Level of Risk?

   ✓ The highest level of risk recorded

   ☐ The lowest level of risk recorded

   ☐ The average of all levels of risk recorded

   ☐ Green, yellow, and red

   ☐ Yellow

5. What will you communicate to the transport coordinating physician? Use the SBARR format.

Item	Verbalize	Description and example
S – situation	"This is my chief concern"	*I am calling about a 30-min-old, 2100 g, 34-week-GA infant who required 30% supplemental oxygen at birth and now has mild respiratory distress, cannot be fed, and requires IV dextrose or OG feeds.*
B – background	"I want you to know"	*Heart rate is 160 bpm, respiratory rate 70, SpO2 92% in 30% oxygen by T-piece, and axillary temperature is 37°C. Infant has mild subcostal retractions, grunting with handling, and decreased breath sounds. The pulses are palpable in the 4 extremities and blood pressure was 58/32 mean of 41. Tone and activity normal. The blood glucose was just done and is 3.2 mmol/L.* *We are preparing to initiate an infusion of D10%W at 3 mL/kg/h and have inserted a nasogastric tube.* *We will obtain a CBC with differential, blood culture, blood gas, and a chest and abdomen radiograph.* *This infant is 34 weeks with respiratory distress and has 2 non-red flag items suggesting infection, so ampicillin and gentamycin have been ordered.*
A – assessment	"This is the infant's condition"	*Baby is stable. His risk level is red because despite the mild respiratory distress, he is preterm, and he has suspected infection requiring antibiotics. We cannot sustain the level of care at our level 1 centre.*
R – recommendation	"I need"	*We need the transport team.*
R – read back/ response	"Are there any questions?"	*Do you have any other suggestions for care?*

Respiratory

3

Educational objectives

Upon completion of this chapter, you will be able to:

- Identify infants who require respiratory support or interventions.
- Apply the Acute Care of at-Risk Newborns (ACoRN) Respiratory Sequence.
- Determine oxygen requirements and select an appropriate oxygen delivery method.
- Use the Respiratory Score to organize care and monitor status on the basis of severity of respiratory distress.
- Recognize the need for, and how to initiate, respiratory support.
- Perform basic interpretation of chest radiographs and blood gas results.
- Recognize and manage the common causes of respiratory distress.
- Recognize when to exit the Respiratory Sequence to other ACoRN sequences.

Key concepts

1. Establishment of ventilation and prevention of hypoxia are required for successful transition from fetal to neonatal circulation.
2. Oxygenation is critical for cellular, tissue, and organ function.
3. Infants with increasing oxygen requirements require close observation and may require additional interventions.
4. Hyperoxia ($SpO2 > 95\%$ in infants receiving supplemental oxygen) is associated with oxygen toxicity.
5. The most common cause of cardiorespiratory failure in the newborn is hypoxemia, which is corrected with adequate oxygenation and ventilation.
6. Processes that interfere with the inflation and subsequent ventilation of a newborn's lungs cause respiratory distress.
7. The goal of early detection and intervention for respiratory distress is to optimize oxygenation and ventilation.
8. Severe respiratory distress is a precursor to respiratory failure.
9. A low, irregular respiratory rate with respiratory distress can be an early indication of respiratory failure.
10. Infants with severe respiratory distress, apnea, or gasping require immediate intubation and ventilation.
11. Preterm infants have poor respiratory reserve and may require earlier intervention.
12. Respiratory distress may be a sign of infection requiring immediate treatment.

Skills

- Blood gas interpretation
- Chest radiograph interpretation
- Assessment and delivery of oxygen needs
- Provision of respiratory support (i.e., continuous positive airway pressure [CPAP], intubation, mechanical ventilation)
- Management of pneumothorax

The objectives when caring for infants with respiratory problems are to ensure that oxygenation and ventilation are adequate, to provide early support and intervention as required to maintain function, and to prevent further deterioration.

The Respiratory Sequence is the first area of concern in the ACoRN Primary Survey. Its priority reflects the critical importance of establishing and maintaining adequate oxygenation and ventilation in the management of the unwell or at-risk newborn.

Transient or ongoing respiratory disorders are among the most common conditions encountered in neonatal care, particularly in preterm infants. Understanding transitional physiology and attention to the early signs and symptoms of respiratory insufficiency will often prevent destabilization or deterioration.

Neonatal respiratory problems

A delay or inability to complete the normal pulmonary transition to extrauterine life results in neonatal respiratory problems. Common examples include:

- Transient tachypnea of the newborn (TTN), when reabsorption of alveolar fluid is delayed.
- Respiratory distress syndrome (RDS), when surfactant is deficient and alveoli do not stay inflated after alveolar fluid is reabsorbed.
- Aspiration syndromes, when small airways and alveoli become obstructed by meconium, blood, or amniotic fluid.
- Pneumonia, when lungs become infected.
- Persistent pulmonary hypertension of the newborn (PPHN), when smooth muscle in the pulmonary vasculature does not relax and pulmonary pressures remain high, causing cyanosis from right to left or bidirectional shunting at the patent ductus arteriosus (PDA) and patent foramen ovale (PFO).
- Pneumothorax, when lungs suffer external compression from air trapped between the lung and chest wall.
- Pulmonary hypoplasia, when lungs are small and underdeveloped due to a space-occupying lesion in the chest (e.g., congenital diaphragmatic hernia [CDH]) or prolonged, severe oligohydramnios.

ACoRN Respiratory Sequence

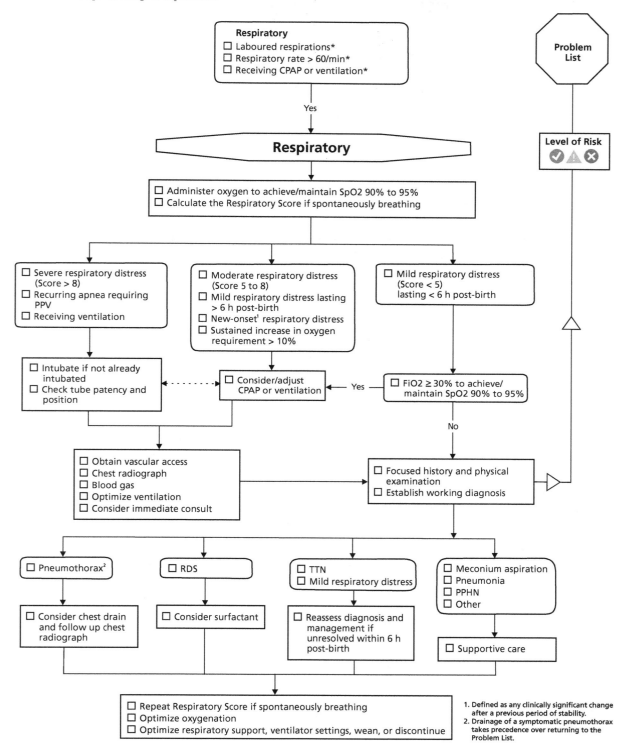

Respiratory
- ☐ Laboured respirations*
- ☐ Respiratory rate > 60/min*
- ☐ Receiving CPAP or ventilation*

Problem List

Yes

Respiratory

Level of Risk

- ☐ Administer oxygen to achieve/maintain SpO2 90% to 95%
- ☐ Calculate the Respiratory Score if spontaneously breathing

- ☐ Severe respiratory distress (Score > 8)
- ☐ Recurring apnea requiring PPV
- ☐ Receiving ventilation

- ☐ Moderate respiratory distress (Score 5 to 8)
- ☐ Mild respiratory distress lasting > 6 h post-birth
- ☐ New-onset[1] respiratory distress
- ☐ Sustained increase in oxygen requirement > 10%

- ☐ Mild respiratory distress (Score < 5) lasting < 6 h post-birth

- ☐ Intubate if not already intubated
- ☐ Check tube patency and position

- ☐ Consider/adjust CPAP or ventilation

Yes

- ☐ FiO2 ≥ 30% to achieve/maintain SpO2 90% to 95%

No

- ☐ Obtain vascular access
- ☐ Chest radiograph
- ☐ Blood gas
- ☐ Optimize ventilation
- ☐ Consider immediate consult

- ☐ Focused history and physical examination
- ☐ Establish working diagnosis

- ☐ Pneumothorax[2]

- ☐ RDS

- ☐ TTN
- ☐ Mild respiratory distress

- ☐ Meconium aspiration
- ☐ Pneumonia
- ☐ PPHN
- ☐ Other

- ☐ Consider chest drain and follow up chest radiograph

- ☐ Consider surfactant

- ☐ Reassess diagnosis and management if unresolved within 6 h post-birth

- ☐ Supportive care

- ☐ Repeat Respiratory Score if spontaneously breathing
- ☐ Optimize oxygenation
- ☐ Optimize respiratory support, ventilator settings, wean, or discontinue

1. Defined as any clinically significant change after a previous period of stability.
2. Drainage of a symptomatic pneumothorax takes precedence over returning to the Problem List.

Abbreviations: CPAP - continuous positive airway pressure, FiO2 - fraction of inspired oxygen, h - hours, min - minute, PPHN - persistent pulmonary hypertension of the newborn, PPV - positive pressure ventilation, RDS - respiratory distress syndrome, SpO2 - peripheral oxygen saturation, TTN - transient tachypnea of the newborn

Alerting Signs

An infant who shows one or more of the following Alerting Signs enters the ACoRN Respiratory Sequence:

> **Respiratory**
> ☐ Laboured respirations*
> ☐ Respiratory rate > 60/min*
> ☐ Receiving CPAP or ventilation*

*Laboured respirations**

An infant with laboured respirations is also described as having respiratory distress, difficulty breathing, or increased work of breathing. The signs of laboured respirations are:

- **Nasal flaring**—Outward flaring movements of the nostrils on inspiration in an attempt to move more air into the lungs.
- **Grunting**—Audible sounds produced as the infant exhales against a partially closed glottis in an effort to maintain end-expiratory pressure and increase functional residual capacity.
- **Intercostal and subcostal retractions**—Retractions of the intercostal and subcostal spaces due to increased negative pressure within the chest. Mild retractions involve the intercostal spaces only; moderate retractions involve the intercostal and subcostal spaces.
- **Sternal retractions**—Paradoxical backward movements of the sternum on inspiration caused by increased negative pressure within the chest. Involvement of the intercostal, subcostal, and sternal spaces is considered severe.

Gasping is an ominous sign of cerebral hypoxia characterized by deep, single or stacked, slow, and irregular breaths, indicating a terminal respiratory rhythm. Gasping is an Alerting Sign for the Resuscitation Sequence and not an indication of laboured breathing.

*Respiratory rate > 60 breaths/min**

The normal newborn respiratory rate is 40 to 60 breaths/min. Tachypnea, a respiratory rate greater than 60 breaths/min, usually indicates an intrathoracic process causing respiratory difficulty or distress. Tachypnea is often the first and most subtle sign of respiratory distress in infants with mildly decreased respiratory function.

*Receiving CPAP or ventilation**

This Alerting Sign identifies infants who are receiving ongoing respiratory support via either CPAP or ventilation. Any infant receiving positive inspiratory pressure (PIP) and positive end-expiratory pressure (PEEP) qualifies as receiving ventilation, irrespective of whether it is being delivered manually or by ventilator, through an endotracheal tube (ETT; invasively) or via nasal prongs or mask (noninvasively).

Infection commonly presents with respiratory signs in the newborn. All three Alerting Signs in the Respiratory Sequence have an asterisk (*) to remind ACoRN providers to check (✓) Infection in the Problem List.

Core Steps

Infants entering the Respiratory Sequence will have had monitoring established and some interventions performed as part of the Consolidated Core Steps. ACoRN providers should continually reassess airway patency and adequacy of respiratory drive in infants with respiratory Alerting Signs. The Core Steps in the Respiratory Sequence are to:

- Administer oxygen as needed to achieve and maintain a SpO2 of 90% to 95%, based on pulse oximetry, and
- Calculate the Respiratory Score for all spontaneously breathing infants.

Oxygen administration

Oxygen can be administered to a spontaneously breathing infant during resuscitation and stabilization in different ways (Figure 3.1).

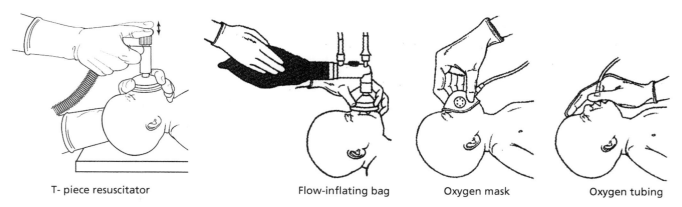

| T- piece resuscitator | Flow-inflating bag | Oxygen mask | Oxygen tubing |

Figure 3.1. Oxygen administration.

Source: American Academy of Pediatrics, American Heart Association, Canadian Paediatric Society. Neonatal Resuscitation Textbook, 6th edition, 2011.

Oxygen administration during resuscitation

- Apply the T-piece resuscitator, flow-inflating bag, oxygen mask, or oxygen tubing/prongs to the infant's face.
- Use a flow rate of 10 L/min.

- A T-piece resuscitator or flow-inflating bag delivers the oxygen concentration set on the blender if there is a seal between the infant's face and the mask. When there is a seal, either device may also deliver CPAP, depending on the set flow rate.
- A T-piece resuscitator or flow-inflating bag held close to the infant's face but without a seal functions like an oxygen mask or oxygen tubing by diluting flow with room air and cannot deliver the oxygen concentration set on the blender.

Oxygen administration during stabilization

Administering oxygen to a spontaneously breathing infant during stabilization requires a less user-dependent system and, because these infants require oxygen for longer periods, it should, ideally, be humidified. Options include:

- Low-flow nasal prongs
- An oxygen hood or incubator
- Heated, humidified high-flow nasal cannula therapy (H3FNC)

Low-flow nasal prongs (Figure 3.2) are not the preferred method of oxygen delivery during stabilization because oxygen is easily diluted by room air as the infant breathes or cries. The rate and depth of respiration, and the precise amount of oxygen the infant is receiving, cannot be reliably determined.

- 100% oxygen is administered at a flow rate of up to 1 L/min. As it is not humidified, higher flows can irritate and dry the nasal mucosa.
- Oxygen flow is adjusted up or down to achieve SpO2 between 90% and 95%.

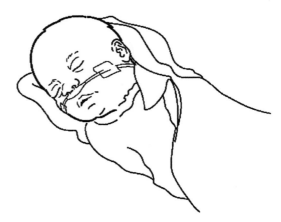

Figure 3.2. Infant with nasal prongs.

An **oxygen hood**, placed over the infant's head, contains the breathing environment (Figure 3.3).

- Blended humidified oxygen/air is administered at the concentration set on the blender.
- A gas flow greater than 7 L/min prevents CO_2 accumulation.
- An exact amount of delivered oxygen can be determined using an oxygen analyzer placed close to the infant's mouth and adjusted via the oxygen blender to achieve the desired SpO2 between 90% and 95%.
- Gas entering the hood should be warmed to 32°C to 34°C and humidified.

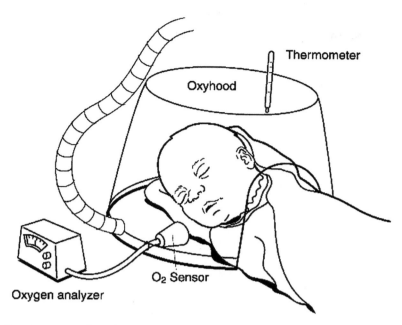

Figure 3.3. Infant in oxygen hood.

Incubators manufactured after 1990 can administer high oxygen concentrations, humidity, and warmth and have built-in oxygen analyzers that continuously adjust the oxygen flow to maintain a pre-set concentration. Older incubators or incubators with the port-hole doors opened frequently are not able to maintain set oxygen concentrations.

H3FNC (Figure 3.4) administers blended oxygen at flows of 1 L/min to 8 L/min via special prongs.

- Gas is humidified to prevent irritation and drying of the nasal mucosa.
- Oxygen can be titrated up or down to maintain a SpO2 of 90% to 95%.
- Higher flow rates can wash out dead space in the infant's upper airway, which allows accurate assessment of the oxygen content being delivered to the alveoli.
- Theoretical concerns exist about the pressure generated by high flow rates, with current systems being unable to measure pressures delivered. High pressures may increase the risk of air leaks and become more likely when exhalation is impaired, such as when cannulae are greater than half the diameter of an infant's nares or migrate too far into the nares and when an infant's mouth is closed.

Knowing whether an infant's oxygen requirements are increasing or decreasing over time is important. When delivering oxygen via oxygen hood or incubator, an oxygen analyzer can trend requirements. When delivering oxygen via H3FNC, requirements can be trended by recording oxygen blender set-points. It is not possible to measure oxygen delivery or trend requirements using low-flow nasal prongs.

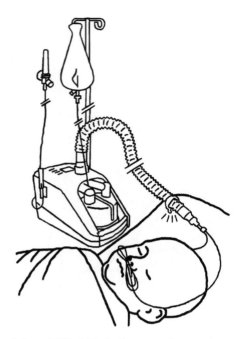

Figure 3.4. Infant with heated, humidified high-flow nasal cannula.

Oxygen delivery

Oxygen delivery to an infant's organs depends on cardiac output (discussed in Chapter 4, Cardiovascular) and the oxygen content (CaO2) in the circulating blood. Factors affecting the blood's ability to carry oxygen include:

- Oxygen saturation (SpO2 or SaO2)
- Hemoglobin (Hb) concentration
- Oxygen dissolved in plasma (PO2 or PaO2)

If these factors are known, the amount of oxygen carried to the infant's tissues can be calculated using this formula:

$$CaO2 = (SaO2 \times Hb \times 1.34 \text{ g/mL}) + 0.003 \text{ (PaO2)}$$

Most of the oxygen carried in blood is bound to Hb in an approximate ratio of bound to dissolved oxygen of 40:1. The amount of oxygen bound to Hb or the oxygen saturation is measured using pulse oximetry.

Pulse oximetry

Pulse oximetry is frequently used to monitor an infant's oxygenation because it is noninvasive, easy to use, and provides immediate readings in a continuous display. SpO2 closely reflects SaO2. Applying the probe to an infant's right hand or wrist measures pre-ductal oxygen saturation, which reflects the oxygen content of blood coming from the lungs and going to the brain.

Safe oxygen saturation levels for infants

While the ideal oxygen saturation range for infants, particularly preterm infants, is unclear, levels of 90% to 95% are generally recommended for newborns receiving supplemental oxygen. Oxygen saturation values greater than 95% are associated with oxygen toxicity, which can cause tissue and organ damage. The lower an infant's gestational age (GA), the greater the risk for oxygen toxicity. Term infants with hypoxic ischemic injury are also at high risk.

When Hb levels and cardiac function are normal, oxygen saturations in the normal range indicate adequate oxygen delivery to tissues and organs which, in turn, prevents the development of acidosis and pulmonary vasoconstriction. However, while oxygen saturation monitoring provides a good indication of how effective respiratory interventions have been in oxygenating the blood, it is not an indicator of effective breathing or ventilation.

Hemoglobin concentration

Adequate Hb levels are essential for oxygen delivery. In the face of severe anemia, cyanosis may not be detectable because approximately 50 g of deoxygenated Hb is required for an infant to appear cyanotic on inspection. An anemic infant with a Hb of 100 g/L, for example, would not appear cyanotic until the SpO2 dropped to 50%. When significant anemia is present, hypoxemic infants may appear pale rather than cyanotic. Blood transfusion can be lifesaving in cases with decreased oxygen carrying capacity secondary to anemia.

Partial pressure of oxygen

PO2 is a measure of the partial pressure exerted by oxygen molecules dissolved in plasma. As PO2 increases, more oxygen is bound to Hb, until saturation is complete. PaO2 indicates how well the lungs are transferring oxygen to blood. The relationship between SO2 and PO2 is shown in Figure 3.5.

As PO2 increases, saturation also rises rapidly, resulting in more oxygen bound to Hb and available for transport in circulating blood. When SO2 rises above 95%, large changes in PO2 cause minimal additional increases in saturation. This hyperoxic state increases risk for oxygen toxicity.

In newborns, fetal Hb binds oxygen with greater affinity than adult Hb. This is represented by a shift in the oxyhemoglobin dissociation curve to the left for fetal Hb.

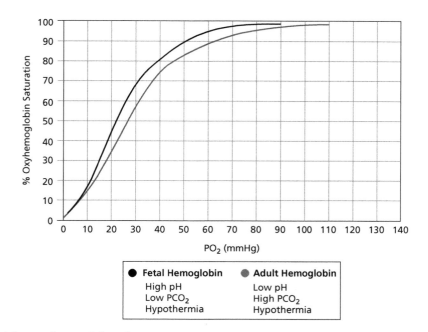

Figure 3.5. The oxyhemoglobin dissociation curve.

Calculation of the Respiratory Score

Infants who have difficulty inflating and ventilating their lungs show increased work of breathing and develop respiratory distress. Judging the severity of respiratory distress is a skill acquired with experience. The Respiratory Score (Table 3.1) assists ACoRN providers in recognizing the signs and symptoms of distress that need assessment. It is used in all infants who are breathing spontaneously, including those being treated with CPAP or noninvasive positive pressure ventilation (PPV). The Respiratory Score is not intended for infants who are intubated and receiving ventilation.

Table 3.1 lists the six components of the Respiratory Score with their descriptors. Each component is scored from 0 to 2.

- The first three components help to quantify the degree of respiratory distress.
- The oxygen requirement reflects the extent of lung recruitment.
- Breath sounds on auscultation reflect the success of lung ventilation.
- The degree of prematurity has been included as the leading modifier of an infant's ability to cope with respiratory distress. The more premature the infant, the earlier and quicker decompensation will occur.

Table 3.1.
The Respiratory Score

Score	0	1	2
Respiratory rate	40 to 60/min	60 to 80/min	> 80/min
Retractions	None	Intercostal or subcostal retractions (or both)	Intercostal, subcostal, and sternal retractions
Grunting	None	With stimulation	Continuous at rest
Oxygen requirement*	None	≤ 30%	> 30%
Breath sounds on auscultation	Easily heard throughout	Decreased	Barely heard
Prematurity	> 34 weeks	30 to 34 weeks	< 30 weeks
		Respiratory Score	__/12

Adapted from Downes JJ, Vidyasagar D, Boggs TR, Morrow GM. Respiratory distress syndrome of newborn infants. I. New clinical scoring system (RDS score) with acid-base and blood-gas correlations. Clin Pediatr 1970; 9(6):325–331.

**Note:* An infant receiving oxygen before an O2 analyzer is set up or in an open oxygen delivery system is assigned a score of 1.

An infant in respiratory failure cannot maintain work of breathing and signs of respiratory distress for long and may score lower than expected as they fatigue. If not stabilized effectively, they may present with new onset gasping or apnea.

The Respiratory Score is the sum of the six component items. It is used by itself or in conjunction with other clinical factors to organize care of the infant presenting with:

- Recurring apnea that requires PPV,
- Mild respiratory distress that lasts longer than 6 h post-birth,

- New-onset respiratory distress in a previously asymptomatic infant, and
- A sustained increase in oxygen requirement more than 10% above baseline, for 10 min or longer, to keep oxygen saturations within the target range.

The Respiratory Score is also used to track changes in the severity of the respiratory distress over time in infants who are not intubated.

Organization of Care

In the ACoRN Respiratory Sequence, Organization of Care is based on severity of respiratory distress as defined by the Respiratory Score and is modified by the presence of additional clinical factors.

Mild respiratory distress is defined as:

- A Respiratory Score less than 5, with signs starting at birth *and* lasting less than 6 h.

Moderate respiratory distress is defined as:

- A Respiratory Score of 5 to 8.

Included in this arm of the Organization of Care are infants with:

- Mild respiratory distress that lasts longer than 6 h post-birth, or
- New-onset respiratory distress in a previously asymptomatic infant, or
- A sustained increase in oxygen requirement more than 10% above baseline, for 10 min or longer, to keep oxygen saturations within the target range.

These infants are at risk of progressing to respiratory failure without support. Infants with persistent or new-onset respiratory distress may be symptomatic due to other causes, such as infection. A sustained increase in oxygen requirement indicates decreasingly effective oxygenation and may indicate impaired ventilation as well.

Other factors that increase risk of an infant's being unable to sustain adequate oxygenation and ventilation include:

- Prematurity
  o Infants with a GA less than 27 weeks require respiratory support.
  o Infants with a GA less than 32 weeks or a birth weight less than 1500 g usually require respiratory support.
  o Infants born less than 34 weeks GA, whose antenatal steroid coverage is incomplete, may require respiratory support.
- Baseline oxygen requirements greater than 30% indicate that an infant's respiratory reserves are low.

Severe respiratory distress is defined as:

- A Respiratory Score greater than 8.

Included in this arm of the Organization of Care are infants:

- With recurring apnea that requires PPV, or
- Who are already receiving ventilation due to respiratory failure during resuscitation or a previous passage through the Respiratory Sequence.

These infants require immediate intervention to prevent further deterioration and even death.

Response

Mild respiratory distress

Infants with mild respiratory distress lasting less than 6 h post-birth require close observation and regular monitoring using the Respiratory Score. They may require supplemental oxygen to maintain blood oxygen levels within the target SpO2 range of 90% to 95%.

Any of the following signs suggest that an infant is no longer meeting criteria for mild respiratory distress and should prompt the ACoRN provider to reassess and increase respiratory support:

- Persistence of respiratory signs beyond 6 h of age
- A worsening Respiratory Score
- A sustained increase in oxygen requirement of greater than 10% from baseline for 10 min or more
- An oxygen requirement of 30% or greater to maintain saturations within the target range. In an infant who is not receiving respiratory support, this indicates atelectasis (loss of lung volume) and inability to sustain adequate oxygenation.

Additional respiratory support should be considered, particularly for preterm infants or term infants with other risk factors.

In infants with mild respiratory distress, a further sepsis work-up and antibiotics are required only if they meet criteria in the ACoRN Infection Sequence (see Chapter 10, Infection).

Moderate respiratory distress

Infants who are breathing spontaneously but experiencing moderate respiratory distress will benefit from support with CPAP, which prevents atelectasis by stabilizing the small airways and chest wall at end-expiration. CPAP can delay or prevent the progression to severe respiratory distress and eventual respiratory failure. A sustained increase in oxygen requirements in an infant with moderate respiratory distress usually indicates a loss of lung volume and the need to increase the level of respiratory support provided. Increasing the CPAP level should help to stabilize lung volumes and improve oxygenation. Higher CPAP levels may increase the risk for pneumothorax. Administering CPAP pressures greater than 8 cmH2O or switching to noninvasive PPV (biphasic respiratory support) should be decided in consultation with your referral centre.

In the extreme preterm infant with RDS, improving lung function may require the administration of surfactant.

Continuous positive airway pressure

CPAP (Figure 3.6) decreases the need for endotracheal intubation and mechanical ventilation in infants with moderate respiratory distress and good respiratory drive. CPAP must be administered and monitored by on-site, trained personnel, in settings resourced to provide additional respiratory support, especially if escalation in care is anticipated. The purpose of CPAP is to:

- Improve arterial PO2 to reduce inspired oxygen concentration in infants with respiratory distress who do not require mechanical ventilation,
- Stabilize respiratory function on extubation from mechanical ventilation, and
- Treat obstructive apnea in some preterm infants.
  - CPAP reduces mixed and obstructive apnea. It has no effect on central apnea.

CPAP is contraindicated in infants with:

- Inadequate respiratory drive (i.e., irregular breathing or apnea),
- Impaired spontaneous breathing (e.g., as in central nervous system disorders),
- Significant agitation or who cannot tolerate CPAP, and
- Conditions where air swallowing is undesirable (e.g., gastrointestinal obstruction, necrotizing enterocolitis, congenital diaphragmatic hernia [CDH]).

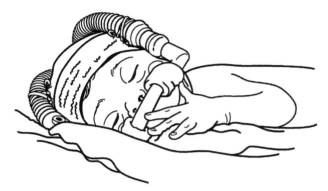

Figure 3.6. Infant on CPAP.

Severe respiratory distress

Infants with severe respiratory distress, recurrent apnea, or gasping require immediate intubation and ventilation to prevent respiratory failure. If a care provider with intubation skills is not present, use of a laryngeal mask airway should be considered.

Intubation

Intubation should not be delayed for intravenous (IV) access and premedication in infants requiring urgent or emergent care (e.g., during resuscitation). However, newborns should be premedicated whenever possible because laryngoscopy and intubation are painful procedures that can cause hypertension, increased intracranial pressure, bradycardia, and hypoxia. Premedication provides analgesia and can lessen hemodynamic consequences. A typical premedication regimen includes combining atropine and opiates (e.g., morphine or fentanyl) with a short-acting paralyzing agent (e.g., succinylcholine). The paralytic should only be administered by a care provider who is familiar with its use and skilled in neonatal intubation.

In the event of a sudden deterioration in an intubated infant, airway patency should be assessed. The **DOPE** acronym can help identify and troubleshoot possible causes.

D . . . Displaced ETT? Has the infant accidentally extubated or is the ETT in the right main stem bronchus? Ensuring that the ETT is not displaced from its proper position involves:
- Making certain that it is at the same measurement mark at the lip or nares as when inserted,
- Using an exhaled CO_2 detector to determine whether the tube is inserted in the airway, not the esophagus,
- Auscultating for presence and symmetry of breath sounds in the chest but not over the stomach area (this may not be a reliable sign in small infants), and
- Inspecting the tube position using a laryngoscope.

O . . . Obstructed airway or ETT? Kinked or blocked by secretions?

P . . . Pneumothorax or other critical diagnosis? Other possible causes include pulmonary interstitial emphysema, or atelectasis.

E . . . Equipment working and ventilation optimized?

Mechanical ventilation

Administering mechanical ventilation (cycled positive inspiratory pressure [PIP] with PEEP) stabilizes the infant's small airways and chest wall, expands the lungs during inspiration by delivering a tidal volume at a set respiratory rate, and prevents atelectasis at end-expiration.

Ventilation is delivered via an ETT:

* Manually, using a T-piece resuscitator or self- or flow-inflating bag, or
* Using a ventilator.

The indications for ventilation include:

* Ineffective respiration with decreased respiratory drive (irregular breathing or apnea),
* Severe respiratory distress (Respiratory Score greater than 8),
* Moderate respiratory distress (Respiratory Score 5 to 8) with unsatisfactory blood gases (pH $\leq$ 7.25 and $PCO_2 \geq 55$),
* Increasing Respiratory Score, increasing oxygen requirements despite CPAP (or both),
* The decision to administer surfactant,
* Use as an alternative to CPAP for infants requiring transport.

Mechanical ventilation must be administered and monitored by on-site, trained personnel in settings resourced to provide respiratory support, especially if escalation in care is anticipated.

Next Steps

The Next Steps in the Respiratory Sequence should include obtaining a focused history and conducting a physical examination.

For infants with moderate to severe respiratory distress, Next Steps also include obtaining vascular access, ordering diagnostic tests and imaging (e.g., blood gases and a chest radiograph), optimizing ventilation, and requesting an expert consult.

Focused history

Important information to gather for a focused respiratory history includes:

Antepartum

* Confirm GA and accuracy of dates
* Prenatal ultrasound findings, for evidence of conditions that impair lung function, such as CDH, congenital pulmonary airway malformation (congenital cystic adenomatoid malformation), abnormal lung echotexture, and oligohydramnios
* Maternal diabetes, as a risk factor for RDS or cardiac outflow tract anomalies

- Risk factors for congenital pneumonia, including maternal Group B *Streptococcus* (GBS) status, premature rupture of membranes, maternal fever, or chorioamnionitis
- Receipt of antenatal steroids for pulmonary maturation
- Maternal use of medications (e.g., selective serotonin reuptake inhibitors) which may cause tachypnea or PPHN, or illicit substances, particularly narcotics, which can suppress respiratory drive

Intrapartum

- Presence of atypical or abnormal fetal heart rate during labour and delivery
- Meconium-stained amniotic fluid
- Time of rupture of membranes
- Signs of chorioamnionitis (maternal fever, uterine tenderness, fetal tachycardia, foul-smelling vaginal discharge)
- Nature of labour and mode of delivery
- Medications used
- Intrapartum antibiotics for GBS prophylaxis

Neonatal

- Umbilical cord blood gas results (arterial and venous)
- Condition at birth, including Apgar score
- Need for resuscitation, and response
- Timing for onset of symptoms (i.e., present at birth or after a period of normal respiratory function)
- GA and birth weight

Focused physical examination

A focused respiratory examination includes:

Observation

- Laboured respirations (e.g., nasal flaring, retractions, or grunting)
- Colour of skin and mucous membranes (i.e., peripheral versus central cyanosis)
- Respiratory support (e.g., oxygen requirements, size and position of ETT, ventilator settings)

Measurement of vital signs should include respiratory rate, heart rate, temperature, blood pressure, and oxygen saturation.

Examination

- Auscultate both lung fields for equality and nature of breath sounds. Diminished breath sounds unilaterally may signal intubation of the right bronchus, pneumonia, atelectasis, or a pneumothorax or other space-occupying lesion (e.g., a diaphragmatic hernia).
- Listen for grunting, inspiratory stridor, expiratory wheeze, crackles.
- Check for cleft palate or micrognathia (small jaw).
- Pass a nasogastric tube through each nare to rule out choanal atresia.

Diagnostic tests are conducted for all infants entering the Respiratory Sequence *except* term infants with mild respiratory distress lasting less than 6 h.

Vascular access

- Obtain vascular access to administer dextrose solution. Provide fluids and glucose during stabilization and early management. Infants with moderate to severe respiratory distress and those receiving respiratory support cannot be orally fed because of poor oral–motor coordination and risk of aspiration.
- Consider risks for infection and need for antibiotics.

Chest radiograph

Order a chest radiograph to aid diagnosis, help optimize PEEP/CPAP levels for optimal lung volume, and guide further management. (See Appendix B for information on interpretation.)

Blood gas

Blood gases help monitor oxygenation (SaO2 and PaO2), ventilation (PaCO2), and acid base status. (See Appendix B for more information on interpretation.)

- **pH** estimates the blood total acid load, which mostly reflects dissolved CO2 but may also include metabolic acids (e.g., lactic acid).
- **PCO2** indicates how well the lungs are removing CO2 from blood (ventilation).
- **PaO2** (arterial PO2) indicates how well the lungs are transferring oxygen to blood (oxygenation) in relation to % inspired oxygen.
- **Base deficit (BD)** estimates how much metabolic acid is present in the blood. Base excess (BE), the negative value of BD, and bicarbonate are also used to describe acid-base status.

Arterial, capillary, or venous samples are nearly equally useful for determining PCO2, pH, and BD. In acute respiratory illness, blood gases are considered satisfactory when the pH is 7.25 to 7.40 and the PCO2 is 45 mmHg to 55 mmHg. An acidosis (pH ≤ 7.25) with PCO2 at or above 55 indicates poor ventilation (respiratory acidosis).

Optimize ventilation

Optimizing ventilation involves ensuring that:

- The infant is connected to the ventilator,
- The ventilator or manual ventilation equipment is delivering the settings indicated and is not malfunctioning,
- Chest expansion can be observed, and breath sounds are equal and symmetrical,
- The infant breathes in synchrony with the ventilator and work of breathing has decreased, and
- Pulse oximetry and blood gases are within the target range.

Consider immediate consult

Consideration should be given to obtaining immediate consultation for guidance depending on expertise with managing neonatal respiratory disease and the resources available on site. When an infant's needs exceed or are anticipated to exceed site capabilities, early recognition and planning for transport can be lifesaving.

While waiting for diagnostic test results, the ACoRN provider should establish a working diagnosis based on the presentation of mild, moderate, or severe respiratory distress and a Level of Risk category for this infant.

In a spontaneously breathing infant, the ACoRN Respiratory Score is used to monitor an infant's condition and response to interventions over time. It is used to guide the organization of care according to changes in severity.

Oxygen administration should be continuously adjusted to maintain SpO2 levels in target range.

Adjustments to respiratory support (CPAP or ventilator settings) are guided by the infant's condition and response to interventions, chest X-ray and blood gas results, and consultation with your referral centre.

Specific Diagnosis and Management

Formulation of a Specific Diagnosis and Management plan will depend on the provider's experience and knowledge of conditions that present with respiratory distress in the newborn, along with radiographic findings. Common conditions include:

- Pneumothorax and other air leaks
- RDS
- TTN
- Meconium aspiration syndrome (MAS)
- Pneumonia
- PPHN

Specific diagnosis and management planning may require consultation with your referral centre.

Pneumothorax

A pneumothorax (Figure 3.7) occurs when overdistension of an infant's lung results in rupture of the alveoli or terminal bronchioles and release of intrapulmonary air into the pleural space ('air leak'). Clinically, a pneumothorax may occur when there is:

- rapid improvement in lung compliance after surfactant therapy,
- delivery of excessive airway pressures, or
- plugging of small airways causing a ball-valve effect, as in meconium aspiration.

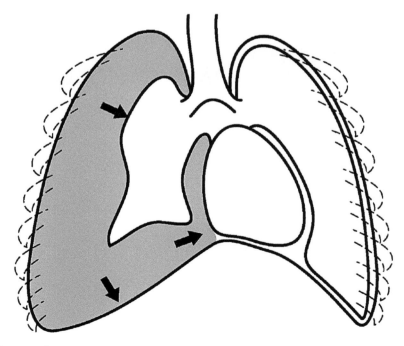

Figure 3.7. Pneumothorax.

Infants at high risk for pneumothorax include those:

- with lung disease (RDS, aspiration syndromes, or hypoplastic lungs), or
- receiving respiratory support, especially high levels of CPAP or mechanical ventilation.

Risk for pneumothorax is highest in the first 24 to 48 h post-birth. A 'spontaneous pneumothorax' can occur in spontaneously breathing infants not receiving respiratory support, usually around the time of initial lung inflation. Pneumothoraces usually present with an acute increase in respiratory distress, oxygen requirements, and CO_2 retention.

A tension pneumothorax may present with sudden onset of cardiovascular collapse as venous return to the heart is impaired.

Chest radiograph

A chest radiograph is the definitive test to diagnose a pneumothorax.

Small pneumothorax:

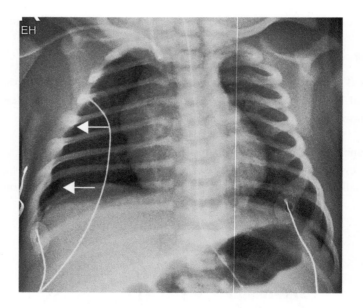

- Hemithorax volume is similar in the affected (right) and unaffected (left) side.
- The affected side (right) is more lucent, and a black rim of air, which contains no lung markings, (arrows) may be noted between the chest wall and the lung tissue.
- The cardiac silhouette is not shifted toward the unaffected side.

A small pneumothorax with minimal respiratory distress and no cardiovascular deterioration can be observed until it resolves spontaneously.

Moderate pneumothorax:

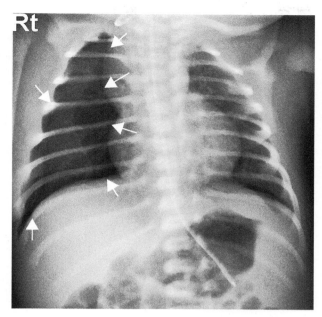

- Hemithorax volume is slightly larger in the affected (right) side than in the unaffected (left) side.
- The affected side (right) is more lucent, and a black rim of air (arrows) is noted between the chest wall, diaphragm, mediastinum, and the lung tissue.
- The cardiac silhouette is slightly shifted toward the unaffected side.

Large (tension) pneumothorax—anteroposterior view:

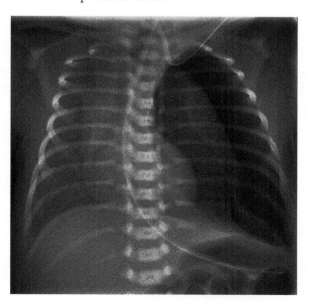

- Hemithorax volume is markedly larger in the affected side (left) than in the unaffected side (right), and the diaphragm may be flattened.
- The affected side is more lucent, and a black rim of air, which contains no lung markings, is noted between the chest wall and the lung tissue.
- The cardiac silhouette is markedly shifted toward the unaffected side.

Large (tension) pneumothorax—lateral view:

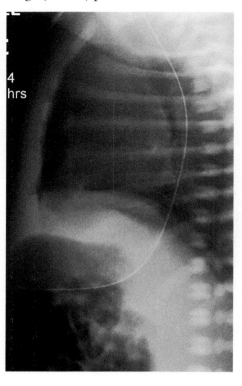

- The pneumothorax is represented by a large anterior lucency and lucency at the level of the diaphragm.
- The diaphragm may be flattened.

Pneumomediastinum and left–sided pneumothorax:

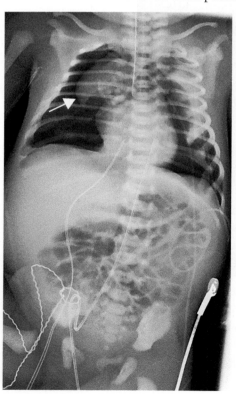

Signs of pneumomediastinum:

- The arrow shows a thymus outlined by air and clearly lifted off the cardiac surface, radiologically referred to as the 'sail' or 'butterfly' sign.
- The heart borders are sharp, the diaphragms are flattened and sharply outlined, indicating air tracking inferiorly down the mediastinum and out along the right and left sides of the diaphragm.

Signs of pneumothorax:

- The entire right hemithorax is hyperlucent, as is the lower edge of the left hemithorax.
- Most of the air is anterior to the lung (the lung 'rim' can only be seen easily inferiorly on the right).
- If a pneumopericardium were present, it would present as a halo seen around the heart.

Chest transillumination

Comparative transillumination of the chest may be useful when an infant is deteriorating rapidly and a chest radiograph cannot be obtained quickly. Transillumination is less sensitive when used in term and late preterm infants.

Transillumination *must* be performed in a darkened environment, using a fibreoptic device (transilluminator) capable of delivering high illumination.

- The transilluminator must be in direct contact with the infant's chest.
- A unilateral pneumothorax is suspected when the halo around the point of contact is significantly larger on one side of the chest compared with the other.

Point-of-care lung ultrasound

Ultrasound assessment for pneumothorax is emerging as a new application of point-of-care ultrasound (POCUS) in the neonatal period. POCUS should be performed by trained individuals. A pneumothorax on ultrasound is characterized by a series of patterns including prominent A-lines, absence of B-lines, absent lung sliding, and possibly a lung point sign.

Management of a symptomatic pneumothorax

A symptomatic pneumothorax, especially one under tension, needs to be drained urgently and takes precedence over returning to the Problem List to address the next ACoRN Sequence.

There are two ways to drain a pneumothorax: needle aspiration or chest tube insertion.

1. **Needle aspiration**

   This procedure should only be undertaken as an emergency in an infant with significant compromise and a positive transillumination or chest radiograph. In severely symptomatic infants, it may be necessary to proceed with needle aspiration before a confirmatory chest radiograph but after ensuring the ETT has not been displaced or obstructed.

   The needle or vascular catheter can be held in place for ongoing removal of air or be connected to an underwater seal. Needle aspiration is usually an interim measure, pending placement of a chest tube.

2. **Chest tube insertion**

   Inserting a chest tube provides continuous drainage of a pneumothorax, allowing re-expansion of the ipsilateral collapsed lung and release of pressure on the heart and other mediastinal structures.

   A chest tube should never be left open to the environment because this would allow air to be drawn back into the pleural space with spontaneous, negative-pressure breathing. Before unclamping the chest tube, it should be connected to a drainage system with an underwater seal or a flutter (Heimlich) valve to prevent air re-entry.

   Initial indications that a chest tube is within the pleural space are:

   - Palpation of the tube between the ribs rather than up the chest wall after the tube insertion
   - Bubbling in the underwater seal at the time of unclamping
   - Condensation and serous drainage in the tube
   - Fluid meniscus moving along the tube
   - Signs of improvement in the infant's oxygenation and perfusion

Drainage of frank blood is unusual and may indicate that a blood vessel has been ruptured.

Definitive confirmation that the chest tube is in the pleural space and the pneumothorax has been drained is obtained by chest radiograph.

Tension pneumothorax, post–drain insertion:

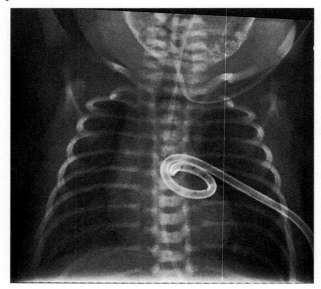

Respiratory distress syndrome

RDS is a condition caused by lack of pulmonary surfactant, a soapy substance that is normally present in mature lungs. Surfactant reduces surface tension within the alveoli, preventing their collapse and allowing them to inflate more easily. Without surfactant, widespread atelectasis (alveolar collapse) results in decreased lung volume and increased work of breathing. The lung surface area for gas exchange is reduced, causing hypoxemia and hypercarbia.

RDS is primarily a disease of preterm infants and its incidence increases with decreasing GA. Risk for RDS also increases in late preterm infants born to mothers with poorly controlled diabetes.

Infants with RDS can present with any degree of respiratory distress and oxygen requirement. Symptoms usually appear shortly after birth and become progressively more severe in the first 72 h if the infant's own respiratory efforts, or the respiratory supports provided, are unable to prevent progressive lung collapse. The natural course of RDS, if not treated with exogenous surfactant, is to slowly improve after 72 h to 5 days. During this period, endogenous surfactant production and release become established.

Mild RDS:

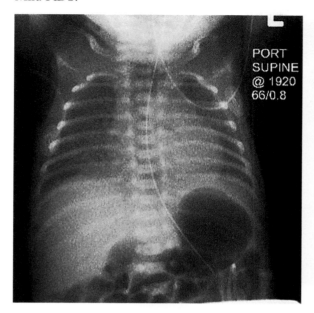

- Normal or slightly decreased lung inflation
- Fairly clear lung fields with slight diffuse haziness
- Diaphragm and heart borders mildly obscured
- Few air bronchograms (airways containing air become visible against collapsed lung) appear longitudinally

Moderate RDS:

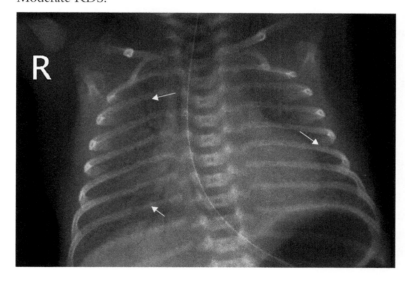

- Moderately decreased lung inflation
- Lung fields diffusely hazy, with a 'ground glass' appearance
- Heart borders and diaphragm greater than 50% obscured
- Air bronchograms more widely seen in upper and lower lobes (arrows)

Severe RDS:

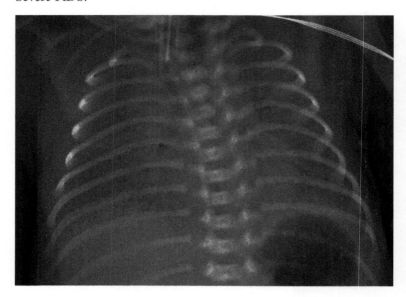

- Decreased lung inflation
- Lung fields diffusely hazy, with a total or near-total 'whiteout' appearance
- Heart borders and diaphragm greater than 50% obscured
- Air bronchograms in upper and lower lobes

Treating infants with RDS who are ventilated includes administering exogenous surfactant as early as possible. Early surfactant use has been shown to reduce pneumothorax, mortality, and other complications of RDS.

Surfactant administration

Exogenous surfactant is administered directly into the infant's trachea and bronchial tree via the endotracheal tube (ETT) or a thin catheter, as shown in Figure 3.8. The usual dose (depending on the brand) is 2.5 mL/kg to 5 mL/kg.

During surfactant administration, infants may develop transient desaturation, bradycardia (or both), due to airway obstruction or vagal stimulation. These effects usually resolve with slowing or halting administration until the infant improves. Sometimes the ventilator settings and the percent of inspired oxygen need to be increased temporarily.

As lung compliance improves following surfactant administration, the pressure required to inflate the lungs (and produce an easy rise of the chest), along with the oxygen required to maintain target saturations, often decrease dramatically. It is important to:

- Closely monitor changes in oximetry readings and serial blood gases,
- Reduce the peak ventilator pressures, as needed, to avoid complications of over-inflation, including pneumothorax, and
- Reduce the oxygen to maintain SpO2 within the desired range.

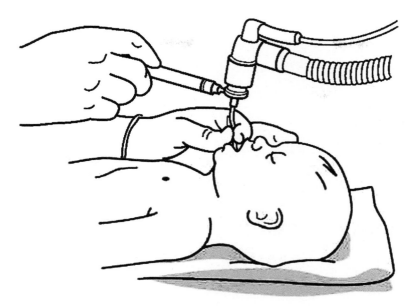

Figure 3.8. Surfactant delivery through endotracheal tube.

An improvement in respiratory status may be temporary and does not eliminate the need for transport to a centre capable of providing higher level neonatal care.

Health care providers administering surfactant must be skilled in neonatal intubation and prepared to deal with the rapid changes in lung compliance and oxygenation during and after surfactant is given. They must also be aware of the potential complications of this treatment. The procedure for and complications of delivering surfactant are also discussed in Appendix A.

Transient tachypnea of the newborn

TTN occurs when lung fluid production does not cease before birth, and there is a delay in clearance of residual lung fluid after birth. It is a primary cause of respiratory distress in term or late preterm infants. TTN is more common in newborns born by Caesarean section (especially when there has been no labour) or after a precipitous vaginal delivery.

Infants with TTN present with mild to moderate respiratory distress and oxygen requirements typically less than 40%. Respiratory distress due to TTN will often improve or resolve over the first few hours post-birth, as residual lung fluid is reabsorbed. TTN has been reported to last as long as 48 to 72 h, but usually shows improvement well before that. When TTN persists beyond 6 h post-birth or worsens within that time frame, other diagnoses need to be considered, including infection and surfactant deficiency or inactivation.

Mild TTN:

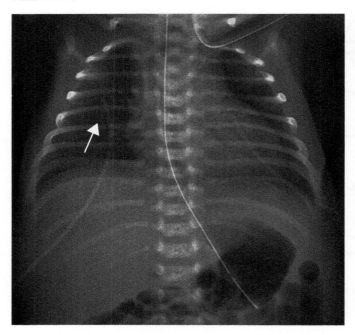

- Normal or increased lung inflation (normal in this example)
- Fairly clear lung fields
- Diaphragm and heart borders are seen throughout
- Increased vascular markings near the heart shadow give lungs a streaky appearance
- Fluid in the major fissure (arrow) may include a small amount of pleural fluid

Severe TTN:

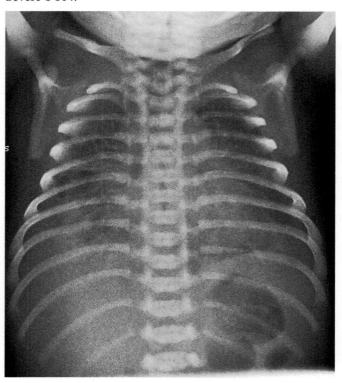

- Same appearance as for mild TTN but with increased haziness of lung fields
- Diaphragm and heart borders are not well seen

Management of TTN is primarily supportive. The goals are to maintain adequate oxygenation and ventilation while lung fluid is reabsorbed. Natural resolution occurs with diuresis. Fluid overload should be avoided with judicious use of IV fluids, if parenteral nutrition and hydration are necessary. Diuretics do not play a role in typical TTN resolution.

Meconium aspiration syndrome

MAS is a spectrum of illness that occurs in post-term, term and, sometimes, late preterm infants (with a functionally mature gastrointestinal tract), who aspirate meconium before or at the time of birth. Respiratory distress in MAS can be mild and transient or severe, leading to respiratory failure with hypoxemia, acidosis, and PPHN. MAS always warrants close observation because even infants who are stable initially can deteriorate and develop refractory PPHN.

Aspirating meconium has three main effects on pulmonary function, resulting in ventilation: perfusion mismatch:

- Large and small airway obstruction
- Surfactant inactivation
- Chemical pneumonitis

Because MAS is a disease that begins with fetal compromise in utero, most cases are not preventable with interventions at birth, such as endotracheal suctioning. Severe MAS is life-threatening and requires prompt, specialized care. The main complications of MAS are respiratory failure, PPHN, and pulmonary air leaks, especially pneumothorax.

Moderate to severe MAS:

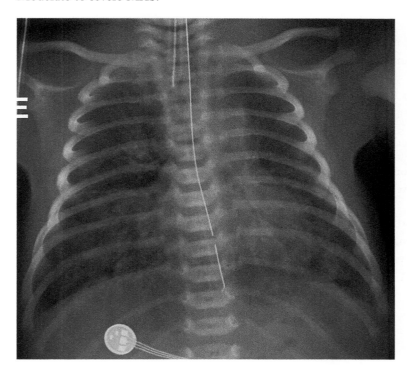

- Normal or increased lung inflation (increased in this example)
- Lung fields show fluffy, patchy, and coarse infiltrates, and asymmetric areas of hyperinflation interposed with areas of atelectasis
- Heart borders and diaphragm are usually significantly obscured by areas of atelectatic lung

Avoiding respiratory failure

The best strategy to avoid respiratory failure is to maintain optimal lung inflation and prevent atelectasis. In infants with moderate respiratory distress associated with MAS, this is best accomplished using CPAP.

Mechanical ventilation for MAS is usually reserved for infants with:

- Escalating oxygen requirements greater than 40% to 50% to maintain SpO2 greater than 90%
- PCO2 greater than 55 or pH less than 7.25.

The acts of intubation and initiation of mechanical ventilation can cause an infant with MAS to react adversely and PPHN to worsen. Premedication for intubation is recommended (see page 59 and Appendix C) and sedation during mechanical ventilation may be needed. Infants with MAS often have low lung compliance and may require high ventilation pressure, increasing the risk for air leaks. Muscle paralysis may be necessary to achieve control of ventilation and oxygenation.

Avoiding PPHN

Infants with MAS are predisposed to PPHN and may have labile pulmonary circulation, dropping their oxygenation in response to stimuli such as excessive handling, painful procedures, bright lights, or loud noises. Once established, PPHN is difficult to treat and may be life-threatening.

The following interventions can help promote stability:

- Shielding the infant's eyes from light
- Speaking in a low voice, and away from the infant's bed
- Minimizing handling
- Nesting
- Providing adequate pain relief
- Considering the need for sedation
- Maintaining pre-ductal SpO2 in the 90% to 95% range
- Documenting and reporting unstable SpO2 and a pre-ductal–post-ductal SpO2 difference

PPHN should be anticipated as a complication of severe MAS. Strategies to minimize PPHN are discussed under the specific management of that disorder.

Avoiding pulmonary air leaks

The best strategy to avoid pulmonary air leaks is to prevent lung overdistension. For infants receiving mechanical ventilation, this is best accomplished by:

- Limiting initial CPAP levels to 5 to 8 cmH2O,
- Avoiding overventilation by maintaining PCO2 above 40 mmHg,
- Considering surfactant administration, and
- Avoiding suctioning of the ETT as much as possible.

Surfactant therapy

Meconium aspiration causes secondary surfactant deficiency. Clinical trials have shown that surfactant replacement therapy can be a beneficial intervention in MAS (see pages 70-71 and Appendix A). However, surfactant must be administered cautiously, avoiding hypoxia and excessive stimulation. The decision to administer surfactant in infants with MAS should be taken with great caution, because these infants can deteriorate due to labile pulmonary hypertension. Consultation with the referral centre is advised.

Pneumonia

Neonatal pneumonia is an infectious infiltrate of the lungs. Pneumonia is usually interstitial and diffuse rather than lobar in appearance. It is more likely to occur in the presence of risk factors for sepsis (e.g., premature rupture of membranes, maternal colonization with GBS, or chorioamnionitis). Infants may or may not be systemically ill at onset, but the clinical course can be fulminant.

Pneumonia:

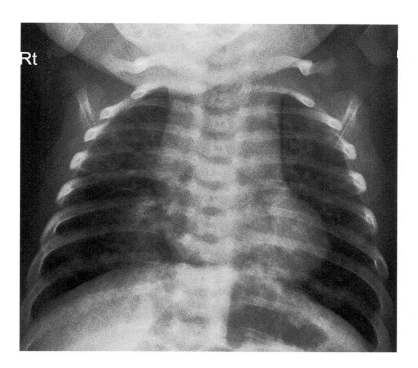

- Radiographic diagnosis is always tentative because the chest radiograph may mimic RDS, TTN, and, occasionally, MAS.
- There may be moderately to markedly increased lung inflation.
- Lung fields may show patchy densities and various degrees of 'whiteout' and air bronchograms.
- Diaphragm and heart borders may be obscured.
- Discrete segmental or lobar involvement may be present but is not common.

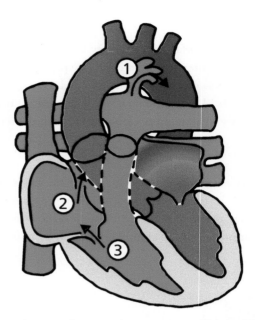

Figure 3.9. Blood flow in persistent pulmonary hypertension of the newborn. 1. Right-to-left shunt via the PDA. 2. Right-to-left shunt via the patent foramen ovale. 3. Functional tricuspid insufficiency and regurgitation due to right ventricular dysfunction.

The inability to rule out pneumonia by clinical or radiographic appearance gives rise to the recommendation to treat all respiratory disease in the newborn lasting longer than 6 h with IV antibiotics. Specific management is guided by the ACoRN Infection Sequence (see Chapter 10).

Persistent pulmonary hypertension of the newborn

PPHN is a disorder of the pulmonary vasculature characterized by failure of the normal drop in pulmonary vascular resistance after birth. PPHN leads to decreased pulmonary blood flow and persistence of the right-to-left shunts that exist in utero. When an infant's pulmonary arterial pressure exceeds systemic blood pressure, and the ductus arteriosus is open, right-to-left shunting is seen clinically as a pre- to post-ductal SpO2 difference with post-ductal hypoxemia (Figure 3.9). When right ventricular strain results in tricuspid valve incompetence and regurgitation of blood into the right atrium, this leads to right-to-left shunting through the foramen ovale. This is seen clinically as pre- *and* post-ductal hypoxemia.

PPHN may have an underlying vascular component of prenatal origin, which includes increased vascular muscularization and reactivity, decreased pulmonary vascularization, or abnormal vascular distribution. PPHN may also be triggered by intra- and post-partum events that cause fetal hypoxia and acidosis. While PPHN is more commonly associated with respiratory conditions such as RDS, MAS, pneumonia, or CDH, it may also occur as a primary disturbance of transition in the absence of parenchymal lung disease.

The diagnosis of PPHN should always be confirmed by an echocardiography to rule out abnormal cardiovascular anatomy.

PPHN is life-threatening and requires prompt, specialized care. Interventions that help decrease the pulmonary arterial pressures during or following transition in infants prone to PPHN include:

- Minimizing handling and disturbance
- Use of sedation when necessary
- Use of paralysis, in consultation, when necessary to meet ventilation needs
- Maintaining oxygenation in the high end of the normal range:
  - PO2 70 mmHg to 90 mmHg, and pre-ductal SpO2 approximately 90% to 95%
- Minimizing atelectasis while avoiding overdistension in infants with moderate to severe respiratory distress, by using CPAP, mechanical ventilation, and/or surfactant therapy in consultation with your referral centre, and
- Avoiding and correcting respiratory and metabolic acidosis to maintain:
  - PH 7.30 to 7.40, and
  - PCO2 40 mmHg to 50 mmHg.

Decreasing pulmonary vascular pressures and maintaining systemic blood pressure are important when managing PPHN. Volume expansion, selective pulmonary vasodilators, and inotropic therapy may be needed to maintain cardiac output and blood pressure. Specific management requires consultation with your referral centre.

Other conditions

Pulmonary hypoplasia

Pulmonary hypoplasia refers to conditions where an infant's lungs are incompletely developed such that the number of patent airways and gas-exchange spaces (alveoli), and corresponding vascular supply, are greatly reduced. Pulmonary hypoplasia may be seen in infants who experienced insufficient lung inflation in utero during early gestation, such as with:

- Severe oligohydramnios, caused by
  - Rupture of the membranes in the second trimester,
  - Renal agenesis, or
  - Urinary outflow obstruction;
- CDH; or
- Neuromuscular disease, with decreased fetal respiration.

Infants with pulmonary hypoplasia present at birth with profound respiratory failure. They have increased risk for PPHN and pneumothorax. This condition is life-threatening and requires prompt, specialized care as advanced forms of ventilation and intensive care result in improved outcomes.

Radiographic findings:

- Small but sometimes clear lung fields
- Bell-shaped chest
- Evidence of a space-occupying lesion (i.e., CDH)

Left–sided CDH:

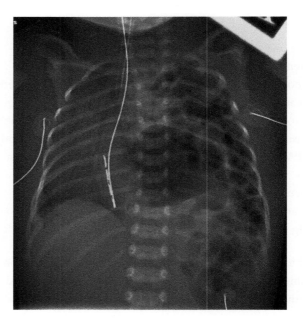

- Stomach bubble is in the abdomen (gastric tube coiled in the chest).
- There is mediastinal shift to the right.
- Air is present in the bowel located within the left chest (diaphragm defect is more common on the left).

Note: Air may not present in the bowel if the infant is intubated immediately after birth (no bag-and-mask ventilation) and administered neuromuscular blockade (unable to swallow air).

Level of Risk: Respiratory
In the ACoRN Respiratory Sequence, level of risk is based on the severity of respiratory distress, oxygen requirements, and the level of respiratory support being administered.

 Green:
- Infant has mild respiratory distress lasting less than 6 hours post- birth, oxygen requirement less than 30% to maintain SpO2 of 90% to 95%, and ongoing monitoring requirements do not exceed site capability

 Yellow:
- Infant is clinically stable but has mild respiratory distress lasting longer than 6 hours post-birth, and oxygen requirements less than 30%, **OR**
- Infant is stable, on CPAP of 8 cmH2O or less, and oxygen requirements less than 30%, **OR**
- Infant is clinically stable with new-onset respiratory distress and oxygen requirements less than 30%, **AND**
- Site can provide appropriate management, investigations, and monitoring for the infant's condition

Infants at a Yellow Level of Risk require increased levels of attention and consultation.

 Red:
- Infant consistently requires more than 30% oxygen to meet target saturations, **OR**
- Infant has sustained increase in oxygen requirement greater than 10% above baseline, which does not improve with stabilization, **OR**
- Infant requires or is receiving ventilation beyond site capacity to manage or monitor safely

Infants at a Red Level of Risk require level 3 care. Transfer is required if needs exceed site capabilities.

Respiratory: Case 1—A dusky baby with mild respiratory distress

A baby girl is born by a Caesarean section at 38 weeks gestation for breech presentation. She was vigorous at birth. You are called to assess her in the recovery room at 30 min of age.

You find her to be dusky in room air, with regular respirations, mild nasal flaring, and audible grunting with stimulation. She has intercostal and mild subcostal retractions. Her heart rate is 120 bpm.

1. What is duskiness?

☐ A bluish discolouration of the of the hands and feet in an otherwise pink baby (acrocyanosis).

☐ An indication for immediate bag-and-mask ventilation.

☐ An 'off colour' that is just not pink.

☐ A bluish discolouration of the body, lips, and mucous membranes (central cyanosis).

☐ A condition that is variably appreciated by different health professionals.

☐ A condition that should prompt the application of a pulse oximeter.

2. Does this baby present with any Alerting Signs for Resuscitation?

☐ Yes   ☐ No

You perform the Core Steps of the Resuscitation Sequence as per Figure 2.3.

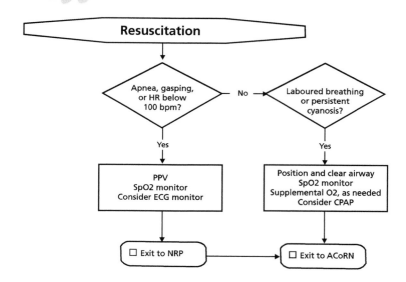

The infant's breathing remains laboured but regular. The respiratory rate is 70 breaths/min and heart rate 140 bpm. Supplemental oxygen is being administered by mask, and you note her colour has improved. The SpO2 is now 93%.

You exit the Resuscitation Sequence.

Your colleague completes the Consolidated Core Steps as you perform the Primary Survey. The baby is appropriately positioned on the over-bed warmer in a nest, the BP reading is normal, and her temperature is 36.8°C axillary.

3. Complete the ACoRN Primary Survey and Consolidated Core Steps, and generate a Problem List.

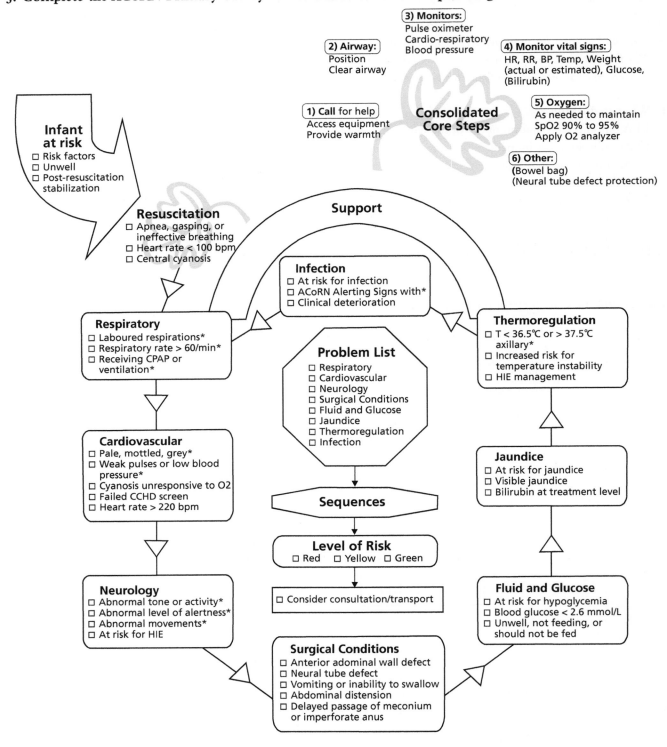

Consolidated Core Steps

1) Call for help:
Access equipment
Provide warmth

2) Airway:
Position
Clear airway

3) Monitors:
Pulse oximeter
Cardio-respiratory
Blood pressure

4) Monitor vital signs:
HR, RR, BP, Temp, Weight
(actual or estimated), Glucose,
(Bilirubin)

5) Oxygen:
As needed to maintain
SpO2 90% to 95%
Apply O2 analyzer

6) Other:
(Bowel bag)
(Neural tube defect protection)

Infant at risk
☐ Risk factors
☐ Unwell
☐ Post-resuscitation stabilization

Resuscitation
☐ Apnea, gasping, or ineffective breathing
☐ Heart rate < 100 bpm
☐ Central cyanosis

Support

Infection
☐ At risk for infection
☐ ACoRN Alerting Signs with*
☐ Clinical deterioration

Respiratory
☐ Laboured respirations*
☐ Respiratory rate > 60/min*
☐ Receiving CPAP or ventilation*

Problem List
☐ Respiratory
☐ Cardiovascular
☐ Neurology
☐ Surgical Conditions
☐ Fluid and Glucose
☐ Jaundice
☐ Thermoregulation
☐ Infection

Thermoregulation
☐ T < 36.5°C or > 37.5°C axillary*
☐ Increased risk for temperature instability
☐ HIE management

Cardiovascular
☐ Pale, mottled, grey*
☐ Weak pulses or low blood pressure*
☐ Cyanosis unresponsive to O2
☐ Failed CCHD screen
☐ Heart rate > 220 bpm

Jaundice
☐ At risk for jaundice
☐ Visible jaundice
☐ Bilirubin at treatment level

Sequences

Level of Risk
☐ Red   ☐ Yellow   ☐ Green

☐ Consider consultation/transport

Neurology
☐ Abnormal tone or activity*
☐ Abnormal level of alertness*
☐ Abnormal movements*
☐ At risk for HIE

Fluid and Glucose
☐ At risk for hypoglycemia
☐ Blood glucose < 2.6 mmol/L
☐ Unwell, not feeding, or should not be fed

Surgical Conditions
☐ Anterior adominal wall defect
☐ Neural tube defect
☐ Vomiting or inability to swallow
☐ Abdominal distension
☐ Delayed passage of meconium or imperforate anus

The infant's blood glucose is not known. She is exhibiting respiratory distress and has not been fed. Her temperature is also unknown.

4. You enter the Respiratory Sequence and perform the Core Steps. Tick all that apply.
- ☐ You ensure the airway is patent, that she has been positioned and suctioned, and that breath sounds are easily heard throughout the lungs on auscultation.
- ☐ You continue to administer oxygen.
- ☐ You change the mode of oxygen administration to an oxygen hood.
- ☐ You administer oxygen by nasal prongs.
- ☐ You titrate the oxygen concentration administered to ensure that SpO2 is 94% to 98%.
- ☐ You calculate the Respiratory Score.

You decide to change the mode of oxygen administration and deliver humidified oxygen via T-piece to help determine the oxygen concentration required to maintain the infant's SpO2 in the 90% to 95% range.

The infant's respiratory rate is 70 breaths/min, she has subcostal (but not sternal) retractions, and she grunts intermittently.

Oxygen is being administered at 25% to achieve SpO2 90% to 95%, and breath sounds are heard throughout the chest.

5. Calculate the Respiratory Score using the following table.

Score	0	1	2
Respiratory rate	40 to 60/min	60 to 80/min	> 80/min
Retractions	None	Intercostal or subcostal retractions (or both)	Intercostal, subcostal, and sternal retractions
Grunting	None	With stimulation	Continuous at rest
Oxygen requirement*	None	≤ 30%	> 30%
Breath sounds on auscultation	Easily heard throughout	Decreased	Barely heard
Prematurity	> 34 weeks	30 to 34 weeks	< 30 weeks
		Respiratory Score	__/12

* Note: An infant receiving oxygen before an O2 analyzer is set up or in an open oxygen delivery system is assigned a score of '1'.

6. What factors determine Organization of Care for this baby?
- ☐ She has severe respiratory distress.
- ☐ She has mild respiratory distress lasting more than 6 h.
- ☐ She has new-onset respiratory distress.
- ☐ She has had an increase in oxygen requirement greater than 10%.
- ☐ She has mild respiratory distress lasting less than 6 h.

The baby requires observation and continued monitoring. The focused history reveals that the mother's pregnancy and delivery were uneventful, there was no maternal fever, membranes were ruptured at birth, and Group B streptococcus screening was negative. The baby looks well despite her respiratory symptoms.

7. **What do you need to keep in mind as you continue to observe this infant? Tick all that apply.**

☐ Mild respiratory distress is often due to transient tachypnea of the newborn and can be expected to resolve over the first 4 h post-birth, as residual lung fluid is reabsorbed.

☐ Further assessment and a chest radiograph may be considered when respiratory distress persists for ≥ 6 h.

☐ Further assessment and a chest radiograph are needed when respiratory distress worsens or oxygen requirements increase over time.

☐ The Primary Survey and Respiratory Score should be repeated for infants with respiratory distress when vital signs are being checked.

☐ A sustained increase in oxygen requirement in the Respiratory Score should be considered clinically acceptable in infants with respiratory distress.

☐ Optimization of oxygenation means targeting the inspired oxygen so that SpO2 remains between 88% and 92%.

Over the next hour, the nurse reports that the infant is no longer grunting, has a respiratory rate of 50 breaths/min, and is alert and active.

The supplemental oxygen is gradually decreased while the SpO2 is monitored continually. At the end of the hour, the infant has a saturation of 93% in room air. Your diagnosis is TTN.

Infection commonly presents with respiratory signs in the newborn. All three Alerting Signs in the Respiratory Sequence have an asterisk (*), to remind ACoRN providers to check (✓) Infection in the Problem List.

In infants with mild respiratory distress, a further sepsis work-up and antibiotics are required only if they meet criteria in the ACoRN Infection Sequence (see Chapter 10, Infection) or exhibit signs of clinical deterioration (e.g., an increase in oxygen requirement or new-onset respiratory distress that was not present at birth).

Respiratory: Case 2—Respiratory distress in a preterm newborn

A 2240-gram baby boy is born vaginally at 34 weeks after 4 h ruptured membranes and preterm labour. He cried at birth and required no resuscitation. His Apgar score was 7 at 1 min and 8 at 5 min. After initial resuscitation, he develops regular but laboured respirations, audible grunting at rest, and intercostal and mild subcostal retractions. His respiratory rate is 72 breaths/min and his heart rate 160 bpm. He requires oxygen to maintain SpO2 in the 90% to 95% range.

The baby is in an incubator with servo control and is receiving 35% oxygen. The pulse oximeter reading is 92%. His respiratory rate is 72 breaths/min, heart rate 160 bpm, and blood pressure by cuff is 48/30, mean 36 mmHg (normal for an infant of 34 weeks gestation). He looks pink and is lying in a semi-flexed posture characteristic of an infant of his GA. He continues to grunt at rest, with intercostal and mild subcostal retractions. You auscultate his chest and find that breath sounds are decreased bilaterally.

You complete the Primary Survey and Consolidated Core Steps.

1. **The Problem List shows which of the following areas of concern?**

Problem List
- ☐ Respiratory
- ☐ Cardiovascular
- ☐ Neurology
- ☐ Surgical Conditions
- ☐ Fluid and Glucose
- ☐ Jaundice
- ☐ Thermoregulation
- ☐ Infection

You enter the Respiratory Sequence as the first sequence in your prioritized Problem List, carry out the Core Steps, and calculate the Respiratory Score:

2. **Calculate the Respiratory Score using the following table.**

Score	0	1	2
Respiratory rate	40 to 60/min	60 to 80/min	> 80/min
Retractions	None	Intercostal or subcostal retractions (or both)	Intercostal, subcostal, and sternal retractions
Grunting	None	With stimulation	Continuous at rest
Oxygen requirement*	None	≤ 30%	> 30%
Breath sounds on auscultation	Easily heard throughout	Decreased	Barely heard
Prematurity	> 34 weeks	30 to 34 weeks	< 30 weeks
		Respiratory Score	__/12

Note: An infant receiving oxygen before an O2 analyzer is set up or in an open oxygen delivery system is assigned a score of 1.

3. **Based on the Respiratory Score, what are the appropriate interventions to consider at this time? Tick all that apply.**
   - ☐ Increase the administered oxygen concentration to 50%.
   - ☐ Consider administering CPAP.
   - ☐ Start preparing for possible intubation, ventilation, and administration of surfactant.
   - ☐ Obtain vascular access.
   - ☐ Request a chest radiograph.
   - ☐ Request a capillary blood gas.

4. **How is CPAP likely to benefit this infant? Tick all that apply.**
   - ☐ By stabilizing the small airways and chest wall.
   - ☐ By preventing atelectasis at end-expiration.
   - ☐ By decreasing the need for endotracheal intubation and mechanical ventilation in infants with moderate respiratory distress and good respiratory drive.
   - ☐ By preventing and treating central apnea.
   - ☐ CPAP might reduce the oxygen concentration needed in infants with respiratory distress.

5. What clinical indicators would suggest CPAP is being effective?

☐ Less severe retractions.

☐ Stable or decreasing oxygen requirements.

☐ A lower Respiratory Score.

☐ Increased grunting.

A colleague gathers supplies for an IV and calls radiology for a chest radiograph. Ventilation is optimized at present. You start a 'to-do' list and add blood gas to it. You feel the baby is stable on CPAP and before calling the tertiary referral centre, you gather more history.

The mother is a 24-yo primigravida with an unremarkable past medical and family history. She had an uneventful pregnancy until the onset of labour at 34 weeks. On admission, her cervix was 7 cm dilated and contractions were occurring every 3 min. In discussion with the regional centre, it was decided that transfer would be unsafe because delivery was imminent. Intrapartum antibiotic prophylaxis was suggested, and 1 dose of penicillin G was given 4 h before birth. Membranes had ruptured 5 h before birth.

Currently the infant is on CPAP of 5 cmH2O, 35% oxygen, and his SpO2 is stable at around 92%. Respiration is less laboured. The respiratory rate is 60 breaths/min. Heart rate, blood pressure, and temperature remain within normal limits.

You exit the Respiratory Sequence and return to the ACoRN Problem List to address Fluid and Glucose, Jaundice, and Thermoregulation. There are several Alerting Signs with an *, indicating that you will also have to address the Infection Sequence.

After addressing the Core Steps, Organization of Care, and Response in the other sequences, you tackle the 'to-do' list and draw the required blood work (gas, CBC and differential, blood culture, and glucose). You also prepare to administer antibiotics while waiting for the chest radiograph results.

The chest radiograph becomes available and is shown here.

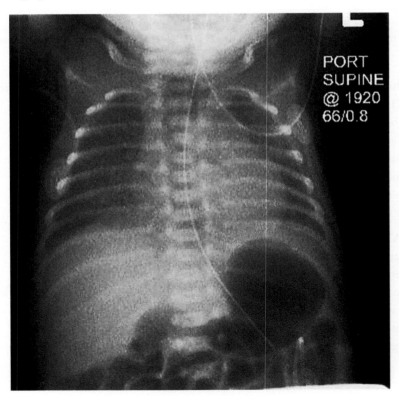

6. Identify features seen in this infant's chest radiograph.

☐ Fluid in the right horizontal fissure.

☐ The heart borders are easy to see.

☐ The hemidiaphragms are partially obscured.

☐ The lung fields have a 'grainy' or 'ground glass' appearance, volumes are low.

☐ Lots of air bronchograms extend past the cardiac silhouette.

☐ A stomach air bubble cannot be seen.

The blood gas (venous) results are as follows: pH 7.20   pCO2   68   pO2 38 BE −4

7. How would you interpret the blood gas?

☐ Respiratory acidosis   ☐ Respiratory alkalosis

☐ Metabolic acidosis   ☐ Metabolic alkalosis

After obtaining blood work, the baby's FiO2 rises to 45% with intercostal, subcostal, and sternal retractions, continuous grunting, and reduced air entry. His respiratory rate is 90 bpm.

Given the changes in this baby, you repeat the Primary Survey, re-enter the Respiratory Sequence, and recalculate the Respiratory Score.

8. Calculate the Respiratory Score using the following table.

Score	0	1	2
Respiratory rate	40 to 60/min	60 to 80/min	> 80/min
Retractions	None	Intercostal or subcostal retractions (or both)	Intercostal, subcostal, and sternal retractions
Grunting	None	With stimulation	Continuous at rest
Oxygen requirement*	None	≤ 30%	> 30%
Breath sounds on auscultation	Easily heard throughout	Decreased	Barely heard
Prematurity	> 34 weeks	30 to 34 weeks	< 30 weeks
		Respiratory Score	__/12

*Note: An infant receiving oxygen before an O2 analyzer is set up or in an open oxygen delivery system is assigned a score of 1.

9. Based on the Respiratory Score, how would you manage this baby?

☐ Place him skin-to-skin.

☐ Wait for the transport team to arrive.

☐ Prepare your team for intubation.

☐ Place a chest tube.

☐ Feed the baby.

The baby is intubated at first attempt using rapid sequence intubation medications. You are providing PPV via T-piece, using pressures of 20/6. You see chest movement and hear good air entry, with positive end-tidal carbon dioxide response. The FiO2 remains at 45%.

10. What specific management would you consider? Tick all that apply.

☐ Place the baby on a mechanical ventilator.

☐ Provide surfactant.

☐ Extubate to CPAP.

☐ Repeat the chest radiograph.

☐ Obtain further consultation.

The history, physical examination, and chest radiograph findings lead you to make a working diagnosis of moderate respiratory distress due to RDS.

11. What is this baby's Level of Risk?

☐ Green   ☐ Yellow   ☐ Red

Bibliography

American Association for Respiratory Care. Clinical Practice Guideline: Selection of an oxygen delivery device for neonatal and pediatric patients; 2002 revision and update. Respir Care J 2002;47(6):707–16: www.rcjournal.com/cpgs/soddnppcpg-update.html (Accessed May 1, 2019).

American Academy of Pediatrics, American Heart Association, Canadian Paediatric Society. Textbook of Neonatal Resuscitation, 7th ed. Elk Grove Village, IL: AAP; 2016.

Ardell S, Pfister RH, Soll R. Animal derived surfactant extract versus protein free synthetic surfactant for the prevention and treatment of respiratory distress syndrome. Cochrane Database Syst Rev 2015;8:CD000144.

Carbajal R, Eble B, Anand KJ. Premedication for tracheal intubation in neonates: Confusion or controversy? Semin Perinatol 2007;31(5):309–17.

Davis DJ, Barrington KJ, Canadian Paediatric Society, Fetus and Newborn Committee. Recommendations for neonatal surfactant therapy. Paediatr Child Health 2005;10(2):10–16; Updated 2015: www.cps.ca/en/documents/position/neonatal-surfactant-therapy

De Paoli AG, Davis PG, Faber B, Morely CJ. Devices and pressure sources for administration of nasal continuous positive airway pressure (NCPAP) in preterm neonates. Cochrane Database Syst Rev 2008;1:CD002977.

Downes JJ, Vidyasagar D, Boggs TR, Morrow GM. Respiratory distress syndrome of newborn infants. I. New clinical scoring system (RDS score) with acid-base and blood gas correlations. Clin Pediatr 1970; 9(6):325–31.

Goldsmith JP, Karotkin EH, Gutham S, Keszler M. Assisted Ventilation of the Neonate: Evidence-based Approach to Newborn Respiratory Care, 6th ed. Philadelphia, PA: Saunders/Elsevier; 2016.

Hagen E, Chu A, Lew C. Transient tachypnea of the newborn. NeoReviews 2017;18(3):e141–8.

Keszler M. State of the art in conventional mechanical ventilation. J Perinatol 2009;29(4): 262–75.

Konduri GG, Kim UO. Advances in the diagnosis and management of persistent pulmonary hypertension of the newborn. Pediatr Clin North Am 2009;56(3):579–600.

Kotecha SJ, Adappa R, Gupta N, Watkins WJ, Kotecha S, Chakraborty M. Safety and efficacy of high-flow nasal cannula therapy in preterm infants: A meta-analysis. Pediatrics 2015;136(3):542–53.

Morley CJ, Davis PG. Continuous positive airway pressure: Scientific and clinical rationale. Curr Opin Pediatr 2008;20(2):119–24.

Myers TR. AARC Clinical practice guideline: Selection of an oxygen delivery device for neonatal and pediatric patients–2002 revision and update. Respir Care 2002;47(6):707–16: www.aarc.org/wp-content/uploads/2014/08/06.02.707.pdf (Accessed May 13, 2019).

Ng E, Shah V; Canadian Paediatric Society, Fetus and Newborn Committee. Guidelines for surfactant replacement in neonates. Paediatr Child Health 2021;26(1): https://www.cps.ca/en/documents/position/guidelines-for-surfactant-replacement-therapy-in-neonates

Nowadzky T, Pantoja A, Britton JR. Bubble continuous positive airway pressure, a potentially better practice, reduces the use of mechanical ventilation among very low birth weight infants with respiratory distress syndrome. Pediatrics 2009;123(6):1534–40.

Saugstad OD, Aune D. Optimal oxygenation of extremely low birth weight infants: A meta-analysis and systematic review of the oxygen saturation target studies. Neonatology 2014;105(1):55–63.

Silverman WA, Andersen DH. A controlled clinical trial of effects of water mist on obstructive respiratory signs, death rate and necropsy findings among premature infants. Pediatrics 1956;17(1):1–10.

Stevens TP, Harrington EW, Blennow M, Soll RF. Early surfactant administration with brief ventilation vs. selective surfactant and continued mechanical ventilation for preterm infants with or at risk for respiratory distress syndrome. Cochrane Database Syst Rev 2007;4:CD003063.

Sweet DG, Carnielle V, Greisen G, et al. European consensus guidelines on the management of respiratory distress syndrome–2019 update. Neonatology 2019;115:432–50.

Sweet DG, Halliday HL. The use of surfactants in 2009. Arch Dis Child Educ Pract Ed 2009;94(3):78–83.

van Kaam AH, Rimensberger PC. Lung-protective ventilation strategies in neonatology: What do we know—what do we need to know? Crit Care Med 2007;35(3):925–31.

Answer key: Respiratory Case 1—A dusky baby with mild respiratory distress

1. What is duskiness?

☐ A bluish discolouration of the of the hands and feet in an otherwise pink baby (acrocyanosis).

☐ An indication for immediate bag-and-mask ventilation.

☐ An 'off colour' that is just not pink.

☐ A bluish discolouration of the body, lips, and mucous membranes (central cyanosis).

✓ A condition that is variably appreciated by different health professionals.

✓ A condition that should prompt the application of a pulse oximeter.

Duskiness is a term commonly used to describe cyanosis in the newborn. It is an imprecise term, variably appreciated by health professionals. To avoid confusion, specific terms such as 'central cyanosis' or 'acrocyanosis' should be used.

Central cyanosis is a bluish discolouration of the torso, lips, and mucous membranes, while acrocyanosis is a bluish discolouration of the hands and feet in an otherwise pink baby. Central cyanosis is an indication for resuscitation and should prompt the application of a pulse oximeter.

2. Does this baby present with any Alerting Signs for Resuscitation?

✓ Yes ☐ No

Although her breathing is laboured, it appears to be effective because her heart rate is greater than 100 bpm and respiration is regular. However, cyanosis is one of the Alerting Signs for Resuscitation and this baby was described as 'dusky', so cyanosis must be considered. The Resuscitation Sequence prompts you to position the baby appropriately, clear the airway, apply a SpO2 monitor and oxygen or CPAP, as necessary. The Resuscitation Sequence is the beginning of NRP. With a stable heart rate and effective breathing, the sequence prompts the provider to exit to ACoRN and continue with stabilization efforts.

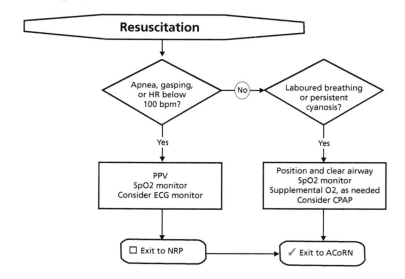

Resuscitation
☐ Apnea, gasping, or ineffective breathing
☐ Heart rate < 100 bpm
✓ Central cyanosis

3. **Complete the ACoRN Primary Survey and Consolidated Core Steps, and generate a Problem List.**

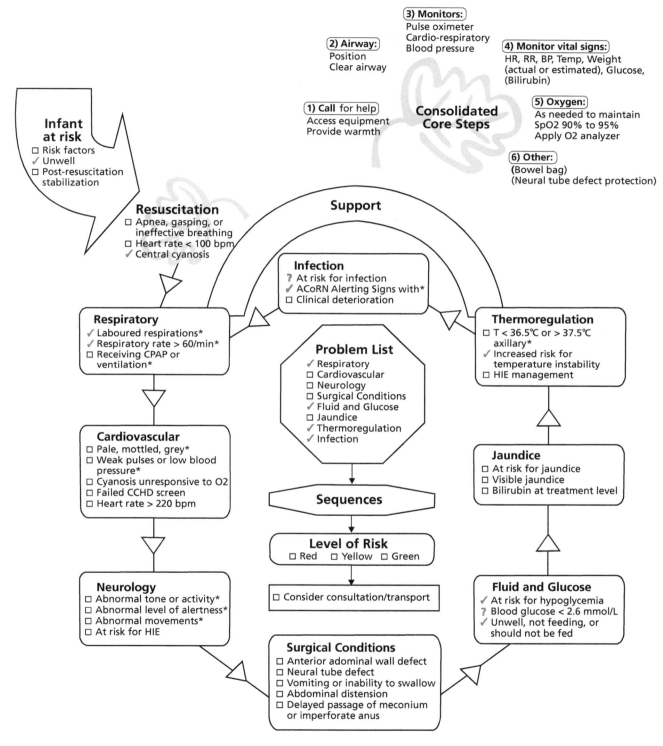

Infant at risk
- ☐ Risk factors
- ✓ Unwell
- ☐ Post-resuscitation stabilization

Resuscitation
- ☐ Apnea, gasping, or ineffective breathing
- ☐ Heart rate < 100 bpm
- ✓ Central cyanosis

Consolidated Core Steps

1) Call for help:
Access equipment
Provide warmth

2) Airway:
Position
Clear airway

3) Monitors:
Pulse oximeter
Cardio-respiratory
Blood pressure

4) Monitor vital signs:
HR, RR, BP, Temp, Weight (actual or estimated), Glucose, (Bilirubin)

5) Oxygen:
As needed to maintain SpO2 90% to 95%
Apply O2 analyzer

6) Other:
(Bowel bag)
(Neural tube defect protection)

Support

Respiratory
- ✓ Laboured respirations*
- ✓ Respiratory rate > 60/min*
- ☐ Receiving CPAP or ventilation*

Infection
- ? At risk for infection
- ✓ ACoRN Alerting Signs with*
- ☐ Clinical deterioration

Thermoregulation
- ☐ T < 36.5°C or > 37.5°C axillary*
- ✓ Increased risk for temperature instability
- ☐ HIE management

Problem List
- ✓ Respiratory
- ☐ Cardiovascular
- ☐ Neurology
- ☐ Surgical Conditions
- ✓ Fluid and Glucose
- ☐ Jaundice
- ✓ Thermoregulation
- ✓ Infection

Cardiovascular
- ☐ Pale, mottled, grey*
- ☐ Weak pulses or low blood pressure*
- ☐ Cyanosis unresponsive to O2
- ☐ Failed CCHD screen
- ☐ Heart rate > 220 bpm

Jaundice
- ☐ At risk for jaundice
- ☐ Visible jaundice
- ☐ Bilirubin at treatment level

Sequences

Level of Risk
- ☐ Red ☐ Yellow ☐ Green

☐ Consider consultation/transport

Neurology
- ☐ Abnormal tone or activity*
- ☐ Abnormal level of alertness*
- ☐ Abnormal movements*
- ☐ At risk for HIE

Fluid and Glucose
- ✓ At risk for hypoglycemia
- ? Blood glucose < 2.6 mmol/L
- ✓ Unwell, not feeding, or should not be fed

Surgical Conditions
- ☐ Anterior adominal wall defect
- ☐ Neural tube defect
- ☐ Vomiting or inability to swallow
- ☐ Abdominal distension
- ☐ Delayed passage of meconium or imperforate anus

The infant exhibits two of the Alerting Signs for the Respiratory Sequence. Her blood glucose is not known, and she is at risk for hypoglycemia because she is exhibiting respiratory distress and has not been fed. The infant's temperature is also unknown, and she is at risk for temperature instability.

4. You enter the Respiratory Sequence and perform the Core Steps.

    ☐ You ensure the airway is patent, that she has been positioned and suctioned, and that breath sounds are easily heard throughout the lungs on auscultation.

    ✓ You continue to administer oxygen.

    ☐ You change the mode of oxygen administration to an oxygen hood.

    ☐ You administer oxygen by nasal prongs.

    ☐ You titrate the oxygen concentration administered to ensure SpO2 is 94% to 98%.

    ✓ You calculate the Respiratory Score.

The Core Steps in the Respiratory Sequence include administration of oxygen to maintain saturations at 90% to 95% and calculation of the Respiratory Score.

Ensuring the baby's airway is patent and breath sounds are audible throughout the lung fields is essential and is part of the Consolidated Core Steps that are completed at the same time as the Primary Survey.

You could certainly change the mode of oxygen administration to one that is easier to both maintain and assess the concentration of oxygen delivered (i.e., oxyhood or incubator), although this step is not a priority right now.

5. Calculate the Respiratory Score using the following table.

Score	0	1	2
Respiratory rate	40 to 60/min	60 to 80/min	> 80/min
Retractions	None	Intercostal or subcostal retractions (or both)	Intercostal, subcostal, and sternal retractions
Grunting	None	With stimulation	Continuous at rest
Oxygen requirement*	None	≤ 30%	> 30%
Breath sounds on auscultation	Easily heard throughout	Decreased	Barely heard
Prematurity	> 34 weeks	30 to 34 weeks	< 30 weeks
		Respiratory Score	4/12

*Note: An infant receiving oxygen before an O2 analyzer is set up or in an open oxygen delivery system is assigned a score of 1.

The baby's Respiratory Score is 4, consistent with mild respiratory distress.

6. What factors determine the Organization of Care for this baby?

    ☐ She has severe respiratory distress.

    ☐ She has mild respiratory distress lasting more than 6 h.

    ☐ She has new-onset respiratory distress.

    ☐ She has had an increase in oxygen requirement greater than 10%.

    ✓ Has mild respiratory distress lasting less than 6 h.

The Organization of Care for a baby with mild respiratory distress involves ongoing observation and continued monitoring, with specific attention to the concentration of oxygen required to maintain saturations within normal limits. A focused history and physical exam should be completed.

7. **What do you need to keep in mind as you continue to observe this infant?**
   - ☐ Mild respiratory distress is often due to transient tachypnea of the newborn and can be expected to resolve over the first 4 h post-birth, as residual lung fluid is reabsorbed.
   - ✓ Further assessment and a chest radiograph may be considered when respiratory distress persists for ≥ 6 h.
   - ✓ Further assessment and a chest radiograph are needed when respiratory distress worsens or oxygen requirements increase over time.
   - ✓ The Primary Survey and Respiratory Score should be repeated for infants with respiratory distress when vital signs are being checked.
   - ☐ A sustained increase in oxygen requirement in the Respiratory Score should be considered clinically acceptable in infants with respiratory distress.
   - ☐ Optimization of oxygenation means targeting the inspired oxygen so that SpO2 remains between 88% and 92%.

Respiratory distress due to TTN will often improve or resolve over the first few hours post-birth, as residual lung fluid is reabsorbed. TTN has been reported to last as long as 48 to 72 h but usually shows improvement well before that.

When TTN persists beyond 6 h post-birth or worsens within that time frame, other diagnoses need to be considered, including infection and surfactant deficiency or inactivation. Further assessment and a chest radiograph may be needed to make a diagnosis.

A sustained increase in oxygen requirements is a sign that the infant no longer meets the criteria for mild respiratory distress and should prompt reassessment and an increase in respiratory support.

Optimization of oxygenation means targeting the inspired oxygen so that SpO2 remains between 90% and 95%.

Ongoing assessment of respiratory status is paramount. Until the infant has stabilized, it is reasonable to repeat the Primary Survey and recalculate the Respiratory Score each time vital signs are done.

Answer key: Respiratory Case 2—Respiratory distress in a preterm newborn

1. **The Problem List shows which of the following areas of concern?**

Problem List
- ✓ Respiratory
- ☐ Cardiovascular
- ☐ Neurology
- ☐ Surgical Conditions
- ✓ Fluid and Glucose
- ✓ Jaundice
- ✓ Thermoregulation
- ✓ Infection

2. Calculate the Respiratory Score using this table.

Score	0	1	2
Respiratory rate	40 to 60/min	60 to 80/min	> 80/min
Retractions	None	Intercostal or subcostal retractions (or both)	Intercostal, subcostal, and sternal retractions
Grunting	None	With stimulation	Continuous at rest
Oxygen requirement*	None	≤ 30%	> 30%
Breath sounds on auscultation	Easily heard throughout	Decreased	Barely heard
Prematurity	> 34 weeks	30 to 34 weeks	< 30 weeks
		Respiratory Score	8/12

*Note: An infant receiving oxygen before an O2 analyzer is set up or in an open oxygen delivery system is assigned a score of 1.

This preterm infant has a Respiratory Score of 8, consistent with moderate respiratory distress.

3. Based on the Respiratory Score, what are the appropriate interventions to consider at this time?

☐ Increase the administered oxygen concentration to 50%.
✓ Consider administering CPAP.
☐ Start preparing for possible intubation, ventilation, and administration of surfactant.
✓ Obtain vascular access.
✓ Request a chest radiograph.
✓ Request a blood gas.

There is no need to increase the oxygen at this time because the baby's saturations are within normal limits. With moderate respiratory distress, the administration of CPAP is recommended. Because this baby will not be fed, it is important to initiate IV access (for fluid maintenance and, potentially, for antibiotic administration). This can be put on your 'to-do' list with a chest radiograph and a blood gas, which are also appropriate after initiating CPAP. You may, after discussion with the team, decide to wait to draw blood work until the baby has been on CPAP for 30 min. This would allow you to refer to the 'to-do' list and draw all the required blood work at once. When adding 'recalculate Respiratory Score' to the 'to-do' list, you realize that if the baby's respiratory distress worsens, you may need to augment support (i.e., intubation and administration of surfactant).

4. How is CPAP likely to benefit this infant?

✓ By stabilizing the small airways and chest wall.
✓ By preventing atelectasis at end-expiration.
✓ By decreasing the need for endotracheal intubation and mechanical ventilation in infants with moderate respiratory distress and good respiratory drive.
☐ By preventing and treating central apnea.
✓ CPAP might reduce the oxygen concentration needed in infants with respiratory distress.

The purpose of CPAP is to:

- Improve arterial PO2 to reduce inspired oxygen concentration in infants with respiratory distress who do not require mechanical ventilation.
- Stabilize respiratory function on extubation from mechanical ventilation.

- Treat obstructive apnea in some preterm infants.
  - CPAP reduces mixed and obstructive apnea. It has no effect on central apnea.

CPAP will stabilize the small airways in the lungs and the chest wall. It prevents atelectasis at the end of expiration and can decrease the need for mechanical ventilation. The concentration of oxygen needed may also be reduced.

CPAP is not first-line treatment for central apnea.

5. What clinical indicators would suggest CPAP is being effective?
- ✓ Less severe retractions.
- ✓ Stable or decreasing oxygen requirements.
- ✓ A lower Respiratory Score.
- ☐ Increased grunting.

An improvement in respiratory status indicates that CPAP is effective. Increased grunting is not a sign of respiratory improvement and would indicate that CPAP is ineffective.

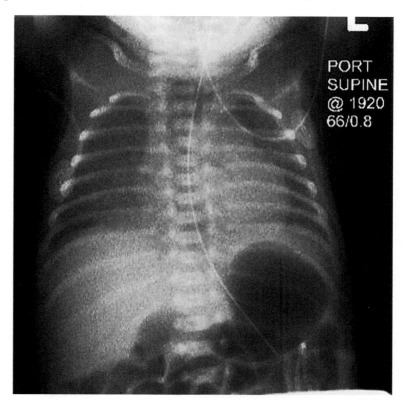

6. Identify features seen in this infant's chest radiograph.
- ☐ Fluid in the right horizontal fissure.
- ☐ The heart borders are easy to see.
- ✓ The hemidiaphragms are partially obscured.
- ✓ The lung fields have a 'grainy' or 'ground glass' appearance, volumes are low.
- ☐ Lots of air bronchograms extend past the cardiac silhouette.
- ☐ A stomach air bubble cannot be seen.

From the chest radiograph, the heart borders and hemi-diaphragm at the right base are partially obscured. Air bronchograms are present in right upper chest. The lung fields appear homogeneously grainy with the texture of ground glass and are inflated to 7.5 ribs (low volumes). The stomach bubble is visible in the lower right corner of the film.

7. How do you interpret the blood gas?

✓ Respiratory acidosis   ☐ Respiratory alkalosis

☐ Metabolic acidosis   ☐ Metabolic alkalosis

The blood gas shows respiratory acidosis with hypoxemia (↓ pH ↑ pCO2 ↓ pO2 BE is within normal limits).

8. Calculate the Respiratory Score using the following table.

Score	0	1	2
Respiratory rate	40 to 60/min	60 to 80/min	> 80/min
Retractions	None	Intercostal or subcostal retractions (or both)	Intercostal, subcostal, and sternal retractions
Grunting	None	With stimulation	Continuous at rest
Oxygen requirement*	None	≤ 30%	> 30%
Breath sounds on auscultation	Easily heard throughout	Decreased	Barely heard
Prematurity	> 34 weeks	30 to 34 weeks	< 30 weeks
		Respiratory Score	10/12

Note: An infant receiving oxygen before an O2 analyzer is set up or in an open oxygen delivery system is assigned a score of 1.

The baby now has a Respiratory Score of 10, consistent with severe respiratory distress. His score has progressed despite CPAP.

9. Based on the Respiratory Score, how would you manage this baby?

☐ Place him skin-to-skin.

☐ Wait for the transport team to arrive.

✓ Prepare your team for intubation.

☐ Place a chest tube.

☐ Feed the baby.

This baby's respiratory status has worsened despite CPAP therapy and he now requires urgent intubation. If no one at your site has the ability to intubate, insertion of a laryngeal mask airway should be considered.

There is no evidence of a pneumothorax on the chest radiograph, so no need to insert a chest tube. Severe respiratory distress is a contraindication for feeding. You will need to calculate the infant's fluid requirements based on weight and age, as identified in Fluid and Glucose Sequence, Chapter 7.

While skin-to-skin care has been shown to decrease respiratory rate and effort in mild distress, this infant has severe distress and requires intubation. A discussion with the parents to update them regarding the baby's status and explain the treatment course is needed.

10. **What specific management would you consider?**

    ? Place baby on a mechanical ventilator.

    ✓ Provide surfactant.

    ☐ Extubate to CPAP.

    ✓ Repeat the chest radiograph.

    ✓ Obtain further consultation.

Despite being intubated, this baby requires high levels of oxygen administration. The baby also needs a chest X-ray to confirm that the ETT is in the appropriate location and will then require a dose of surfactant. Depending on his response to surfactant, the baby may continue to require mechanical ventilation or may be able to be extubated. These decisions are best made in consultation with the tertiary referral centre. If the baby requires transport to a higher level of care, extubation may be delayed to ensure adequate airway control during transport.

The baby will require ongoing assessment and monitoring. The Primary Survey and Respiratory Score should be repeated, along with vital signs.

11. **What is this baby's Level of Risk?**

    ☐ Green   ☐ Yellow   ✓ Red

The Level of Risk for this baby is Red. He meets all of the criteria for this risk classification because he:

- Consistently requires more than 30% oxygen to meet target saturations, **OR**
- Has sustained increase in oxygen requirement greater than 10% above baseline, which does not improve with stabilization, **OR**
- Requires or is receiving ventilation beyond site capacity to manage or monitor safely.

Cardiovascular

4

Educational objectives

Upon completion of this chapter, you will be able to:

- Identify infants who require cardiovascular stabilization.
- Apply the Acute Care of at-Risk Newborns (ACoRN) Cardiovascular Sequence.
- Assess adequacy of circulation and end-organ perfusion.
- Recognize and manage circulatory shock.
- Recognize and manage cyanosis.
- Know how to perform and interpret a critical congenital heart disease (CCHD) screen.
- Recognize and manage supraventricular tachycardia (SVT).
- Recognize when to exit the Cardiovascular Sequence to other ACoRN sequences.

Key concepts

1. Shock, cyanosis unresponsive to oxygen, and tachycardia all indicate cardiovascular instability.
2. Initially, infants with underlying congenital heart disease (CHD) can appear well.
3. Routine screening for CCHD identifies infants who require assessment to rule out severe or cyanotic CHD.
4. The underlying cause of shock can be difficult to ascertain at presentation, but all causes are characterized by underperfusion of vital organs. Always consider volume expansion while establishing a diagnosis.
5. Cardiovascular instability and shock may be the initial presentation of sepsis. These infants should be treated with antibiotics as soon as possible after stabilizing the systems identified by the ACoRN Primary Survey.
6. Cyanosis and shock may both be present with duct-dependent CHD.
7. Prostaglandin E1 (PGE1) is the life-saving treatment in duct-dependent CHD.
8. Consider SVT when an infant's heart rate (HR) is more than 220 bpm.

Skills

- Clinical assessment of circulation
- Appropriate administration of cardiovascular medications
- Performing a hyperoxia test
- CCHD screening

The key function of the cardiovascular system is to deliver oxygen to the tissues.

- Oxygen delivery depends on the oxygen content of blood and the cardiac output.
- The oxygen content of blood depends on hemoglobin concentration and the oxygen saturation (SO2) of hemoglobin.

- Cardiac output depends on stroke volume (the volume ejected by each cardiac contraction) and HR.
- Stroke volume depends on preload (filling), cardiac contractility, and afterload (vascular resistance affecting the ability of the heart to pump blood forward).

Decreased oxygen delivery to the tissues due to respiratory causes is addressed in the ACoRN Respiratory Sequence. Decreased oxygen delivery to the tissues in the ACoRN Cardiovascular Sequence is caused by one or more of the following mechanisms:

- Insufficient circulating blood volume or oxygen-carrying capacity (anemia).
- Poor heart muscle function (myocardial dysfunction).
- Anatomical abnormalities of the heart and great vessels (cyanotic and acyanotic CHD).
- Abnormal heart rhythms (tachyarrhythmia or bradyarrhythmia).

In a well infant, bradycardia due to increased vagal tone is benign. Bradyarrhythmias caused by conduction disorders are uncommon in newborns and fall outside the scope of ACoRN.

Hypoxia is the failure of oxygenation at the tissue level, when oxygen delivery is impaired or tissues are unable to use oxygen effectively. Hypoxia must be differentiated from hypoxemia, which is a decrease in the partial pressure of oxygen in the blood. Hypoxia may not present in infants with a degree of low oxygen tension (hypoxemia) or low hemoglobin saturation (desaturation) when those factors can be compensated for by increasing cardiac output. The components of oxygen delivery are shown in Figure 4.1.

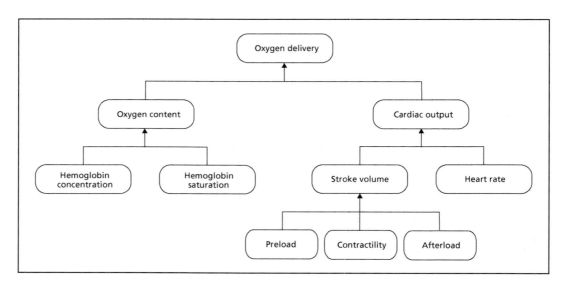

Figure 4.1. Components that determine oxygen delivery to the tissues.

With hypoxia, **lactate** is the end product of the anaerobic breakdown of glucose in tissues. Anaerobic metabolism does not require oxygen to liberate energy from glucose but is inefficient for producing adenosine triphosphate. Rarely, lactic acidosis may occur in the absence of hypoxia or hypoperfusion, such as in disorders of mitochondrial function. While the normal value of lactate is below 2 mmol/L, the clinical significance of blood lactate between 2 mmol/L and 5 mmol/L is often uncertain. Lactate levels greater than 5 mmol/L should always be considered clinically significant.

Shock is an unstable cardiovascular state in which cardiac output cannot meet the oxygen and energy requirements of vital organs, leading to deteriorating organ function. Shock is a medical emergency. Infants in shock require immediate stabilization, including cardiorespiratory support and management with medications, based on underlying physiology.

Recognizing the Alerting Signs for the ACoRN Cardiovascular Sequence and intervening early and appropriately can mitigate risk and improve infant outcomes.

ACoRN Cardiovascular Sequence

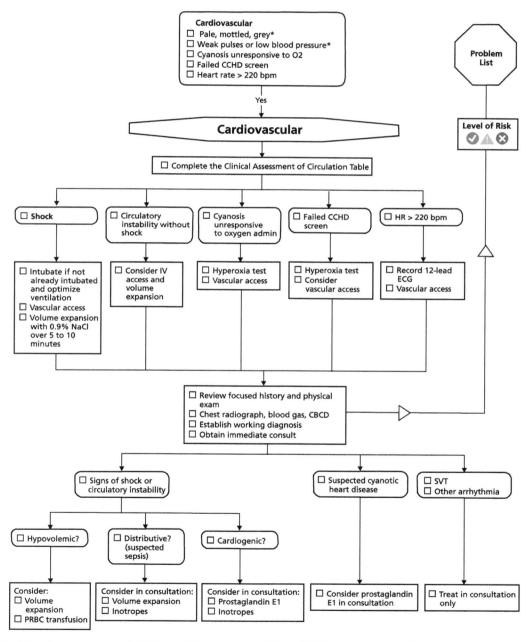

Abbreviations: bpm - beats per minute, CBCD - complete blood count and differential, CCHD - critical congenital heart disease, ECG - electrocardiogram, HR - heart rate, IV - intravenous, NaCl - normal saline, O2 - oxygen, PRBC - packed red blood cells, SVT - supraventricular tachycardia

Alerting Signs

An infant showing one or more of the following Alerting Signs enters the ACoRN Cardiovascular Sequence:

> **Cardiovascular**
> ☐ Pale, mottled, grey*
> ☐ Weak pulses or low blood pressure*
> ☐ Cyanosis unresponsive to O2
> ☐ Failed CCHD screen
> ☐ Heart rate > 220 bpm

Being **pale, mottled, or grey** is a critically important sign because it indicates inadequate end-organ perfusion and serious circulatory instability. For such infants, assume shock or impending shock.

Weak pulses are also important, particularly when the femoral or peripheral pulses are difficult to palpate. **Low blood pressure (BP)** can be a sign of low vascular tone, volume, or decreased cardiac output. This Alerting Sign must be interpreted and addressed with caution. Ten percent of normal, stable infants have a mean BP below the 10th percentile. Conversely, infants can have normal BP despite low cardiac output. Blood pressure must be interpreted in context with other indicators of end-organ perfusion.

Cyanosis that is unresponsive to oxygen identifies infants with clinical cyanosis or hemoglobin desaturation despite the administration of 100% oxygen. This is an important sign of congenital cyanotic heart disease, especially when it occurs in the absence of respiratory distress. Cyanosis only becomes readily apparent when desaturated hemoglobin levels reach 50 g/L. Therefore, the infant with a hemoglobin of 200 g/L would only appear cyanosed when SpO2 levels dropped below 75%, and the infant with a hemoglobin of 150 g/L would not be visibly cyanosed until SpO2 dropped to 67%. When significant anemia is present, hypoxemic neonates may appear pale rather than cyanosed. Figure 4.2 explains respiratory and cardiac mechanisms of cyanosis.

(A)

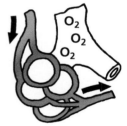 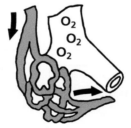 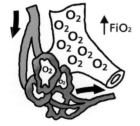

Healthy lung (alveoli well inflated), room air, blood past the alveolus is red.

Alveoli poorly inflated, room air, blood past the alveolus is cyanotic (purple-blue).

Alveoli poorly inflated, on supplemental oxygen, blood past the alveolus is red.

Figure 4.2. Differentiating cyanosis of cardiac and respiratory origins. **A: In cyanosis of respiratory origin**, all of the blood pumped by the right ventricle goes through the lungs before being pumped by the left ventricle to the body.

(B)

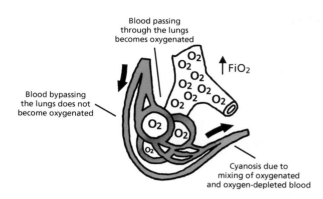

Blood passing through the lungs becomes oxygenated

↑FiO$_2$

Blood bypassing the lungs does not become oxygenated

Cyanosis due to mixing of oxygenated and oxygen-depleted blood

Figure 4.2.B: In **cyanosis of cardiac origin**, the SpO$_2$ level depends on the proportion of oxygenated blood versus deoxygenated blood.

Suspicion of cyanosis requires confirmation by pulse oximetry.

Assessing skin colour is challenging and made more difficult by factors such as lighting, temperature, and infant skin tone. Appearing 'dusky' or 'not pink' are key signs of central cyanosis but can be missed.

A CCHD screen should be performed for all term and late preterm newborns at 24 to 36 h of age. A **failed CCHD screen** requires prompt investigation. A failed screen occurs when the SpO$_2$ in an infant's right hand or either foot is less than 90% on a single reading. The infant also fails when SpO$_2$ is between 90% and 94% in the right hand and foot, OR when the difference between the right hand and foot is more than 3% on 3 separate readings taken 1 h apart. Early diagnosis of CCHD is crucial because delays in detection and management increase risk for morbidity and mortality.

Examples of lesions detectable using pulse oximetry screening

Most consistently cyanotic

- Hypoplastic left heart syndrome
- Pulmonary atresia with intact ventricular septum
- Total anomalous pulmonary venous return
- Tetralogy of Fallot
- Transposition of the great arteries
- Tricuspid atresia
- Truncus arteriosus

May be cyanotic

- Coarctation of the aorta
- Double outlet right ventricle
- Ebstein's anomaly
- Interrupted aortic arch
- Defects with single ventricle physiology

Source: Michael Narvey, Kenny Wong, Anne Fournier; Canadian Paediatric Society, Fetus and Newborn Committee. Pulse oximetry screening in newborns to enhance detection of critical congenital heart disease. Paediatrics & Child Health 2017;22(8):494–498.

Routine screening with pulse oximetry is safe, noninvasive, easy to perform, and widely available. It has been shown to enhance detection of CCHD, with a reported specificity of 99.9% and a moderately high sensitivity (76.5%).

The CCHD screening protocol endorsed by the CPS is intended for use in asymptomatic newborns in nonacute care settings.

CCHD screening is performed by placing one pulse oximeter probe on the right hand and one on either foot and recording the readings. The results of screening are reported using the algorithm shown in the following figure. The screening test is declared a 'pass' or a 'fail'.

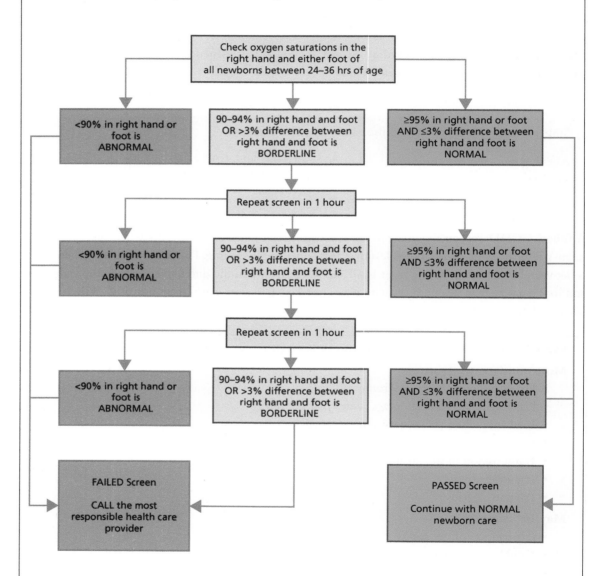

Figure 4.3. How to perform a CCHD screen.

Source: Michael Narvey, Kenny Wong, Anne Fournier; Canadian Paediatric Society, Fetus and Newborn Committee. Pulse oximetry screening in newborns to enhance detection of critical congenital heart disease. Paediatrics & Child Health 2017;22(8):494–498.

When an infant's **HR is greater than 220 bpm**, the ACoRN provider should consider tachyarrhythmia. Infants who are distressed can have HRs of 160 bpm to 200 bpm (sinus tachycardia), but rarely have HRs over 220 bpm.

SVT should be suspected when HR is greater than 220 bpm with lack of variability, in episodes that start and stop suddenly.

Core Steps

The essential Core Step in the ACoRN Cardiovascular Sequence is to assess the presence and degree of cardiovascular instability, using Table 4.1: Clinical Assessment of Circulation. The goal is to identify infants who are critically ill and require accelerated stabilization, including immediate multisystem support to optimize end-organ perfusion and oxygenation.

Tone, activity, and alertness

Abnormal tone, activity, and level of alertness are critical signs of inadequate cerebral perfusion in the ACoRN Cardiovascular Sequence. Conversely, having normal tone, being active and alert, and looking well indicate adequate cerebral perfusion.

Altered levels of tone, activity, and alertness, as signs of cardiovascular instability, may be confounded by co-morbid conditions such as neurologic injury or infection.

Critical perfusion

Being pale, mottled, or grey are critical signs of inadequate end-organ perfusion. Being pale but well perfused is not a sign of circulatory instability.

Pulses

Assessing pulses is an acquired skill. ACoRN providers should routinely palpate brachial and femoral pulses in healthy infants to become familiar with their characteristics, and regularly compare upper and lower limb pulses.

Table 4.1.
Clinical Assessment of Circulation

Sign	Stable	Unstable
Abnormal tone, activity, or level of alertness	Normal tone, active, alert, and looking well	Decreased tone, listless, lethargic
Critical perfusion	Well perfused, pink, and peripherally warm	Pale, mottled, grey
Pulses	Easy to palpate	Weak, absent, or femoral pulses weaker than right brachial pulses
Mean blood pressure	≥ gestational age (in weeks)	< gestational age (in weeks)
Capillary refill time	≤ 3 sec centrally	> 3 sec centrally
Skin temperature	Peripherally warm	Peripherally cool
Heart rate	100 to 180 bpm	> 180 bpm
Hourly urine output (if older than 24 h)	≥1 mL/kg/h	< 1 mL/kg/h
Shock is present when signs of critical perfusion (red box) coexist in an infant with decreased tone, activity, and alertness (red box), in the absence of an alternative explanation.		

Weak or low amplitude pulses may be an indicator of inadequate perfusion.

> When a diminished femoral pulse is found, confirmation (by a second individual or a repeated attempt) is strongly recommended.

In coarctation of the aorta, the infant's femoral (and other lower extremity) pulses are either much weaker, or absent, compared with upper-right extremity (brachial, ulnar, or radial) pulses.

Blood pressure

Considered alongside mean BP, the systolic BP provides information on the contractility of the heart and the output of the left ventricle. A drop in systolic BP indicates reduced stroke volume due to altered left ventricular preload, contractility, or afterload. The diastolic BP provides information on the resting pressure of blood against vessel walls. A drop in diastolic BP indicates decreasing vascular resistance or blood volume. Diastolic hypotension is a common cause of low mean BP in preterm infants.

> In otherwise well infants, treatment should not be guided by BP measurement alone.

Capillary refill time

Capillary refill time (CRT) is measured by pressing the skin of the infant's sternum and foot or hand for 5 sec, then counting the seconds it takes for the skin to refill with capillary blood. The normal CRT is less than 3 sec in both central and peripheral locations. Record the CRT in seconds (e.g., '4 sec' or 'less than 2 sec') rather than using terms such as 'prolonged'.

> While a CRT of greater than 3 to 4 sec is a reliable sign of circulatory deterioration, a normal CRT test should not, by itself, be relied upon to rule out serious illness.

Skin temperature

Warm skin, including feet and hands, suggests good skin perfusion. Cool feet and hands compared with a warm trunk may be a sign of low peripheral perfusion. This indicator can be masked when newborns are cared for on a radiant warmer.

> Cool feet and hands and peripheral cyanosis (acrocyanosis) are common during transition and can be caused by sluggish peripheral circulation, peripheral vasomotor instability, or cold stress.

Heart rate

The normal HR in term newborns is between 100 bpm and 140 bpm. In premature newborns, HR is normally between 120 bpm and 160 bpm. Heart rate can be impacted by medications, pain, agitation, and temperature. An HR that is persistently greater than 180 bpm should be investigated.

A lower resting HR (80–100 bpm) in the sleeping term infant is common in the first few days post-birth and is not by itself concerning.

Urine output

Normal urine production depends on adequate blood perfusion to the kidneys. Low urine output can be a sign of insufficient circulation but only after 24 h of age, as many infants do not void in the first 12 to 24 h.

Organization of Care

Care in the ACoRN Cardiovascular Sequence is organized based on whether the infant has:

- Shock,
- Circulatory instability without shock,
- Cyanosis unresponsive to O2,
- A failed CCHD screen, or
- A HR greater than 220 bpm.

Shock

Infants are identified by the Clinical Assessment of Circulation Table (Table 4.1) as having shock when abnormal neurologic signs (decreased tone, activity, or alertness) are present in the context of low perfusion (pale, mottled, or grey). These signs of shock may also co-exist in infants presenting with severe cyanosis or tachycardia.

> An infant with signs of shock is critically ill by definition, and the management of shock is a medical emergency. When shock is suspected, immediate supportive measures must be instituted, regardless of cause.

Circulatory instability without shock

These infants are identified by the Clinical Assessment of Circulation Table (Table 4.1) as having weak pulses, low BP, prolonged CRTs, cool extremities, or a HR greater than 180 bpm, but without having altered neurologic status. In infants older than 24 h, urine output may be less than 1 mL/kg/h.

Infants who have signs of circulatory instability may become critically ill and need ongoing monitoring and support.

Cyanosis unresponsive to O2

A low SpO2 or arterial PO2 is needed to confirm the presence and degree of central cyanosis. With significant arterial desaturation, oxygen delivery to the tissues is compromised and metabolic acidosis develops. Table 4.2 shows how different levels of SpO2 are tolerated.

Table 4.2.
How are differing degrees of desaturation tolerated?

SpO2	Degree of desaturation	Tolerance
> 75%	Mild to moderate	Usually well tolerated
65% to 75%	Marked	Less well tolerated, especially when infants are unwell or anemic
< 65%	Severe	Poorly tolerated

Infants with profound cyanosis may also show decreased tone, reduced activity and level of alertness, or other signs of shock. These infants need to be stabilized first under the **Shock** arm of the Cardiovascular Sequence.

Failed CCHD screen

Newborns who fail their CCHD screen may be clinically stable, have cyanosis outside the visual threshold, and may or may not show other signs of circulatory instability. These infants may become critically ill and need urgent assessment.

Heart rate greater than 220 bpm

An infant with a HR greater than 220 bpm at rest is suspected to have SVT.

Most inpatient newborns with new onset SVT can tolerate a HR of up to 250 bpm for several hours, allowing time for consultation before initiating medical treatment. Without treatment, a sustained tachyarrhythmia eventually progresses to heart failure. Outpatient infants with SVT generally have signs of decompensation at time of presentation to hospital.

Infants with a sustained tachyarrhythmia may show low tone, reduced activity, and decreased alertness, or other signs of shock. Such effects are secondary to reduced cardiac contractility and low cardiac output. These infants need to be stabilized first under the **Shock** arm of the Cardiovascular Sequence.

Response

Shock

The goal when treating shock is to decrease demands on the cardiovascular system while optimizing organ perfusion and oxygen delivery. To stabilize an infant with shock:

- Intubate immediately (if the infant is not already intubated),
- Optimize ventilation, and
- Initiate vascular access and volume expansion. Administer an initial bolus of 10 mL/kg of 0.9% NaCl over 5 to 10 min. Further volume expansion will depend on response and suspected cause of shock.

Circulatory instability without shock

Vascular access and volume expansion with 10 mL/kg of 0.9% NaCl over 15 to 30 min may be considered for infants who have more than one sign of circulatory instability.

Cyanosis

An infant with cyanosis unresponsive to oxygen is suspected to have CCHD.

- Make sure that cyanosis is not caused by respiratory distress or inadequate ventilation, as per the ACoRN Respiratory Alerting Signs. In neonates with a cardiac cause for cyanosis, the Respiratory Score is usually low.
- Perform a hyperoxia test:
  o Place an oximeter on the right wrist or hand (pre-ductal) and record the SpO2. If possible, place a second oximeter on either foot (post-ductal) and record the SpO2 simultaneously. If a second

oximeter is not available, record a sequential SpO2 on either foot with the same oximeter. Note any difference in pre-ductal and post-ductal values.

- o Increase the inspired oxygen to 100% to see whether SpO2 increases.
- o When the infant has received inspired oxygen of 100% for 15 to 20 min, record the pre- and post-ductal SpO2.
- o Note whether there has been any fluctuation in SpO2 during the test, and whether a difference in pre- and post-ductal SpO2 has increased or decreased.
- o Gradually decrease the inspired oxygen from 100% to see whether SpO2 decreases.
- o If an arterial line is being used for blood sampling, record whether it is pre- or post-ductal. Remember that only right arm samples are pre-ductal; umbilical arterial samples are post-ductal. Record the PaO2 at an inspired oxygen of 100%.
- Failure to achieve a significant rise in SpO2 (greater than 10%) or a rise in PaO2 of greater than 20 mmHg to 30 mmHg during the hyperoxia test suggests cyanotic heart disease with a fixed right-to-left shunt. An SpO2 of 95% or higher or a PaO2 of 100 mmHg or higher at any time suggests that cyanotic heart disease is unlikely.
- After completing the hyperoxia test, administered oxygen should be decreased to a level where the SpO2 is stable and does not decline further.
- Infants with cyanosis unresponsive to oxygen should have vascular access whether they have signs of circulatory instability or not.
- Urgent consultation with a paediatric cardiologist is required.

Failed CCHD screen

Most newborns who fail CCHD screening are stable but need to be evaluated to rule out a critical congenital heart defect. Complete clinical assessment by the most responsible health care provider and a paediatrician (if one is available at the centre) is required. Assessment should include cardiac auscultation, 4-limb BPs, and chest radiograph. Assessment should also include a hyperoxia test when SpO2 is less than 90%. In those infants where cardiac illness cannot be ruled out, echocardiogram and referral to a paediatric cardiologist are required.

Heart rate greater than 220 bpm

High pulse rates obtained by a pulse oximeter or non-invasive BP device are not always accurate, and cardiorespiratory monitors sometimes double-count. When responding to an infant with a reported HR greater than 220 bpm:

- Confirm the HR. A 12-lead electrocardiogram (ECG) should be performed.
- When tachycardia is intermittent, try to obtain rhythm strips when the infant's rhythms are tachycardic and normal—and especially when transitioning between the 2 rates. (A rhythm strip is obtained by pressing 'print' on some cardiorespiratory monitors, but such readings are no substitute for a 12-lead ECG.)
- Scan and send the ECG to the consulting paediatric cardiologist.
- Assess the infant for decreased end-organ perfusion.
- Initiate vascular access.

Next Steps

Next Steps in the ACoRN Cardiovascular Sequence are to obtain a focused history, conduct a physical exam, order diagnostic tests, establish a working diagnosis, and obtain an urgent consultation (if not already done).

Focused history

Essential information to gather during a focused cardiovascular history includes the following:

Antepartum

- Family history of CHD or associated genetic syndromes (e.g., trisomies, Marfan syndrome, Noonan syndrome)
- Genetic screens or testing
- Fetal ultrasound diagnosis of cardiac abnormalities
- Fetal arrhythmia
- Maternal conditions such as diabetes or collagen vascular disease
- Maternal medication use (e.g., selective serotonin reuptake inhibitors or serotonin–norepinephrine reuptake inhibitors)
- Infections or exposure to teratogens in early pregnancy

Intrapartum

- Indicators of fetal compromise (e.g., abnormal intermittent auscultation, atypical or abnormal electronic fetal monitoring tracing and/or fetal acidosis)
- Excessive blood loss per vagina
- Presence of nuchal cord
- Acute neonatal blood loss (e.g., cord avulsion, incomplete cord clamp)
- Risk factors for sepsis or evidence of chorioamnionitis

Neonatal

- Onset of symptoms (at birth or during the first week of life)
- Disinterest in or fatigue during feeds
- Excessive weight gain or loss
- Diaphoresis with feeds

Focused physical examination

In addition to the examination conducted during the ACoRN Primary Survey, a focused cardiovascular examination should include the following:

Observation

- Colour
- Level of alertness and activity

- Resting posture and tone
- Respiratory effort and rate (e.g., increased due to pulmonary congestion)
- Dysmorphic features suggestive of chromosomal abnormalities (trisomy 21, 13, or 18), or genetic syndromes. Genetic abnormalities significantly increase the risk for CHD.

Examination

- Check 4-limb BPs. It is normal for the BP to be slightly higher in the legs than the arms. Systolic BPs that are greater than 10 mm to 15 mm higher in the right arm compared with the left arm or legs is abnormal and may indicate coarctation of the aorta.
- Check for peripheral edema.
- Compare temperature of the infant's feet and hands with temperature over the trunk.
- Compare pulses palpated in the upper and lower extremities.
- Palpate for an active precordium or high cardiac impulse over the sternum (right ventricle) or apex (left ventricle), which suggests CHD. Less common signs are a palpable 'second heart' sound or 'thrill'—a palpable murmur that is always abnormal.
- Auscultate for abnormal heart sounds and murmurs, keeping these considerations in mind:
  o Soft murmurs at the apex or over the large vessels are common in well term newborns.
  o A murmur can be transitional **or** a sign of cardiac disease.
  o Severe CHD can exist without a murmur.
  o A 'galloping' rhythm can indicate heart failure.
- Check for hepatomegaly (i.e., the infant's liver is palpable 3 cm or more below the right costal margin).
  o In lung disease with hyperinflation, the liver may be displaced downward.
  o In cardiac disease, hepatomegaly can indicate heart failure.

Diagnostic tests

- Chest radiograph, blood gas, and complete blood count and differential (CBCD).

Chest radiograph

The most helpful view is supine and anteroposterior, including the upper abdomen to determine the position of the stomach. A stomach bubble on the right side of the abdomen suggests *situs inversus* of abdominal organs, which can be associated with structural cardiac abnormalities. There are 5 questions to ask when viewing infant chest radiographs for cardiovascular assessment:

1. Is the heart size normal, large, or small?
2. Is the heart shape normal or abnormal?
3. Are the lung vascular markings normal, increased, or decreased?
4. Is the heart oriented toward the left side of the chest?
5. Is the stomach in the normal position?

Examples

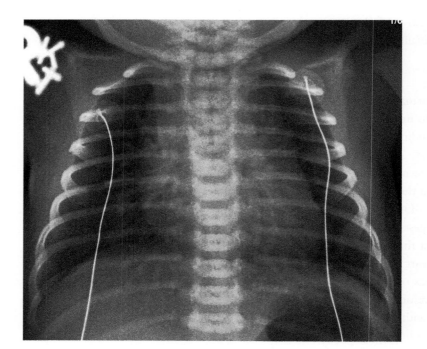

Normal chest radiograph: Normal heart size, shape, and position, normal superior mediastinum and vascular markings, and stomach in the normal position.

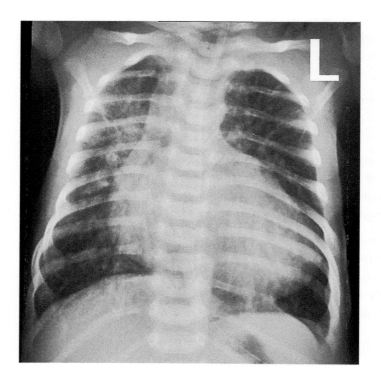

Abnormal chest radiograph: Enlarged heart, 'egg-shaped', narrow mediastinum (due to the anterior/posterior relationship of the great vessels) and increased vascular markings. The stomach is not visible in this image of an infant with transposition of the great arteries (TGA). This cardiac shape is commonly referred to as 'egg on a string'.

Case courtesy of Dr Hani Salam, Radiopaedia.org, rID: 13517

Blood gases

Metabolic acidosis is indicated by a pH of less than 7.25 and an increase in base deficit in venous, arterial, or capillary blood. The clinical significance of a base deficit less than 10 mEq/L is often uncertain. A base deficit greater than 10 mEq/L to 12 mEq/L is clinically significant because it may indicate insufficient tissue perfusion and oxygenation. The combination of metabolic acidosis and high lactate levels (greater than 5) is called lactic acidosis. Acidosis may produce hemodynamic instability because of reduced cardiac contractility, vasodilation, and impaired responsiveness to catecholamines.

Infants with developing heart failure also experience difficulty with gas exchange due to lung congestion, which is indicated by an increased PCO2 and respiratory acidosis.

Complete blood count

The normal hemoglobin range in term infants is 150 g/L to 220 g/L, and the normal hematocrit is 0.45 to 0.65. A low hemoglobin at birth may indicate blood loss:

- When the blood loss is acute, there are signs of shock.
- When the blood loss is chronic, there is anemia without shock.

Polycythemia (hematocrit greater than 0.65 on a venous sample) can lead to hyperviscosity with sluggish peripheral perfusion. These infants may have exaggerated acrocyanosis.

Specific Diagnosis and Management

Signs of shock or cardiovascular instability

While shock can be recognized clinically using ACoRN's Alerting Signs, specific metabolic indicators of shock, such as lactic acidosis, may precede clinical signs while the infant's cardiovascular system is still compensating.

Monitoring clinical and metabolic signs with shock or cardiovascular instability is vitally important. For example, a rapidly resolving metabolic acidosis without a bicarbonate infusion is a promising indicator of improvement.

There are three main categories of shock.

Hypovolemic shock

This type of shock occurs when there is reduced circulating blood volume due to acute blood loss occurring before birth (e.g., in feto–maternal or acute twin-to-twin transfusion), during birth (e.g., vasa praevia), or after birth (e.g., a ruptured cord or massive subgaleal hemorrhage). Note that vaginal bleeding from placental abruption or placenta praevia is almost exclusively maternal in origin. A feto-maternal hemorrhage is suspected when there are decreased fetal movements and an electronic fetal heart tracing has a sinusoidal pattern. A Kleihauer–Betke test quantifies fetal cells in the maternal circulation.

Fetal blood loss can also occur with partial cord occlusion (e.g., with a nuchal cord) that interrupts venous flow into the fetus to a greater degree than the arterial flow from the fetus to the placenta. This imbalance is caused by the thin-walled vein being occluded by compression before the two thick-walled arteries. The occlusion happens just before birth, when descent of the fetal head causes a loop of umbilical cord to tighten around the neck. While often not clinically significant, relative hypovolemia can result and present with pallor post-resuscitation.

In acute blood loss, the infant's hemoglobin concentration will be low. However, the drop in hemoglobin concentration may not reflect the magnitude of hemorrhage before hemodilution occurs.

Hypovolemic shock due to leaking of intravascular fluid into the tissues ('third-spacing') is less common.

The treatment for hypovolemic shock is to restore the circulating blood volume, initially with normal saline boluses, in aliquots of 10 mL/kg. The infant's response, in terms of an improvement in circulation, should be documented after each bolus. In the case of massive blood loss, transfusion of blood will be necessary.

Remember that even massive blood loss can be concealed, such as with a feto-maternal hemorrhage or subgaleal hemorrhage. Subgaleal hemorrhages most commonly occur after applying instrumentation (e.g., vacuum or forceps) to the fetal head at time of birth. They are associated with a rapidly expanding subgaleal space and increasing head circumference. When untreated, a subgaleal hemorrhage can progress to shock and death.

The decision to transfuse blood must take into consideration the clinical condition of the infant, the potential complications associated with blood products, and the ability to obtain parental consent. The choice between uncross-matched O-negative blood or cross-matched type-specific blood depends on the urgency of transfusion. A specific policy should be in place at every institution describing the procedure to access blood products urgently, defining the circumstances for use of uncross-matched blood, and how to proceed when parents refuse this intervention.

Distributive shock

This type of shock occurs when blood vessels lose their normal vascular tone or have increased permeability. One example of distributive shock is septic shock.

> In early distributive shock, the overriding feature is vasodilatation. The infant is pink and appears well perfused but is hypotensive (the 'warm phase'). This clinical presentation can be deceptive and lead to delayed diagnosis of shock. At a later stage, blood is redirected away from the periphery toward the vital organs, and the hypotensive infant appears grey and mottled (the 'cold phase').

In septic shock, there may be a history of preterm labour, prolonged rupture of membranes, maternal fever, or inadequate intrapartum prophylaxis for Group B *Streptococcus* (GBS). However, the absence of these risk factors does not preclude the diagnosis of sepsis in a clinically unwell infant. Infants with septic shock have multisystem failure and high mortality. Urgent management includes volume expansion, antibiotics (after blood cultures have been obtained), and inotropic support. Inotropes increase the force of contraction of the heart and vasoconstrict peripheral blood vessels. Their use should always be guided by level 3 consultation.

Cardiogenic shock

This type of shock occurs when the heart pumps inadequately due to functional or structural impairment of heart function. Functional impairment occurs in perinatal hypoxic injury (i.e., due to myocardial ischemia), severe respiratory failure with pulmonary hypertension, septicemia, and cardiomyopathies. Functional impairment may also be secondary to cardiac arrhythmias. Many infants with cardiogenic shock respond to basic interventions during resuscitation and stabilization but may also require ongoing circulatory support with inotropic drugs.

Structural impairment occurs in CHD (cyanotic or acyanotic). These conditions ultimately require surgical intervention. Cardiogenic shock due to CHD should be suspected when:

- There is no history of adverse perinatal events;
- Symptoms worsen during the time the ductus arteriosus closes, hours to days after birth ('duct dependence'); or
- Shock co-exists with absent lower limb pulses, or with signs of heart failure (such as cardiomegaly, pulmonary edema, and hepatomegaly).

The left heart obstructive lesions that most commonly present with shock in a previously well infant are as follows.

Hypoplastic left heart syndrome

Onset of symptoms occurs a few hours to days after birth, with pallor or grey skin tone, mottling, and cyanosis (pulmonary and systemic venous blood mixes in the right ventricle), poor peripheral pulses, and a single second heart sound. A murmur may or may not be present. Chest radiograph shows cardiomegaly, and there is evidence of right ventricular hypertrophy on ECG. Figure 4.4. shows pre- and post-ductal closure.

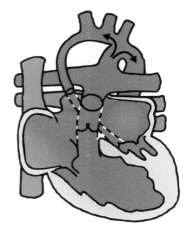

Hypoplastic left heart: when the ductus arteriosus is open, systemic cardiac output can be supported by the right ventricle.

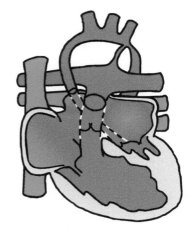

Hypoplastic left heart: when the ductus arteriosus starts closing, the systemic cardiac output can no longer be supported by the right ventricle.

Figure 4.4. The hypoplastic left heart.

Coarctation of the aorta (including interrupted aortic arch)

Onset of symptoms occurs a few hours to days after birth. Although femoral pulses may be palpable on the initial newborn examinations, they then become diminished, delayed, or absent as the ductus arteriosus closes. There may be a murmur, cardiomegaly on chest radiograph, and right ventricular hypertrophy on ECG. CCHD screening prior to hospital discharge may not identify newborns with coarctation of the aorta. See Figure 4.5.

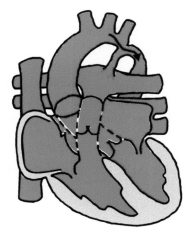 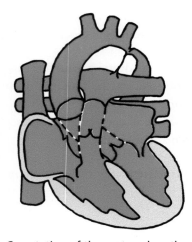

Coarctation of the aorta: when the ductus arteriosus is open, blood is able to flow in the aortic arch and descending aorta despite the coarctation.

Coarctation of the aorta: when the ductus arteriosus is closed, the obstuction at the level of the coarctation is further narrowed. This markedly decreases blood flow to the descending aorta (lower extremities ± left arm.)

Figure 4.5. Coarctation of the aorta.

Hypoplastic left heart syndrome, interrupted aortic arch, and severe coarctation are duct-dependent, and the closure of the ductus is fatal if not prevented or reversed using PGE1 (see Appendix C, Medications). In these cases of left-sided obstructive lesions, the ductus must be kept open to ensure ongoing systemic flow through the aorta.

> Every centre that delivers infants should be able to access PGE1 in an emergency, but this medication should only be administered with paediatric cardiologist guidance. Adverse reactions to PGE1 include apnea and vasodilation leading to hypotension and hyperthermia. Anticipate the need to intubate and initiate volume expansion as part of management. The infant's clinical response to PGE1 must be monitored, documented, and communicated to the paediatric cardiologist. All cases need urgent transfer to a tertiary or quaternary care centre.

Suspected cyanotic heart disease

Cyanosis unresponsive to oxygen occurs when an increasing proportion of blood in the systemic circulation has not been oxygenated in the lungs.

In persistent pulmonary hypertension of the newborn (PPHN), small muscular branches of the pulmonary arteries fail to relax, increasing resistance and pressure in the pulmonary artery, the right ventricle, and the right atrium (Figure 4.6). Some of the blood being pumped to the lungs by the right side of the heart is diverted (shunted) through the ductus arteriosus to the post-ductal aorta and across the foramen ovale to the left atrium. Increased pressure in the right ventricle leads to tricuspid regurgitation. When these shunts are present, the oxygen content of blood returning from the lungs to the left side of the heart is diluted in the left atrium and diluted again in the post-ductal aorta.

PPHN is usually associated with lung disease but can also occur as a primary condition. PPHN can be reversible or irreversible, depending on cause.

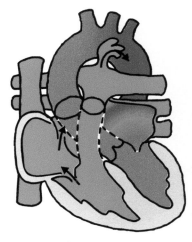

Oxygenated blood returning from the lungs to the left atrium is mixed with blood shunted from the right atrium. Further shunting occurs via the ductus arteriosus, from the pulmonary artery to the aorta.

Figure 4.6. Persistent pulmonary hypertension of the newborn.

An infant's responsiveness to oxygen and ventilation in respiratory disease and PPHN indicates that the mechanism of cyanosis is functional rather than anatomic. Management strategies aim to improve ventilation/perfusion matching (V/Q matching) by preventing alveolar collapse (using positive end-expiratory pressure [PEEP] or continuous positive airway pressure [CPAP]), expanding collapsed alveoli, and increasing the concentration of inspired oxygen to better oxygenate alveoli that are only partially ventilated.

Pulmonary vascular resistance can be very labile in PPHN, and thus, oxygen saturation can fluctuate even with small changes in ventilation or inspired oxygen. This is why SpO2 lability needs to be documented when performing a hyperoxia test in cyanosis (described on pages 106-7).

In cyanotic heart disease, structural abnormalities of the heart or large blood vessels result in a fixed mechanism of cyanosis that is unresponsive to increased FiO2. Although cyanosis due to cyanotic heart disease ultimately needs surgical management, its medical stabilization is critically important.

Certain structural abnormalities of the heart or large blood vessels result in cyanosis because there is:

- Separation between the right- and left-sided circuits (e.g., TGA),
- Right-to-left shunting of deoxygenated blood away from the lungs (e.g., tricuspid or pulmonary atresia), or
- Mixing of already oxygenated blood with deoxygenated blood (e.g., total anomalous pulmonary venous return [TAPVR]).

In transposition of the great arteries (TGA), there is full separation between the right- and left-sided circuits. The aorta arises from the right ventricle and the pulmonary artery arises from the left ventricle (Figure 4.7). These infants are usually visibly cyanosed from birth.

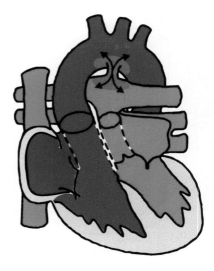

The right and left circulations are separated. Survival is not possible unless there is communication between the left and right atrium; emergency atrial septostomy may be required. In addition, keeping the ductus arteriosus open allows further mixing of oxygenated and deoxygenated blood.

Figure 4.7. Transposition of the great arteries.

The only way that survival is possible when the right- and left-sided circuits are anatomically separated is:

- If oxygenated blood returning to the left atrium is able to flow unrestricted to the right atrium through an interatrial communication (shunt), *and*
- If blood ejected from the right ventricle into the aorta is able to mix with blood being ejected from the left ventricle into the pulmonary artery through the patent ductus.

Maintaining patency of the ductus arteriosus is the critical first step in stabilizing these infants. However, both shunts are necessary in TGA, so keeping the ductus arteriosus open may not be enough to ensure adequate oxygenation. If the interatrial shunt is restrictive, an atrial septostomy at the tertiary referral centre may be necessary. This procedure improves cyanosis by increasing the volume of left atrial oxygenated blood that mixes with the right atrial deoxygenated blood. Urgent transfer to a tertiary/quaternary facility with paediatric cardiology support is critical.

In tricuspid atresia, deoxygenated blood in the right side of the heart is shunted away from the lungs (right-to-left shunting) through an interatrial shunt (Figure 4.8). This deoxygenated blood mixes with oxygenated blood in the left side of the heart. The only path for blood to flow into the pulmonary system is via the patent ductus arteriosus.

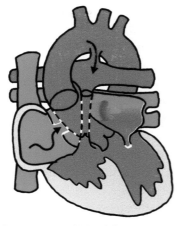

Deoxygenated blood from the right
atrium flows into left atrium via the
foramen ovale, mixing with oxygenated
blood. Keeping the ductus arteriosus
open maintains blood flow to the lungs,
improving oxygenation.

Figure 4.8. Tricuspid atresia.

Infants with right-sided obstructive lesions (e.g., tricuspid atresia, pulmonary atresia, or critical pulmonary stenosis) are often stable initially and may not be visibly cyanosed, but pulse oximetry testing will detect abnormal SpO2 levels. These infants can remain clinically stable until ductal closure triggers acute deterioration. This highlights the importance of CCHD screening for all infants to detect critical cardiac lesions before they become symptomatic. Infants with right-sided obstructive lesions require administration of PGE1 for ductal patency.

In total anomalous pulmonary venous return (TAPVR), the pulmonary veins do not drain into the left atrium, but rather into a central vein and then into the right atrium (Figure 4.9). Therefore,

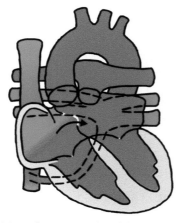

Mixing of oxygenated and deoxygenated
blood in the right atrium in total anomalous
pulmonary venous return. This condition is
difficult to differentiate clinically from PPHN.

Figure 4.9. Total anomalous pulmonary venous return.

oxygenated blood from the pulmonary veins and systemic deoxygenated blood mix in the right atrium. The mixed blood then reaches the left atrium (and the systemic circulation) through the patent foramen ovale. At the same time, pulmonary venous drainage may be obstructed, leading to pulmonary congestion and pulmonary hypertension.

Administration of PGE1 is indicated in suspected cyanotic heart lesions. PGE1 maintains ductal patency, improving pulmonary blood flow in right-sided obstructive lesions and allowing oxygenated and deoxygenated blood to mix more effectively in conditions such as TGA. Although administering PGE1 may lead to worsening pulmonary congestion in TAPVR, it is unlikely that this condition will be diagnosed prior to transfer. When PGE1 treatment is effective, the infant's SpO2 and PaO2 rise within 10 to 15 min, and acidosis improves. Lack of response to PGE1 and severe, ongoing cyanosis signal high risk for mortality.

The specific diagnosis of CHD is usually not apparent before echocardiogram and subspecialty assessment. Consultation with a paediatric cardiologist prior to transfer will guide dosing of PGE1 (usually the lowest dose possible to achieve improvement) and identify an acceptable target SpO2.

Supraventricular tachycardia and other tachyarrhythmias

The tachyarrhythmias need to be differentiated from each other (Table 4.3), making consultation with a paediatric cardiologist essential to management decisions.

The most common tachyarrhythmia in newborns is a narrow complex SVT, where HR typically exceeds 220 bpm. In SVT, the infant's heart is beating so fast that filling during diastole can be compromised. In the most common form of neonatal SVT, the re-entry circuit starts in the atrium, passes through the specific conduction system, much of the ventricle, the accessory pathway, and then back to the atrium. Despite its name, SVT involves the whole heart. During SVT, the infant's HR does not vary with physiological changes such as breathing, and there is no beat-to-beat variability. SVT is sudden-onset and is not triggered by external events. Reversion to sinus rhythm is also sudden and can be spontaneous or in response to therapy. SVT may occur in 'runs' lasting minutes to hours. SVT may initially be asymptomatic but if it is sustained and untreated, heart failure and shock will develop over a variable period of time.

SVT can also occur in utero, leading to fetal heart failure or hydrops fetalis, with high mortality and morbidity. Specialized prenatal assessment and monitoring are needed, in conjunction with measures to control fetal HR and prolong gestation.

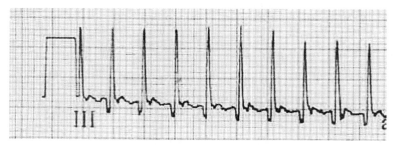

This ECG tracing shows SVT with a HR of 300 bpm. No P waves are visible and the QRS complexes are narrow and uniform.

Atrial flutter is also seen in infants, although less commonly than SVT. With atrial flutter, an infant's atrial rate may be 300 bpm or higher, but the ventricular rate is much slower. The P waves have a characteristic 'sawtooth' or undulating baseline ('flutter waves'), and the atrial rate is different from the ventricular rate because there is a variable heart block, such that not all atrial contractions generate a ventricular contraction. The QRS complexes are narrow. The ventricular rhythm is irregular, and its rate tends to be less than 220 bpm.

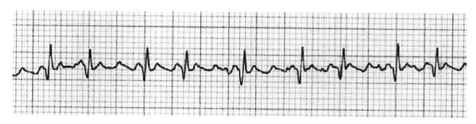

In this tracing, flutter waves are clearly shown, with an atrial rate of approximately 300 bpm. The QRS complexes are narrow. There are 2 to 3 flutter waves for each QRS complex, indicating a variable 2:1 to 3:1 block and an irregular rhythm.

The management of infants with tachyarrhythmias is based on two considerations:

- Clinical stability or instability, and
- Type of arrhythmia.

Table 4.3.
Key features to differentiate common causes of tachycardia

Sinus tachycardia	Supraventricular tachycardia (SVT)	Atrial flutter
HR < 220 bpm	HR 220 to 300 bpm	Atrial rate 300 to 500 bpm (ventricular rate usually < 220)
Gradual onset and cessation	Sudden onset and cessation	HR varies with atrioventricular conduction block (can decrease by half suddenly if 1:1 becomes 2:1 block)
Preserved beat-to-beat variability	No beat-to-beat variability	No atrial beat-to-beat variability
Narrow QRS	Narrow QRS in approximately 90% of cases	Narrow QRS
P waves precede each QRS	P wave relationship to QRS complex is variable. P waves are often not visible during supraventricular tachycardia	P waves with sawtooth pattern are better seen in the inferior and right precordial leads on a 12-lead electrocardiogram. Atrioventricular conduction is variable

When infants with SVT are clinically stable, asymptomatic, or minimally symptomatic, a vagal manoeuvre may be attempted:

- Crush ice inside a plastic bag with water to make a slurry and apply to the infant's face, avoiding contact with the eyes. Hold in place for 15 sec.
- Other vagal manoeuvres such as carotid sinus massage or pressure on the eyeballs are dangerous and should never be used.

When infants with SVT are clinically unstable:

- Intubate and ventilate to support the infant with cardiorespiratory failure.
- Obtain blood gases, including lactate, electrolytes, and serum glucose.
- Consult a paediatric cardiologist for guidance on the use of adenosine or cardioversion.

Intravenous adenosine

The administration of adenosine for SVT should only be undertaken after consultation with, and with the approval of, a paediatric cardiologist. ECG should be monitored continuously throughout administration of adenosine. There should be a 2-min wait and check of vital signs between doses. The recorded strip should be reviewed immediately after conversion to sinus rhythm for concealed pre-excitation, which may be revealed during the first few beats after conversion to sinus rhythm.

Further management of SVT and management of atrial flutter are beyond the scope of ACoRN and will be guided by a paediatric cardiologist after the infant is transferred to the tertiary care centre.

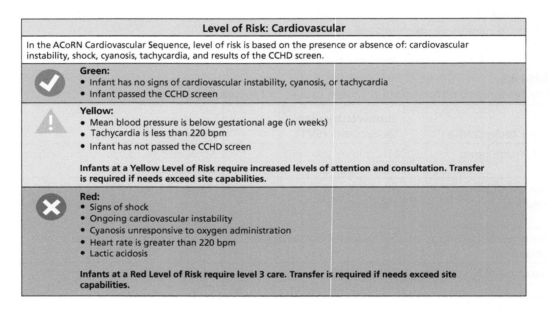

Level of Risk: Cardiovascular

In the ACoRN Cardiovascular Sequence, level of risk is based on the presence or absence of: cardiovascular instability, shock, cyanosis, tachycardia, and results of the CCHD screen.

Green:
- Infant has no signs of cardiovascular instability, cyanosis, or tachycardia
- Infant passed the CCHD screen

Yellow:
- Mean blood pressure is below gestational age (in weeks)
- Tachycardia is less than 220 bpm
- Infant has not passed the CCHD screen

Infants at a Yellow Level of Risk require increased levels of attention and consultation. Transfer is required if needs exceed site capabilities.

Red:
- Signs of shock
- Ongoing cardiovascular instability
- Cyanosis unresponsive to oxygen administration
- Heart rate is greater than 220 bpm
- Lactic acidosis

Infants at a Red Level of Risk require level 3 care. Transfer is required if needs exceed site capabilities.

Cardiovascular: Case 1—Shock or circulatory instability?

You are called STAT to assist with the care of a 14-h-old baby on the postpartum unit. His mother pressed the call button because she was concerned her baby would not wake up for feeds. The nurse responding to the mother's call found the baby to be unresponsive, pale, and grey in colour. He was breathing, and his HR was 175 bpm. His SpO2 was 92%. The nurse quickly took the baby to the radiant warmer in the special care nursery (SCN) and invited his mother to come along.

When you arrive, the staff is completing the ACoRN Primary Survey and the Consolidated Core Steps. The baby's HR is 168 bpm, respiratory rate is 55 breaths/min, but his respirations are shallow; SpO2 is 93%. Blood pressure is 40/22 with a mean of 34 mmHg, and his axillary temperature is 36.2°C. His blood sugar is 6.5 mmol/L. He did not cry in response to the heel poke and is flaccid, with minimal spontaneous movement. The postpartum nurse tells you that he was born at 41 weeks gestation with a birth weight of 3600 g.

You introduce yourself to his mother, who is sitting in a chair across the room, and let her know that the SCN team is moving quickly to help her son and determine what is making him ill. You review the Primary Survey with the team.

1. **Does this baby present with any Alerting Signs for Resuscitation?**

   ☐ Yes   ☐ No

2. **Complete the ACoRN Primary Survey and Consolidated Core Steps, and generate a Problem List.**

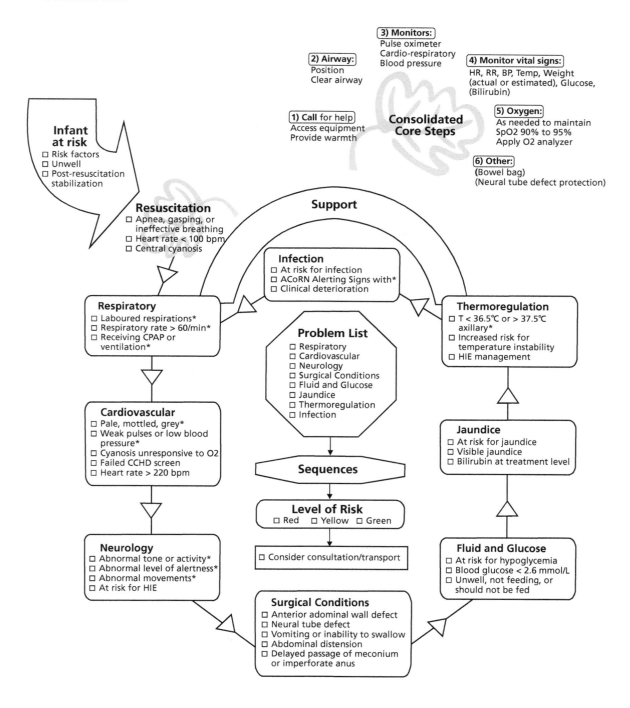

Cardiovascular, Neurology, Fluid and Glucose, Thermoregulation, and Infection are prioritized on your Problem List.

3. **Cardiovascular is the first Sequence identified. Mark applicable Alerting Signs in the following diagram.**

> **Cardiovascular**
> ☐ Pale, mottled, grey*
> ☐ Weak pulses or low blood pressure*
> ☐ Cyanosis unresponsive to O2
> ☐ Failed CCHD screen
> ☐ Heart rate > 220 bpm

The baby remains flaccid and nonresponsive. His colour is mottled and grey. You can feel both brachial and femoral pulses. His CRT is 5 sec centrally, and he feels cool to touch.

4. **As the Core Step in the Cardiovascular Sequence, you complete the Clinical Assessment of Circulation Table. Tick all that apply.**

Sign	Stable	Unstable
Abnormal tone, activity, or level of alertness	☐ Normal tone, active, alert, and looking well	☐ Decreased tone, listless, lethargic
Critical perfusion	☐ Well perfused, pink, and peripherally warm	☐ Pale, mottled, grey
Pulses	☐ Easy to palpate	☐ Weak, absent, or femoral pulses weaker than right brachial pulses
Mean blood pressure	☐ ≥ gestational age (in weeks)	☐ < gestational age (in weeks)
Capillary refill time	☐ ≤ 3 sec centrally	☐ > 3 sec centrally
Skin temperature	☐ Peripherally warm	☐ Peripherally cool
Heart rate	☐ 100 to 180 bpm	☐ > 180 bpm
Hourly urine output (if older than 24 h)	☐ ≥ 1 mL/kg/h	☐ < 1 mL/kg/h
Shock is present when signs of critical perfusion (red box) coexist in an infant with decreased tone, activity, and alertness (red box), in the absence of an alternative explanation.		

5. **From a circulatory perspective, is this infant stable or unstable? Why?**

_____

_____

You continue down the Cardiovascular Sequence.

6. How do you Organize Care for this infant?

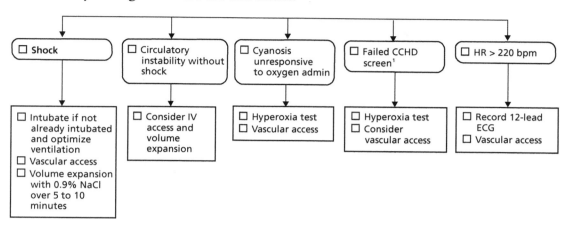

This baby is critically ill, and you determine that you need to intervene quickly to stabilize him. The baby requires intubation and vascular access to support his cardiorespiratory function as part of your initial Response. You ask another team member to insert an IV and initiate a saline bolus while you prepare for intubation.

As part of Next Steps, you know that a focused history, physical examination, diagnostic tests (e.g., blood work, chest radiograph), and timely consultation are priority interventions. The nurse has been tasked to gather more information from the mother about her pregnancy, birth, and the baby's condition prior to his deterioration. She has also called the baby's father to come in to be with his wife and son.

The mother is 38 yo, and this is her third child. She was healthy in pregnancy, and the only medications she took were prenatal vitamins. She did not have gestational diabetes or hypertension. Her antenatal blood work was normal and her GBS swab was negative. She went into spontaneous labour and delivered shortly after arrival to the hospital. The baby was vigorous at birth, with Apgar scores of 8 at 1 min and 9 at 5 min. There was delayed cord clamping for 2 min, and the baby spent the first 2 h skin-to-skin with his mother in the delivery room.

The mother reports that her baby breastfed well in the delivery room and twice on the postpartum unit at about 6 and 9 h of age. After that the baby seemed 'sleepy' and did not want to breastfeed, but he seemed alright otherwise, so she let him sleep. She became concerned when she couldn't wake him, and he seemed listless and 'off colour'.

Once the baby is intubated and the endotracheal tube secured, and IV access is obtained and a normal saline bolus ordered, you continue with Next Steps and perform a more complete examination.

On examination, there is no dysmorphism or obvious congenital abnormality. His head and neck are normal. His lungs are clear, although you note decreased air entry to his lung bases. His heart sounds are normal, and there are no murmurs. Femoral pulses are palpable bilaterally. His abdomen is soft and non-distended. There is no organomegaly or mass. Genitalia are normal and his anus is patent. His spine is intact, and he has no skin lesions.

7. What additional information would help you determine a working diagnosis for this infant? Tick all that apply.

☐ A stat CBCD.
☐ A chest radiograph.
☐ A blood gas.
☐ Pre- and post-ductal oxygen saturations.
☐ A 12-lead ECG.

    □ A visual examination of the placenta.

    □ Evaluation of the infant's response to volume expansion with 10 mL/kg of 0.9% NaCl solution.

You add those tasks to your 'to-do' list and move out of the Cardiovascular Sequence to address other sequences in the Problem List (Neurology, Fluid and Glucose, Thermoregulation, and Infection). You add Respiratory to your Problem List, now that the baby is intubated. You plan to call for consultation once your chest X-ray (CXR) and blood tests are available.

8. What is this baby's Level of Risk?

    □ Green   □ Yellow   □ Red

By the time you've completed your 'to-do' list, some lab results have arrived.

The complete blood count (CBC) shows hemoglobin of 190 g/L, WBC of 1.5 × 10⁹/L with 0.15 × 10⁹/L neutrophils, 0.20 × 10⁹/L bands and platelets of 110 × 10⁹/L. The venous blood gas shows pH 7.12, PCO2 40 mmHg, base deficit (BD) 15, and lactate of 8 mmol/L. The CXR shows well expanded lungs and normal cardiac silhouette.

After the intravenous bolus of 10 mL/kg of 0.9% NaCl, the baby's mean BP increases to 36 mmHg, but he remains mottled, with a central capillary refill time of 4 to 5 sec.

This baby continues to show signs of shock and cardiovascular instability.

9. What do you think is the cause of this infant's circulatory instability?

    □ Hypovolemic shock due to blood loss.

    □ Distributive shock due to sepsis.

    □ Cardiogenic shock due to hypoxic injury.

    □ Cyanotic CHD.

    □ A tachyarrhythmia.

10. What specific management steps would you consider?

    □ An additional bolus of 10 mL/kg of 0.9% NaCl solution.

    □ 15 mL/kg of Ringer's lactate solution.

    □ 15 mL/kg of O-negative uncross-matched packed red cells.

    □ A 12-lead ECG.

    □ An urgent echocardiogram.

    □ Stat administration of antibiotics after blood cultures are drawn, as indicated in the Infection Sequence.

Cardiovascular: Case 2—Circulatory instability or shock?

You are called to assess a baby girl, born at 39 weeks GA by spontaneous vaginal vertex delivery. The mother had a normal progression of labour and was monitored with intermittent auscultation. No fetal HR abnormalities were detected.

The baby cried at birth, had good tone, and was initially placed on her mother's chest. She was noted to be quite pale, so was taken to the radiant warmer at 1 min of age.

On your arrival at 10 min, the baby is crying and active with good tone and movement but is very pale. Her oxygen saturation is 92% in room air, and the midwife reports that her oxygen saturation has always been within the target range.

1. Complete the ACoRN Primary Survey and Consolidated Cores Steps, marking all appropriate boxes.

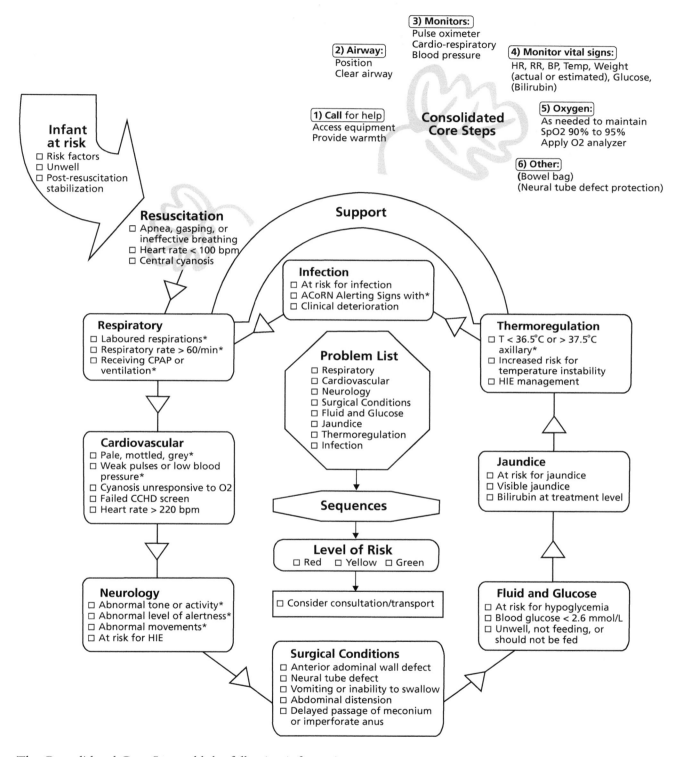

3) Monitors:
Pulse oximeter
Cardio-respiratory
Blood pressure

2) Airway:
Position
Clear airway

4) Monitor vital signs:
HR, RR, BP, Temp, Weight
(actual or estimated), Glucose,
(Bilirubin)

1) Call for help
Access equipment
Provide warmth

Consolidated Core Steps

5) Oxygen:
As needed to maintain
SpO2 90% to 95%
Apply O2 analyzer

6) Other:
(Bowel bag)
(Neural tube defect protection)

Infant at risk
☐ Risk factors
☐ Unwell
☐ Post-resuscitation stabilization

Resuscitation
☐ Apnea, gasping, or ineffective breathing
☐ Heart rate < 100 bpm
☐ Central cyanosis

Support

Infection
☐ At risk for infection
☐ ACoRN Alerting Signs with*
☐ Clinical deterioration

Respiratory
☐ Laboured respirations*
☐ Respiratory rate > 60/min*
☐ Receiving CPAP or ventilation*

Thermoregulation
☐ T < 36.5°C or > 37.5°C axillary*
☐ Increased risk for temperature instability
☐ HIE management

Problem List
☐ Respiratory
☐ Cardiovascular
☐ Neurology
☐ Surgical Conditions
☐ Fluid and Glucose
☐ Jaundice
☐ Thermoregulation
☐ Infection

Cardiovascular
☐ Pale, mottled, grey*
☐ Weak pulses or low blood pressure*
☐ Cyanosis unresponsive to O2
☐ Failed CCHD screen
☐ Heart rate > 220 bpm

Jaundice
☐ At risk for jaundice
☐ Visible jaundice
☐ Bilirubin at treatment level

Sequences

Level of Risk
☐ Red   ☐ Yellow   ☐ Green

Neurology
☐ Abnormal tone or activity*
☐ Abnormal level of alertness*
☐ Abnormal movements*
☐ At risk for HIE

☐ Consider consultation/transport

Fluid and Glucose
☐ At risk for hypoglycemia
☐ Blood glucose < 2.6 mmol/L
☐ Unwell, not feeding, or should not be fed

Surgical Conditions
☐ Anterior adominal wall defect
☐ Neural tube defect
☐ Vomiting or inability to swallow
☐ Abdominal distension
☐ Delayed passage of meconium or imperforate anus

The Consolidated Core Steps add the following information.

The baby's HR is 195 bpm and regular; respiratory rate is 50 breaths/min when the baby is quiet. You have difficulty feeling brachial or femoral pulses, and ask one of the staff to get the BP machine. Her estimated weight is 3000 g and temperature is 36.9°C.

The areas of concern you identify are (in prioritized order): Cardiovascular, Fluid and Glucose, Thermoregulation, and Infection.

The baby is alert and cries when examined, her tone is flexed, and she moves all her limbs spontaneously. She remains very pale and you feel weak brachial pulses. Her BP is 38/21, with a mean of 30 mmHg. You find it difficult to assess central capillary refill, due to her pallor. She feels warm to the touch. Her HR is now 190 bpm.

2. As the Core Step in the Cardiovascular Sequence, you complete the Clinical Assessment of Circulation Table. Tick all that apply.

Sign	Stable	Unstable
Abnormal tone, activity, or level of alertness	☐ Normal tone, active, alert, and looking well	☐ Decreased tone, listless, lethargic
Critical perfusion	☐ Well perfused, pink, and peripherally warm	☐ Pale, mottled, grey
Pulses	☐ Easy to palpate	☐ Weak, absent, or femoral pulses weaker than right brachial pulses
Mean blood pressure	☐ ≥ gestational age (in weeks)	☐ < gestational age (in weeks)
Capillary refill time	☐ ≤ 3 sec centrally	☐ > 3 sec centrally
Skin temperature	☐ Peripherally warm	☐ Peripherally cool
Heart rate	☐ 100 to 180 bpm	☐ > 180 bpm
Hourly urine output (if older than 24 h)	☐ ≥ 1 mL/kg/h	☐ < 1 mL/kg/h
Shock is present when signs of critical perfusion (red box) coexist in an infant with decreased tone, activity, and alertness (red box), in the absence of an alternative explanation.		

3. From a circulatory perspective, is this infant stable or unstable? Why?

_____

_____

You continue down the Cardiovascular Sequence.

4. How do you Organize Care for this infant?

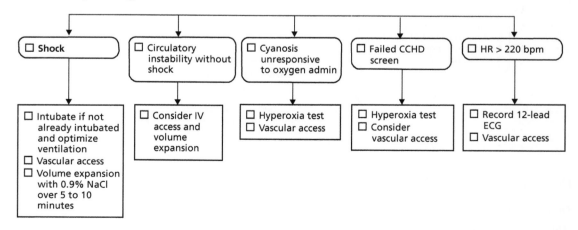

You decide this baby has circulatory instability without shock and plan to insert an IV and give a 10 mL/kg (30 mL) 0.9% NaCl bolus over 20 min. You explain to the baby's parents that you are taking her to the nursery and invite the father to accompany you. As soon as the bolus is done, you will reassess her cardiovascular status.

As part of Next Steps, you collect a focused history and do a physical examination.

The baby's mother is 28 yo, and this was her first pregnancy. Apart from some nausea in early pregnancy, she has been well. All of her antenatal blood work was normal, as were her ultrasounds. Her blood group is O+. There was no gestational diabetes or hypertension. Her GBS screen was negative. Her only medications were Diclectin and pre-natal vitamins. She had spontaneous labour and progressed well to a spontaneous vaginal birth. She had an epidural with good pain control and membranes ruptured 2 h prior to delivery. The midwife noted that the umbilical cord was wrapped tightly twice around the baby's neck, so she needed to clamp and cut the cord before delivering the baby's body.

A quick physical exam reveals no further abnormalities.

5. **What additional information would help you determine a working diagnosis for this infant? Tick all that apply.**
   ☐ A CBCD.
   ☐ A chest radiograph.
   ☐ A blood gas.
   ☐ Pre- and post-ductal oxygen saturations.
   ☐ A 12-lead ECG.
   ☐ A visual examination of the placenta.
   ☐ Evaluation of the infant's response to volume expansion with 10 mL/kg of 0.9% NaCl solution.

While inserting her IV, you send a CBC and do a glucose check. Her blood sugar is 3.2 mmol/L. You decide that you do not need a blood gas or X-ray at this time but will reassess her status after the saline bolus is finished. You think her Level of Risk is Yellow (mean BP below gestational age in weeks). You exit the Cardiovascular Sequence and return to your Problem List to address concerns in the Fluid and Glucose, Thermoregulation, and Infection Sequences.

After 10 mL/kg of 0.9% NaCl solution, the baby's mean BP has increased to 38 mmHg, and her pulses are still slightly weak. Her HR has dropped to 165 bpm. She remains alert and active and is 'pinking up', with a central CRT of 3 sec. You assess that she has responded well to her initial bolus but still has some cardiovascular instability.

The CBC shows hemoglobin of 120 g/L.

6. **What do you think is the cause of this infant's circulatory instability?**
   ☐ Hypovolemia.
   ☐ Distributive shock.
   ☐ Cardiogenic shock.
   ☐ Cyanotic CHD.
   ☐ A tachyarrhythmia.

7. **What specific management steps would you consider?**
   ☐ An additional bolus of 10 mL/kg of 0.9% NaCl solution.
   ☐ 15 mL/kg of Ringer's lactate solution.
   ☐ 15 mL/kg of O-negative uncross-matched packed red cells.
   ☐ A 12-lead ECG.
   ☐ An echocardiogram.

You opt to repeat a bolus of 10 mL/kg of 0.9% NaCl over 15 mins.

At the end of the second bolus, the baby's mean BP is 45 mmHg, her HR is 135 bpm, and her CRT is 2 to 3 sec. She is now well perfused, pink, and peripherally warm, and you palpate her pulses with ease. No risk factors for sepsis were identified on your focus history or physical exam. Your CBCD was not concerning aside from the hemoglobin of 120 g/L.

8. **Indicate the baby's Level of Risk and which criteria helped you make the determination** *at this time.*

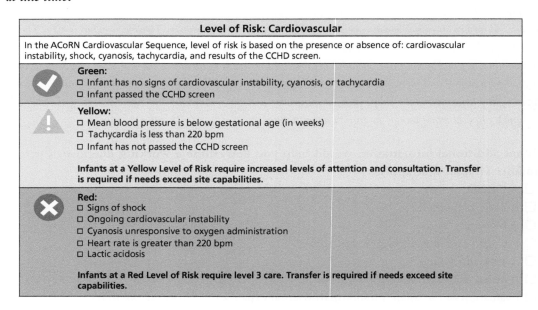

Level of Risk: Cardiovascular
In the ACoRN Cardiovascular Sequence, level of risk is based on the presence or absence of: cardiovascular instability, shock, cyanosis, tachycardia, and results of the CCHD screen.
Green: ☐ Infant has no signs of cardiovascular instability, cyanosis, or tachycardia ☐ Infant passed the CCHD screen
Yellow: ☐ Mean blood pressure is below gestational age (in weeks) ☐ Tachycardia is less than 220 bpm ☐ Infant has not passed the CCHD screen **Infants at a Yellow Level of Risk require increased levels of attention and consultation. Transfer is required if needs exceed site capabilities.**
Red: ☐ Signs of shock ☐ Ongoing cardiovascular instability ☐ Cyanosis unresponsive to oxygen administration ☐ Heart rate is greater than 220 bpm ☐ Lactic acidosis **Infants at a Red Level of Risk require level 3 care. Transfer is required if needs exceed site capabilities.**

Cardiovascular: Case 3—A baby with persistent cyanosis

You are changing the diaper of a 3500-g term baby after helping the mother successfully initiate breastfeeding in the birthing suite. Labour and birth were uncomplicated. As you do this, you notice that the baby appears cyanosed, and his lips are bluish.

You take the baby to the radiant warmer so that you can initiate ACoRN assessment.

Cyanosis is a Resuscitation Alerting Sign, and you enter into the Resuscitation Sequence.

1. **Indicate your course of action in the Resuscitation Sequence.**

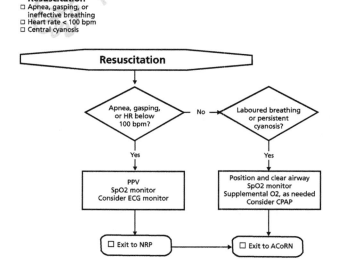

The baby is breathing spontaneously at 54 breaths/min, has an HR of 140 bpm, and SpO2 is 70%.

Cyanosis unresponsive to oxygen therapy, as an isolated sign, requires no further immediate resuscitative efforts. You exit the Resuscitation Sequence and complete the ACoRN Primary Survey.

You call for assistance. A colleague arrives and completes the Consolidated Core Steps. She initiates cardiorespiratory monitoring, adjusts the pulse oximeter on the baby's right wrist, and completes a set of vital signs.

The baby does not appear distressed, is active and alert, and is breathing at a rate of 48 breaths/min. On auscultation, breath sounds are heard bilaterally and the HR remains 140 bpm. His axilla temperature is 36.8°C. The baby remains centrally cyanotic with SpO2 73%, despite receiving free-flow oxygen His blood pressure is 64/32.

2. Complete the ACoRN Primary Survey and Consolidated Core Steps, and generate a Problem List.

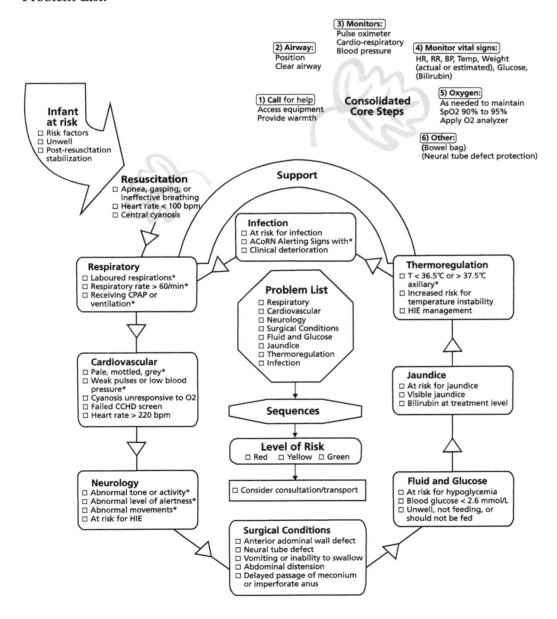

The delivering physician is called back to the room and joins you at the radiant warmer. You review the findings on the Primary Survey and confirm the Problem List. She briefly tries applying CPAP to increase SpO2, but the baby becomes agitated and desaturates further. She asks you to continue 100% oxygen by face mask, and together you move the baby to the nursery. His parents accompany you.

In the nursery, his vital signs remain unchanged. His SpO2 on the nursery monitor is 74%.

You enter the Cardiovascular Sequence as the first sequence on the Problem List. The Core Step in the Cardiovascular Sequence is to complete the Clinical Assessment of Circulation Table. The physician quickly examines the baby to complete the assessment. She reports that he looks well apart from cyanosis, has no unusual features, and has good air entry bilaterally. She says she can't hear a murmur but thinks that the precordium is very active.

His pulses are easy to palpate and his capillary refill is 3 sec. His BP is 65/34 (mean 55 mmHg) and is peripherally and centrally warm. HR is 125 bpm. He has not voided yet.

3. Document your findings in the Clinical Assessment of Circulation Table.

Sign	Stable	Unstable
Abnormal tone, activity, or level of alertness	☐ Normal tone, active, alert, and looking well	☐ Decreased tone, listless, lethargic
Critical perfusion	☐ Well perfused, pink, and peripherally warm	☐ Pale, mottled, grey
Pulses	☐ Easy to palpate	☐ Weak, absent, or femoral pulses weaker than right brachial pulses
Mean blood pressure	☐ ≥ gestational age (in weeks)	☐ < gestational age (in weeks)
Capillary refill time	☐ ≤ 3 sec centrally	☐ > 3 sec centrally
Skin temperature	☐ Peripherally warm	☐ Peripherally cool
Heart rate	☐ 100 to 180 bpm	☐ > 180 bpm
Hourly urine output (if older than 24 h)	☐ ≥ 1 mL/kg/h	☐ < 1 mL/kg/h
Shock is present when signs of critical perfusion (red box) coexist in an infant with decreased tone, alertness, and activity (red box), in the absence of an alternative explanation.		

4. Does this baby have shock? Explain why or why not.

_____

_____

_____

5. How will you Organize Care using the Cardiovascular Sequence? Mark the Cardiovascular Sequence excerpt based on the baby's clinical status.

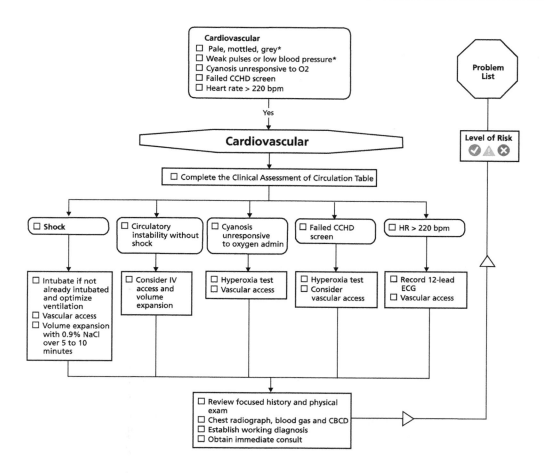

6. What are the two mechanisms of cyanosis in an infant? Which is the most likely in this case?

_____

_____

_____

You Organize Care based on persistent cyanosis and prepare to complete a hyperoxia test. You ensure the baby is receiving 100% O2 by face mask for 20 min. Because it is difficult to obtain an arterial blood sample in your site, you opt to monitor the baby's response using saturations (SpO2). While the hyperoxia test is being completed, the physician speaks with the parents and reviews the baby's chart to obtain a focused history. No significant information is gathered from the focused history.

While doing the hyperoxia test, you work through the other sequences on the Problem List.

After 20 mins, the baby's saturations remain 73–77%. There is no difference between pre- and post-ductal readings.

7. How would you interpret the hyperoxia test results?

☐ The SpO2 increased and you no longer are concerned that the infant has a congenital cyanotic heart defect.

☐ The SpO2 did not increase the requisite 5% to 10%, and this suggests a congenital cyanotic heart defect.

☐ The SpO2 did not increase the requisite 10% or more, and this suggests a congenital cyanotic heart defect.

☐ The PaO2 did not increase the requisite 20 to 30 mmHg, and this suggests a congenital cyanotic heart defect.

Based on the results of the hyperoxia test and the physical examination, the working diagnosis is a congenital cyanotic heart defect.

The physician asks you to start an intravenous of D10W and prepare for a prostaglandin (PGE1) infusion. She orders a chest radiograph and blood work (blood gas, CBC).

Having formulated a working diagnosis and management plan, you exit the Cardiovascular Sequence and complete the remaining sequences in the Problem List.

An urgent call is made to the referral tertiary centre to discuss the baby and arrange transport. The physician speaks with the paediatric cardiologist who recommends an infusion of PGE and weaning the oxygen to maintain SpO2 70–75%. You prepare the IV infusion and ask for a chest X-ray. Blood gases and CBCD are drawn.

The chest radiograph is completed and ready for viewing.

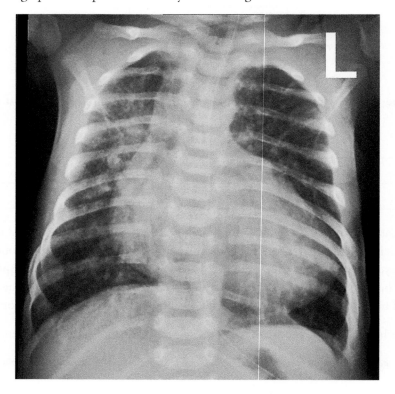

8. Identify main features on this baby's chest radiograph here.

Heart size

_____

Heart shape

_____

Lung vascular markings

_____

Heart on R or L side of chest?

☐ Right / ☐ Left

Is stomach in normal position?

☐ Yes / ☐ No

9. Interpret the following venous blood gas results (high, low, or normal)?

pH: 7.28

☐ High   ☐ Low   ☐ Normal

PCO2: 40 mmHg

☐ High   ☐ Low   ☐ Normal

PO2: 35 mmHg

☐ High   ☐ Low   ☐ Normal

BD: 9

☐ High   ☐ Low   ☐ Normal

The paediatric cardiologist recommends a PGE1 infusion starting at 0.05 mcg/kg/min.

10. Calculate how you would prepare the PGE1 infusion.

_____

_____

11. What adverse effects of PGE1 should you be monitoring for?

_____

_____

12. What is the Level of Risk for this baby?

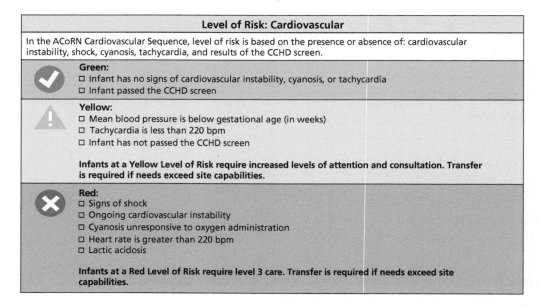

Level of Risk: Cardiovascular
In the ACoRN Cardiovascular Sequence, level of risk is based on the presence or absence of: cardiovascular instability, shock, cyanosis, tachycardia, and results of the CCHD screen.
Green: ☐ Infant has no signs of cardiovascular instability, cyanosis, or tachycardia ☐ Infant passed the CCHD screen
Yellow: ☐ Mean blood pressure is below gestational age (in weeks) ☐ Tachycardia is less than 220 bpm ☐ Infant has not passed the CCHD screen **Infants at a Yellow Level of Risk require increased levels of attention and consultation. Transfer is required if needs exceed site capabilities.**
Red: ☐ Signs of shock ☐ Ongoing cardiovascular instability ☐ Cyanosis unresponsive to oxygen administration ☐ Heart rate is greater than 220 bpm ☐ Lactic acidosis **Infants at a Red Level of Risk require level 3 care. Transfer is required if needs exceed site capabilities.**

The baby is started on a PGE1 infusion and transferred to the referral centre. Arrangements are made to transfer the mother as soon as possible to allow her to be close to her baby.

An echocardiogram performed upon arrival confirmed the diagnosis of TGA with a ventricular septal defect present. A few days later, an arterial switch procedure was performed. The baby was discharged home after 2 weeks.

Bibliography

Brooks PA, Penny DJ. Management of the sick neonate with suspected heart disease. Early Hum Dev 2008;84(3):155–9.

Brown KL, Ridout DA, Hoskote A, Verhulst L, Ricci M, Bull C. Delayed diagnosis of congenital heart disease worsens preoperative condition and outcome of surgery in neonates. Heart 2006;92(9):1298–302.

Carcillo JA, Fields AI, American College of Critical Care Medicine Task Force Committee Members. Clinical practice parameters for hemodynamic support of pediatric and neonatal patients in septic shock. Crit Care Med 2002;30(6):1365–78.

Dempsey EM, Barrington KJ. Evaluation and treatment of hypotension in the preterm infant. Clin Perinatol 2009;36(1):75–85.

Fanaroff J, Fanaroff A, eds. Klause and Fanaroff's Care of the High-Risk Neonate, 6th ed. Philadelphia, PA: W.B. Saunders; 2012.

Fleming S, Gill P, Jones C, et al. The diagnostic value of capillary refill time for detecting serious illness in children: A systematic review and meta-analysis. PLoS One 2015;10(9):e0138155.

Fleming S, Gill PJ, Van den Bruel A, Thompson M. Capillary refill time in sick children: A clinical guide for general practice. Br J Gen Pract 2016;66(652):587.

Hendson L, Shah V, Trkulja S; Canadian Paediatric Society, Fetus and Newborn Committee. Selective serotonin reuptake inhibitors or serotonin-norepinephrine reuptake inhibitors in pregnancy: Infant and childhood outcomes. In press: www.cps.ca/en/documents/position/SSRI-infant-outcomes

Johnson BA, Ades A. Delivery room and early postnatal management of neonates who have prenatally diagnosed congenital heart disease. Clin Perinatol 2005;32(4):921–46.

Mahle WT, Newburger JW, Matherne GP, et al. American Heart Association Congenital Heart Defects Committee of the Council on Cardiovascular Disease in the Young, Council on Cardiovascular Nursing, and Interdisciplinary Council on Quality of Care and Outcomes Research; American Academy of Pediatrics Section on Cardiology and Cardiac Surgery; Committee on Fetus and Newborn. Role of pulse oximetry in examining newborns for congenital heart disease: A scientific statement from the AHA and AAP. Pediatrics 2009;124(2):823–36.

Narvey M, Wong K, Fournier A, CPS Fetus and Newborn Committee. Pulse oximetry screening in newborns to enhance detection of critical congenital heart disease. Paediatr Child Health 2017;22(8):494–8.

Park MK. Pediatric Cardiology for Practitioners, 6th ed. Philadelphia, PA: Elsevier Saunders; 2014.

Penny DJ, Shekerdemian LS. Management of the neonate with symptomatic congenital heart disease. Arch Dis Child Fetal Neonatal Ed 2001;84(3):F141–5.

Thangaratinam S, Brown K, Zamora J, Khan KS, Ewer AK. Pulse oximetry screening for critical congenital heart defects in asymptomatic newborn babies: A systematic review and meta-analysis. Lancet 2012;379(9835):2459–64.

Answer key: Cardiovascular Case 1—Shock or circulatory instability?

1. Does this baby present with any Alerting Signs for Resuscitation?

☐ Yes   ✓ No

This baby does not present with any of the Alerting Signs requiring Resuscitation. He is breathing without evidence of apnea or gasping. Although reported as shallow, his respiratory effort is currently sufficient to maintain an HR above 100 bpm. He is reported as pale and grey but not cyanotic.

If you were uncertain about his respiratory effort or concerned that his colour could represent cyanosis, entering the Resuscitation Sequence is a reasonable choice.

The presence of a stable respiratory rate and a HR above 100 bpm would move you down the right-hand arm of the sequence and direct you to position the baby appropriately, assess the airway, and establish appropriate monitors. These are Consolidated Core Steps provided to all babies entering the ACoRN process.

2. Complete the ACoRN Primary Survey and Consolidated Core Steps, and generate a Problem List.

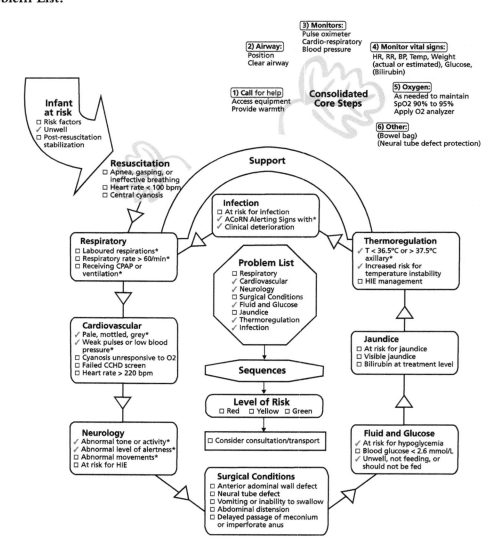

3. **Cardiovascular is the first Sequence identified. Mark applicable Alerting Signs in the following diagram.**

> **Cardiovascular**
> ✓ Pale, mottled, grey*
> ✓ Weak pulses or low blood pressure*
> ☐ Cyanosis unresponsive to O2
> ☐ Failed CCHD screen
> ☐ Heart rate > 220 bpm

4. **As the Core Step in the Cardiovascular Sequence, you complete the Clinical Assessment of Circulation Table.**

Sign	Stable	Unstable
Abnormal tone, activity, or level of alertness	☐ Normal tone, active, alert, and looking well	✓ Decreased tone, listless, lethargic
Critical perfusion	☐ Well perfused, pink, and peripherally warm	✓ Pale, mottled, grey
Pulses	✓ Easy to palpate	☐ Weak, absent, or femoral pulses weaker than right brachial pulses
Mean blood pressure	☐ ≥ gestational age (in weeks)	✓ < gestational age (in weeks)
Capillary refill time	☐ ≤ 3 sec centrally	✓ > 3 sec centrally
Skin temperature	☐ Peripherally warm	✓ Peripherally cool
Heart rate	✓ 100 to 180 bpm	☐ > 180 bpm
Hourly urine output (if older than 24 h)	? ≥ 1 mL/kg/h	? < 1 mL/kg/h
Shock is present when signs of critical perfusion problems (red box) coexist in an infant with decreased tone, alertness, and activity (red box), in the absence of an alternative explanation.		

5. **From a circulatory perspective, is this infant stable or unstable? Why?**

From the Clinical Assessment of Circulation Table, you determine that this baby is unstable. He shows signs of instability (e.g., weak pulses, low mean BP, poor capillary refill) in addition to indicators of critical perfusion problems (grey and mottled) in combination with critical signs of inadequate end organ (cerebral) perfusion (abnormal tone, decreased level of alertness). As he is less than 24 h old, urine output may not be a reliable indicator of volume status yet. It should be monitored.

6. How do you Organize Care for this infant?

✓ Shock	□ Circulatory instability without shock	□ Cyanosis unresponsive to oxygen admin	□ Failed CCHD screen[1]	□ HR > 220 bpm
✓ Intubate if not already intubated and optimize ventilation ✓ Vascular access ✓ Volume expansion with 0.9% NaCl over 5 to 10 minutes	□ Consider IV access and volume expansion	□ Hyperoxia test □ Vascular access	□ Hyperoxia test □ Consider vascular access	□ Record 12-lead ECG □ Vascular access

You base your Response on a provisional diagnosis of **shock**. You will need to intubate him and optimize ventilation. As well, initiation of an IV and a fluid bolus of 10 mL/kg of 0.9% NaCl over 5 to 10 min to mitigate hypoperfusion are indicated.

Ongoing assessment is needed to evaluate whether additional fluid boluses are necessary.

7. What additional information would help you determine a working diagnosis for this infant?

✓ A stat CBCD.

✓ A chest radiograph.

✓ A blood gas.

✓ Pre- and post-ductal oxygen saturations.

□ A 12-lead ECG.

✓ A visual examination of the placenta.

✓ Evaluation of the infant's response to volume expansion with 10 mL/kg of 0.9% NaCl solution.

You will need to determine the origin of the shock (i.e., hypovolemic, distributive, or cardiogenic) to direct your specific diagnosis and management.

If the hemoglobin is low, it may indicate blood loss. When blood loss is acute, there are signs of shock. The white blood cell differential may help to determine whether sepsis is a probable cause of the shock.

A CXR will provide information about the size and shape of the cardiac silhouette and help to determine whether cardiac anomalies exist. It will also show how well the lungs are perfused.

A blood gas will help to determine the presence and type of acidosis. Metabolic acidosis is present when the pH is less than 7.25, and there is an increase in base deficit in venous, arterial, or capillary blood.

A base deficit greater than 10 mEq/L to 12 mEq/L is clinically significant because it may indicate insufficient tissue perfusion and oxygenation. The combination of metabolic acidosis and high lactate levels (greater than 5) is called lactic acidosis.

Infants with developing heart failure also experience difficulty with gas exchange, due to lung congestion, which is indicated by an increased PCO_2 and respiratory acidosis.

A visual inspection of the placenta may help to determine the etiology of the cardiac instability. Evidence of chorioamnionitis would support sepsis as a cause of the baby's status.

An evaluation of the baby's response to the fluid bolus is needed to help determine ongoing management (i.e., the need for an additional bolus).

8. What is this baby's Level of Risk?

☐ Green ☐ Yellow ✓ Red

This baby's Level of Risk is Red because he has signs of shock, cardiovascular instability, and lactic acidosis.

9. What do you think is the cause of this infant's circulatory instability?

☐ Hypovolemic shock due to blood loss.

✓ Distributive shock due to sepsis.

☐ Cardiogenic shock due to hypoxic injury.

☐ Cyanotic CHD.

☐ A tachyarrhythmia.

You found no evidence of significant blood loss, a tachyarrhythmia, or cyanotic heart disease.

The CBC, however, shows leukopenia (WBC—1.5×10^9/L with a marked left shift—hallmark signs of significant sepsis). However, the absence of risk factors does not preclude the diagnosis of sepsis in a clinically unwell infant.

You revisit the Primary Survey and add a tickmark for 'At risk for jaundice' because this baby has acidosis and sepsis, both of which put him at increased risk for developing hyperbilirubinemia.

10. What specific management steps would you consider?

✓ An additional bolus of 10 mL/kg of 0.9% NaCl solution.

☐ 15 mL/kg of Ringer's lactate solution.

☐ 15 mL/kg of O-negative uncross-matched packed red cells.

☐ A 12-lead ECG.

☐ An urgent echocardiogram.

✓ Stat administration of antibiotics after blood cultures are drawn, as indicated in the Infection Sequence.

Infants with septic shock have multisystem failure and high mortality. Urgent management includes volume expansion, antibiotics (after blood cultures have been obtained), and inotropic support. Inotropes, when needed, increase the force of contraction of the heart and vasoconstrict peripheral blood vessels. Their use should always be guided by level 3 consultation.

Answer key: Cardiovascular Case 2—Circulatory instability or shock?

1. **Complete the ACoRN Primary Survey and Consolidated Cores Steps, marking all appropriate boxes.**

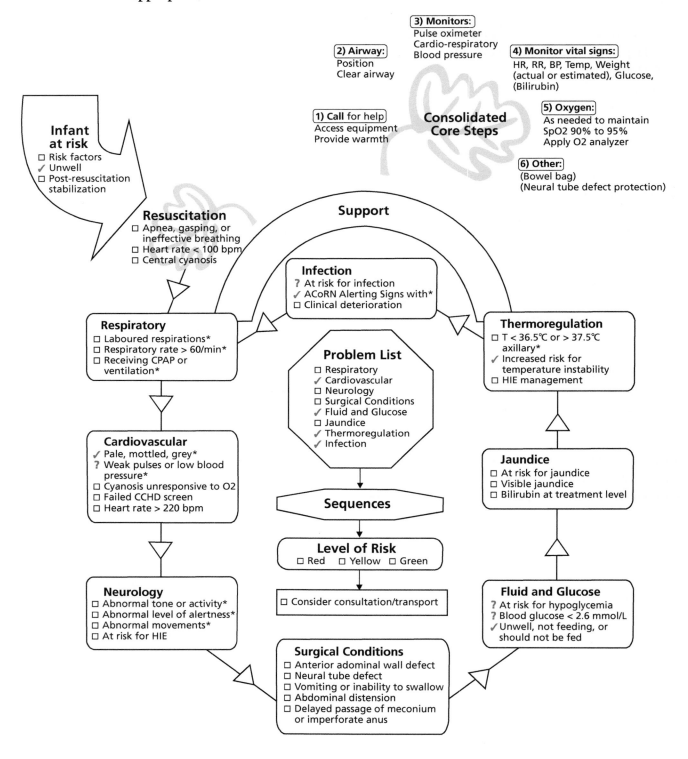

3) Monitors:
Pulse oximeter
Cardio-respiratory
Blood pressure

2) Airway:
Position
Clear airway

4) Monitor vital signs:
HR, RR, BP, Temp, Weight
(actual or estimated), Glucose,
(Bilirubin)

1) Call for help
Access equipment
Provide warmth

Consolidated Core Steps

5) Oxygen:
As needed to maintain
SpO2 90% to 95%
Apply O2 analyzer

6) Other:
(Bowel bag)
(Neural tube defect protection)

Infant at risk
☐ Risk factors
✓ Unwell
☐ Post-resuscitation stabilization

Resuscitation
☐ Apnea, gasping, or ineffective breathing
☐ Heart rate < 100 bpm
☐ Central cyanosis

Support

Infection
? At risk for infection
✓ ACoRN Alerting Signs with*
☐ Clinical deterioration

Respiratory
☐ Laboured respirations*
☐ Respiratory rate > 60/min*
☐ Receiving CPAP or ventilation*

Problem List
☐ Respiratory
✓ Cardiovascular
☐ Neurology
☐ Surgical Conditions
✓ Fluid and Glucose
☐ Jaundice
✓ Thermoregulation
✓ Infection

Thermoregulation
☐ T < 36.5℃ or > 37.5℃ axillary*
✓ Increased risk for temperature instability
☐ HIE management

Cardiovascular
✓ Pale, mottled, grey*
? Weak pulses or low blood pressure*
☐ Cyanosis unresponsive to O2
☐ Failed CCHD screen
☐ Heart rate > 220 bpm

Jaundice
☐ At risk for jaundice
☐ Visible jaundice
☐ Bilirubin at treatment level

Sequences

Level of Risk
☐ Red   ☐ Yellow   ☐ Green

Neurology
☐ Abnormal tone or activity*
☐ Abnormal level of alertness*
☐ Abnormal movements*
☐ At risk for HIE

☐ Consider consultation/transport

Fluid and Glucose
? At risk for hypoglycemia
? Blood glucose < 2.6 mmol/L
✓ Unwell, not feeding, or should not be fed

Surgical Conditions
☐ Anterior adominal wall defect
☐ Neural tube defect
☐ Vomiting or inability to swallow
☐ Abdominal distension
☐ Delayed passage of meconium or imperforate anus

2. As the Core Step in the Cardiovascular Sequence, you complete the Clinical Assessment of Circulation Table.

Sign	Stable	Unstable
Abnormal tone, activity, or level of alertness	✓ Normal tone, active, alert, and looking well	☐ **Decreased tone, listless, lethargic**
Critical perfusion	☐ Well perfused, pink, and peripherally warm	✓ **Pale, mottled, grey**
Pulses	☐ Easy to palpate	✓ Weak, absent, or femoral pulses weaker than right brachial pulses
Mean blood pressure	☐ ≥ gestational age (in weeks)	✓ < gestational age (in weeks)
Capillary refill time	? ≤ 3 sec centrally	? > 3 sec centrally
Skin temperature	✓ Peripherally warm	☐ Peripherally cool
Heart rate	☐ 100 to 180 bpm	✓ > 180 bpm
Hourly urine output (if older than 24 h)	? ≥ 1 mL/kg/h	? < 1 mL/kg/h
Shock is present when signs of critical perfusion problems (red box) coexist in an infant with decreased tone, alertness, and activity (red box), in the absence of an alternative explanation.		

3. From a circulatory perspective, is this infant stable or unstable? Why?

From the Clinical Assessment of Circulation Table, you determine that this baby is unstable (pallor, weak pulses, mean BP less than GA, HR >180 bpm) but has normal tone, activity, and level of alertness. You decide that she has circulatory instability without shock.

4. How do you Organize Care for this infant?

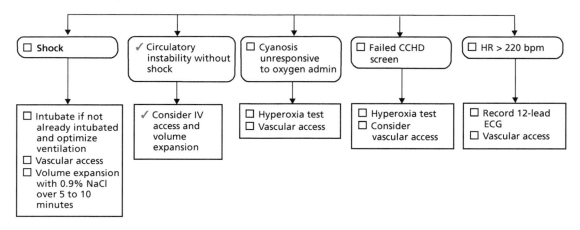

Vascular access and volume expansion with 10 mL/kg of 0.9% NaCl over 20 to 30 min should be considered for infants who have more than one sign of circulatory instability.

5. What additional information would help you determine a working diagnosis for this infant?

- ✓ A CBCD.
- ☐ A chest radiograph.
- ☐ A blood gas.
- ☐ Pre- and post-ductal oxygen saturations.
- ☐ A 12-lead ECG.
- ☐ A visual examination of the placenta.
- ✓ Evaluation of the infant's response to volume expansion with 10 mL/kg of 0.9% NaCl solution.

There is no evidence to support cyanosis unresponsive to oxygen, a tachyarrhythmia, or functional/structural anomalies of the heart at this time. A chest radiograph, blood gas, pre- and post-ductal oxygen saturations, 12-lead ECG, or visual inspection of the placenta are not warranted at this time.

A CBC will identify whether the hemoglobin is low, suggesting blood loss.

6. What do you think is the cause of this infant's circulatory instability?

- ✓ Hypovolemia.
- ☐ Distributive shock.
- ☐ Cardiogenic shock.
- ☐ Cyanotic CHD.
- ☐ A tachyarrhythmia.

As part of your Focused History, you learned that the umbilical cord was wrapped tightly around the baby's neck twice and that the midwife needed to clamp and cut the cord prior to delivering the baby's body.

It is important to note that fetal blood loss can occur when a nuchal cord is present. Occlusion of the umbilical cord occurs just before birth, as the head descends, interrupting umbilical venous flow (blood flowing into the baby) to a greater extent than umbilical arterial flow (blood flowing out of the baby). While often not clinically significant, relative hypovolemia can result and present with pallor post-birth.

The baby's hemoglobin level of 120 g/L also helps to confirm blood loss, because it is less than the normal range for a newborn (150 g/L to 220 g/L).

7. What specific management steps would you consider?

- ✓ An additional bolus of 10 mL/kg of 0.9% NaCl solution.
- ☐ 15 mL/kg of Ringer's lactate solution.
- ☐ 15 mL/kg of O-negative uncross-matched packed red cells.
- ☐ A 12-lead ECG.
- ☐ An echocardiogram.

Because the baby responded to the first fluid bolus, you opt to repeat it and administer a second bolus of 10 mL/kg of 0.9% NaCl over 15 min. You note that her hemoglobin might drop further as her blood volume returns to normal, and that you may need to do a repeat CBC.

Ringer's lactate is no longer recommended as a solution for fluid resuscitation, as per current Neonatal Resuscitation Program (NRP) guidelines. A blood transfusion is not warranted at this time because the hemoglobin, though low, does not meet parameters for administering packed cells.

Again, there is no evidence of arrhythmias or cardiac anomalies. Therefore, neither an ECG nor an echocardiogram is needed at this time.

8. **Indicate the baby's Level of Risk and which criteria helped you make the determination** *at this time.*

Level of Risk: Cardiovascular
In the ACoRN Cardiovascular Sequence, level of risk is based on the presence or absence of: cardiovascular instability, shock, cyanosis, tachycardia, and results of the CCHD screen.

Green:
- ✓ Infant has no signs of cardiovascular instability, cyanosis, or tachycardia
- ☐ Infant passed the CCHD screen

Yellow:
- ☐ Mean blood pressure is below gestational age (in weeks)
- ☐ Tachycardia is less than 220 bpm
- ☐ Infant has not passed the CCHD screen

Infants at a Yellow Level of Risk require increased levels of attention and consultation. Transfer is required if needs exceed site capabilities.

Red:
- ☐ Signs of shock
- ☐ Ongoing cardiovascular instability
- ☐ Cyanosis unresponsive to oxygen administration
- ☐ Heart rate is greater than 220 bpm
- ☐ Lactic acidosis

Infants at a Red Level of Risk require level 3 care. Transfer is required if needs exceed site capabilities.

The baby's condition has improved with assessment and prompt management, and she no longer exhibits signs of cardiovascular instability, cyanosis, or tachycardia. Her Level of Risk is Green. Your team is comfortable to care for her at your site as long as her Level of Risk in the remaining ACoRN Sequences is such that she does not require transfer.

Answer key: Cardiovascular Case 3—A baby with persistent cyanosis

1. Indicate your course of action in the Resuscitation Sequence.

Resuscitation
- ☐ Apnea, gasping, or ineffective breathing
- ☐ Heart rate < 100 bpm
- ✓ Central cyanosis

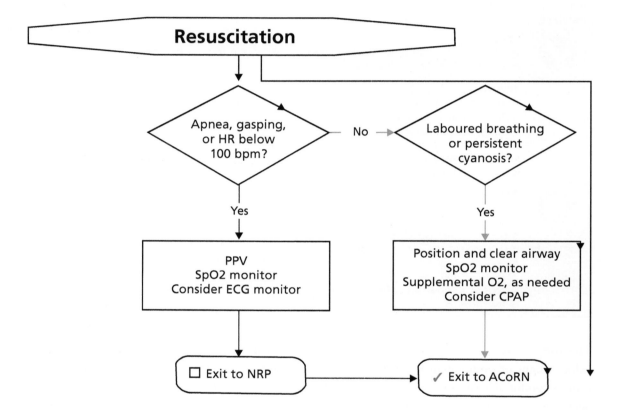

This baby has no apnea or gasping and the HR is above 100 bpm. Because the baby is breathing spontaneously but has persistent cyanosis, you proceed down the right-hand arm of the resuscitation sequence that prompts you to position and clear the baby's airway and initiate supplemental oxygen as needed. This baby has no laboured breathing, and you feel that CPAP is not warranted at this time. You then exit to ACoRN and complete the Primary Survey.

2. Complete the ACoRN Primary Survey and Consolidated Core Steps, and generate a Problem List.

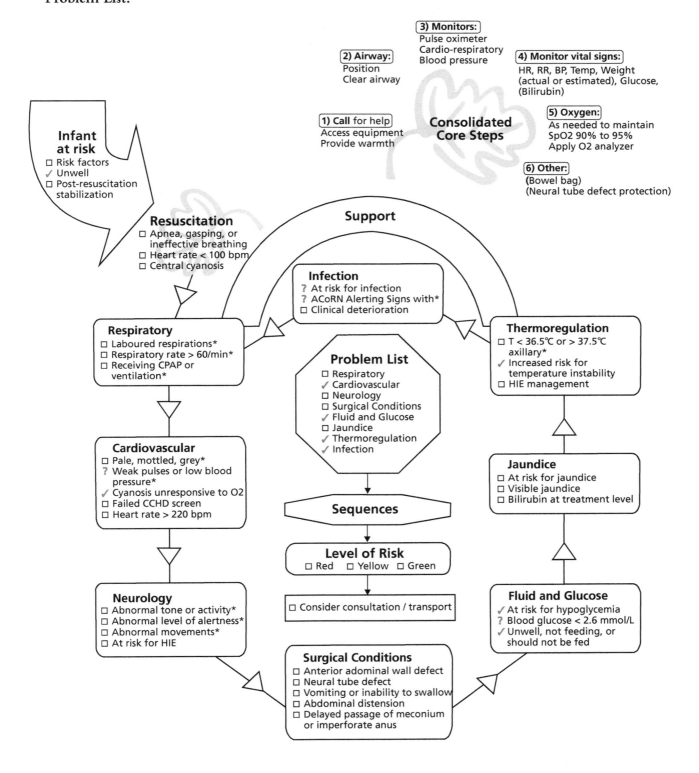

3) Monitors:
Pulse oximeter
Cardio-respiratory
Blood pressure

2) Airway:
Position
Clear airway

4) Monitor vital signs:
HR, RR, BP, Temp, Weight
(actual or estimated), Glucose,
(Bilirubin)

1) Call for help
Access equipment
Provide warmth

**Consolidated
Core Steps**

5) Oxygen:
As needed to maintain
SpO2 90% to 95%
Apply O2 analyzer

6) Other:
(Bowel bag)
(Neural tube defect protection)

**Infant
at risk**
□ Risk factors
✓ Unwell
□ Post-resuscitation
stabilization

Resuscitation
□ Apnea, gasping, or
ineffective breathing
□ Heart rate < 100 bpm
□ Central cyanosis

Support

Infection
? At risk for infection
? ACoRN Alerting Signs with*
□ Clinical deterioration

Respiratory
□ Laboured respirations*
□ Respiratory rate > 60/min*
□ Receiving CPAP or
ventilation*

Problem List
□ Respiratory
✓ Cardiovascular
□ Neurology
□ Surgical Conditions
✓ Fluid and Glucose
□ Jaundice
✓ Thermoregulation
✓ Infection

Thermoregulation
□ T < 36.5℃ or > 37.5℃
axillary*
✓ Increased risk for
temperature instability
□ HIE management

Cardiovascular
□ Pale, mottled, grey*
? Weak pulses or low blood
pressure*
✓ Cyanosis unresponsive to O2
□ Failed CCHD screen
□ Heart rate > 220 bpm

Jaundice
□ At risk for jaundice
□ Visible jaundice
□ Bilirubin at treatment level

Sequences

Level of Risk
□ Red   □ Yellow   □ Green

Neurology
□ Abnormal tone or activity*
□ Abnormal level of alertness*
□ Abnormal movements*
□ At risk for HIE

□ Consider consultation / transport

Fluid and Glucose
✓ At risk for hypoglycemia
? Blood glucose < 2.6 mmol/L
✓ Unwell, not feeding, or
should not be fed

Surgical Conditions
□ Anterior adominal wall defect
□ Neural tube defect
□ Vomiting or inability to swallow
□ Abdominal distension
□ Delayed passage of meconium
or imperforate anus

3. Document your findings in the Clinical Assessment of Circulation Table.

Sign	Stable	Unstable
Abnormal tone, activity, or level of alertness	✓ Normal tone, active, alert, and looking well	☐ **Decreased tone, listless, lethargic**
Critical perfusion	☐ Well perfused, pink, and peripherally warm	? **Pale, mottled, grey**
Pulses	✓ Easy to palpate	? Weak, absent, or femoral pulses weaker than right brachial pulses
Mean blood pressure	✓ ≥ gestational age (in weeks)	☐ < gestational age (in weeks)
Capillary refill time	✓ ≤ 3 sec centrally	☐ > 3 sec centrally
Skin temperature	✓ Peripherally warm	☐ Peripherally cool
Heart rate	✓ 100 to 180 bpm	☐ > 180 bpm
Hourly urine output (if older than 24 h)	? ≥ 1 mL/kg/h	? < 1 mL/kg/h

Shock is present when signs of critical perfusion (red box) coexist in an infant with decreased tone, activity, and alertness (red box), in the absence of an alternative explanation.

Although the baby is unwell, he is active and alert and does not appear distressed in any way.

You find it challenging to score his critical perfusion because the baby appears to be fairly well perfused and warm to the touch but remains cyanotic. You opt to place a **?** in the critical perfusion boxes because he never really 'pinks-up'. You have not measured the baby's urine output.

4. Does this baby have shock? Explain why or why not.

No. Although this baby has some abnormalities on his cardiovascular exam, he does not have decreased tone, activity, or alertness, which suggests his cerebral perfusion is maintained. The presence of cyanosis in an otherwise well-appearing infant without respiratory distress is a common presentation in babies with cyanotic heart disease. They can, however, deteriorate quickly, so prompt assessment utilizing the ACoRN Cardiovascular Sequence and expert consultation is critically important.

5. **How will you Organize Care using the Cardiovascular Sequence? Mark the Cardiovascular Sequence excerpt based on the baby's clinical status.**

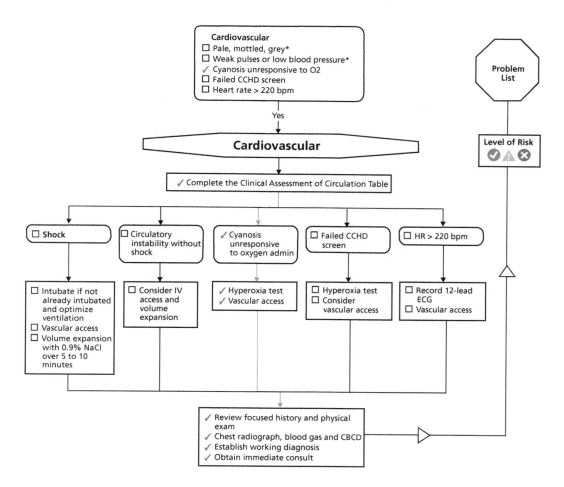

6. **What are the two mechanisms of cyanosis in an infant? Which is the most likely in this case?**
   1) **Respiratory origin**—Cyanosis results from poorly ventilated and/or poorly oxygenated alveoli due to lung disease. This type of cyanosis will respond to oxygenation and ventilation. It is also usually associated with more severe respiratory symptoms, including laboured breathing, retractions, and grunting.
   2) **Cardiac origin**—Deoxygenated blood bypasses the lungs and mixes with oxygenated blood from the lungs. The resultant blood has a low SpO2 and does not respond to more oxygen. Babies with cyanosis of cardiac origin often have no respiratory symptoms.
      The likely cause of this baby's cyanosis is cardiac.

7. **How would you interpret the hyperoxia test results?**
   ☐ The SpO2 increased and you no longer are concerned that the infant has a congenital cyanotic heart defect.
   ☐ The SpO2 did not increase the requisite 5% to10%, and this suggests a congenital cyanotic heart defect.
   ✓ The SpO2 did not increase the requisite 10% or more, and this suggests a congenital cyanotic heart defect.
   ☐ The PaO2 did not increase the requisite 20 to 30 mmHg, and this suggests a congenital cyanotic heart defect.

The hyperoxia test helps to differentiate cyanosis of respiratory or cardiovascular origin on the basis that oxygen administration improves oxygenation in lung disease. Failure to achieve a significant rise in SpO2 (>10% using a pulse oximeter) or an increase in PaO2 >20 to 30 mmHg (on arterial blood gas) after 20 min in 100% oxygen suggests cyanotic CHD with a fixed right-to-left shunt.

8. Identify main features on this baby's chest radiograph.

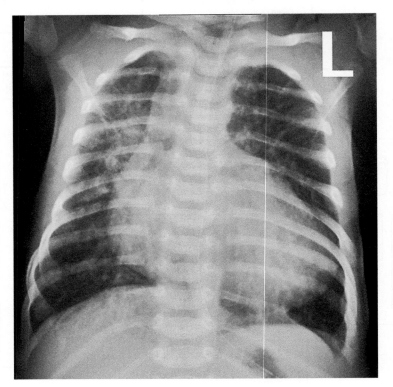

Heart size is large (cardiothoracic ratio > 60%)

Heart is egg-shaped

Lung vascular markings are increased

Heart on R or L side of chest?

□ Right / ✓ Left

Is stomach in normal position?

✓ Yes / □ No

In addition, the mediastinum is narrow, and the cardiac silhouette appears like 'egg on a string'. These characteristics are suggestive of TGA.

9. **Interpret the following venous blood gas results (high, low, or normal)?**

pH: 7.28

☐ High   ✓ Low   ☐ Normal

PCO2: 40 mmHg

☐ High   ☐ Low   ✓ Normal

PO2: 35 mmHg

☐ High   ✓ Low   ☐ Normal

BD: 9

✓ High   ☐ Low   ☐ Normal

This is an example of a metabolic acidosis. The baby has marked oxygen desaturation. Compromised oxygen delivery to the tissues leads to metabolic acidosis.

10. **Calculate how you would prepare the PGE1 infusion.**

PGE1 comes prepared in 500 mcg/mL vials.

Step 1: Dilute to 5 mcg/mL concentration:
    Add 1 mL 500 mcg/mL PGE1 to 99 mL of D5W or NS
    Final concentration = 5 mcg/mL

Step 2: Infusion rate (mL/hr) = $\dfrac{\text{dose (mcg/kg/min)} \times \text{wt (kg)} \times 60 \text{ (min/hr)}}{\text{concentration of PGE1}}$

Infusion rate (mL/hr) = $\dfrac{0.05 \text{ mcg/kg/min} \times 3.5 \text{ kg} \times 60 \text{ min/hr}}{5 \text{ mcg/mL}}$

Infusion rate = 2.1

Run IV of 5 mcg/mL PGE1 at 2.1 mL/hr

This infusion provides 0.05 mcg/kg/min, as recommended by the paediatric cardiologist.

11. **What adverse effects of PGE1 should you be monitoring for?**

Adverse reactions to PGE1 include apnea, hypotension secondary to vasodilation, and fever. The clinical response to prostaglandin must be monitored, documented, and communicated to the tertiary referral centre. The need for respiratory support, including intubation, should be anticipated and appropriate resources immediately available. Volume expansion may also be needed as well as thermoregulatory interventions.

12. **What is the Level of Risk for this baby?**

Red: This baby has cyanosis unresponsive to oxygen administration. The care needs exceed the level of care provided outside of a paediatric tertiary care centre.

Neurology

5

Educational objectives

Upon completion of this chapter, you will be able to:

- Identify infants needing neurologic stabilization.
- Apply the Acute Care of at-Risk Newborns (ACoRN) Neurology Sequence.
- Recognize and assess abnormal tone and activity.
- Recognize and assess abnormal level of alertness.
- Recognize and manage abnormal movements.
- Recognize and manage neonatal encephalopathy.
- Identify hypoxic ischemic encephalopathy (HIE) and manage newborns that may benefit from therapeutic hypothermia.
- Recognize when to exit the Neurology Sequence to other ACoRN Sequences.

Key concepts

1. Abnormal tone or activity, level of alertness, and movements, can occur in many neonatal conditions, some of which require immediate intervention.
2. Symptomatic hypoglycemia can have long-term neurodevelopmental consequences and must be treated as an emergency.
3. Jitteriness must be distinguished from seizures because their significance and management are different.
4. Seizures in the neonate may present as a subtle change in activity.
5. Anticonvulsant therapy should be initiated for seizures, even when their underlying cause has not been determined.
6. Neonatal encephalopathy has multiple etiologies which may or may not result in permanent neurologic impairment.
7. Neonatal encephalopathy due to hypoxic ischemic injury may be associated with pathology in other organs or systems, especially the renal, hepatic, cardiovascular, and respiratory systems.
8. Therapeutic hypothermia decreases mortality and severe long-term neurodevelopmental disabilities in infants with moderate to severe HIE who are born at 35 weeks gestational age or later.
9. Therapeutic hypothermia should be considered, after initial resuscitation and stabilization, in consultation with the referral centre.
10. Neonatal effects from intrauterine exposures (e.g., nicotine, narcotics, or selective serotonin reuptake inhibitors [SSRIs]/serotonin–norepinephrine reuptake inhibitors [SNRIs]) must be considered in newborns who present with unexplained neurologic, respiratory, or gastro-intestinal symptoms.

Skills

- Completion of the Encephalopathy Assessment Table
- Administration of anticonvulsants
- Initiation and management of thermoregulatory interventions for the initial treatment of HIE

Well newborns have regular sleep–wake states and respond appropriately to their environment and handling. They have normal tone and activity, with no abnormal movements. When they cry, they settle with routine comfort measures or feeding. The best indicators of well-being in infants are behavioural: normal alertness and activity, latching and sucking. Infants with neurologic injury usually present with abnormal tone or activity, level of alertness, or movements. They often have abnormal suck, swallow, or other primitive reflexes.

Neurologic abnormalities can be transient, but they can also predict more serious underlying conditions. In the neonate, abnormal neurologic signs may be caused by neurologic, neuromuscular, or systemic conditions, some of which are reversible and/or treatable. An infant who is less responsive or who is 'depressed' after resuscitation requires special attention. Monitoring for early signs of encephalopathy are warranted and prompt management can often prevent or minimize long-term morbidity.

Conditions related to the ACoRN Neurology Sequence may require:

- Urgent specific therapy, such as for symptomatic hypoglycemia, hyperbilirubinemia, or sepsis.
- Early intervention within a specific time frame, such as therapeutic hypothermia for HIE.

Prompt recognition and appropriate intervention are likely to mitigate risks and improve outcomes.

Conditions that cause abnormal tone or activity, level of alertness, or movements, may also compromise breathing, either due to abnormal respiratory muscle activity, poor central respiratory drive, or inability to manage secretions. During seizures, an infant may have periods of apnea or difficulty protecting the airway and may not have a coordinated suck or swallow reflex, thus risking aspiration of milk or secretions.

Neonatal encephalopathy is a condition in term and late preterm infants that describes a constellation of abnormal clinical findings—including a combination of abnormal tone, reflexes, level of alertness, feeding, respiration, and/or seizures—that may evolve over hours or days.

Possible causes of neonatal encephalopathy include:

- HIE
- Central nervous system (CNS) infections, such as Group B *Streptococcus* meningitis or herpes simplex virus (HSV) encephalitis
- Inborn errors of metabolism
- Intracranial hemorrhage.

HIE is the most common cause of neonatal encephalopathy. The clinical signs of HIE evolve over the first several hours and even days after birth.

ACoRN Neurology Sequence

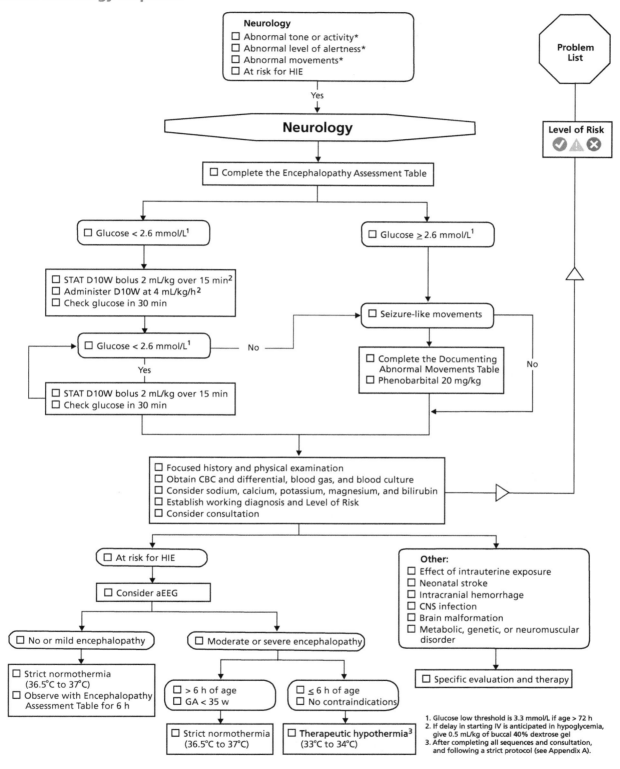

Neurology
- ☐ Abnormal tone or activity*
- ☐ Abnormal level of alertness*
- ☐ Abnormal movements*
- ☐ At risk for HIE

Yes ↓

Problem List

Level of Risk
✓ ⚠ ✕

Neurology

☐ Complete the Encephalopathy Assessment Table

☐ Glucose < 2.6 mmol/L[1]   ☐ Glucose ≥ 2.6 mmol/L[1]

- ☐ STAT D10W bolus 2 mL/kg over 15 min[2]
- ☐ Administer D10W at 4 mL/kg/h[2]
- ☐ Check glucose in 30 min

☐ Glucose < 2.6 mmol/L[1] —No→ ☐ Seizure-like movements

Yes ↓

- ☐ STAT D10W bolus 2 mL/kg over 15 min
- ☐ Check glucose in 30 min

- ☐ Complete the Documenting Abnormal Movements Table
- ☐ Phenobarbital 20 mg/kg

No

- ☐ Focused history and physical examination
- ☐ Obtain CBC and differential, blood gas, and blood culture
- ☐ Consider sodium, calcium, potassium, magnesium, and bilirubin
- ☐ Establish working diagnosis and Level of Risk
- ☐ Consider consultation

☐ At risk for HIE

☐ Consider aEEG

☐ No or mild encephalopathy   ☐ Moderate or severe encephalopathy

- ☐ Strict normothermia (36.5°C to 37°C)
- ☐ Observe with Encephalopathy Assessment Table for 6 h

- ☐ > 6 h of age
- ☐ GA < 35 w

- ☐ ≤ 6 h of age
- ☐ No contraindications

☐ Strict normothermia (36.5°C to 37°C)

☐ **Therapeutic hypothermia[3]** (33°C to 34°C)

Other:
- ☐ Effect of intrauterine exposure
- ☐ Neonatal stroke
- ☐ Intracranial hemorrhage
- ☐ CNS infection
- ☐ Brain malformation
- ☐ Metabolic, genetic, or neuromuscular disorder

☐ Specific evaluation and therapy

1. Glucose low threshold is 3.3 mmol/L if age > 72 h
2. If delay in starting IV is anticipated in hypoglycemia, give 0.5 mL/kg of buccal 40% dextrose gel
3. After completing all sequences and consultation, and following a strict protocol (see Appendix A).

Abbreviations: aEEg - amplitude-integrated electroencephalography, CBC - complete blood count, CNS - central nervous system, D10W - dextrose 10% in water, GA - gestational age, h - hour, HIE - hypoxic ischemic encephalopathy, min - minutes, w - weeks

Alerting Signs

An infant who shows one or more of the following Alerting Signs enters the ACoRN Neurology Sequence:

> **Neurology**
> ☐ Abnormal tone or activity*
> ☐ Abnormal level of alertness*
> ☐ Abnormal movements*
> ☐ At risk for HIE

*Abnormal tone or activity**

Newborns with normal activity have regular sleep–wake states and respond appropriately to their environment and handling. When they cry, they settle with routine comfort measures or feeding.

Tone is the normal tension in, or resistance to, stretch of a healthy muscle. It is assessed by observing resting posture and examining resistance to movement. There is a natural increase in tone with increasing gestational age (GA). A term infant with normal tone has flexion of arms and legs at rest.

Infant tone is clinically assessed by observing tone at rest and examining for:

- Resting posture, resistance to movement and return to resting position,
- Range of motion in several joints, such as the knee, elbow or shoulder joints,
- Extensor and flexor tone of the neck while being pulled to sit, and
- Posture while being suspended ventrally.

You may decide not to examine the last two components when the infant is unstable or when birth injury is suspected.

Resting posture

Resting posture is evaluated by observation when the infant is supine. The degree of flexion at rest increases with GA. The arms and legs of a term infant should be flexed (right panel of the following diagram). The normal degree of flexion, seen at rest in a preterm infant, will be shifted to the left.

A newborn with decreased tone adopts a less flexed position, which may indicate neurologic compromise (left panel of diagram).

Popliteal angle

To evaluate the popliteal angle, the infant is placed supine, with pelvis flat on the examination surface. Use one hand to fully flex the hip joint while extending the lower leg with the other: feel the resistance to passive movement. The angle at the knee is measured, as per the following drawings.

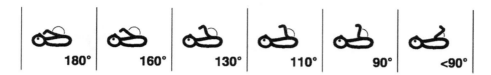

A term infant with good tone has a popliteal angle less or equal to 90°, while a hypotonic or preterm infant has an angle greater than 90°. It is worth noting that breech positioning in utero can also cause a transient popliteal angle greater than 90° in term infants.

Pull-to-sit manoeuvre

The pull-to-sit manoeuvre demonstrates active neck flexor and extensor tone and is used to assess term infants. It must be performed with the head in the midline plane.

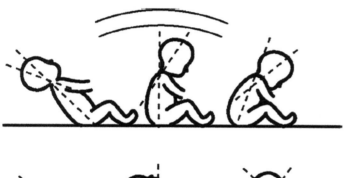

With **normal tone**, an infant's head is balanced over the torso in the sitting position.

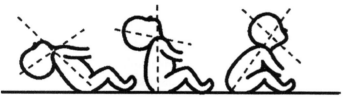

With **increased extensor tone**, an infant's head is hyperextended and cannot drop forward.

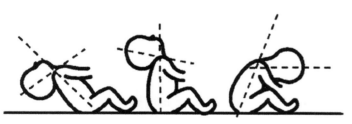

With **decreased tone**, an infant's head lags in extension and then drops forward.

Ventral suspension

To evaluate ventral suspension, an infant is in the prone position with chest resting on the examiner's palm. Posture is observed as the infant is lifted off the examining surface. The continuum of tone in a term infant, from poor (left) to normal (third and fourth panel) to increased (right) is shown in the following diagram.

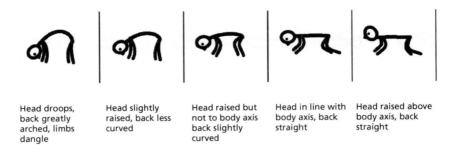

| Head droops, back greatly arched, limbs dangle | Head slightly raised, back less curved | Head raised but not to body axis back slightly curved | Head in line with body axis, back straight | Head raised above body axis, back straight |

Abnormal tone is typically described as 'decreased' (hypotonia) or 'increased' (hypertonia).

- The hypotonic infant is often described as 'floppy' (having low tone) or 'flaccid' (having very low tone). Hypotonia may or may not be associated with weakness or low activity. Weakness is assessed by observing the infant's cry, facial expressions, sucking, Moro reflex, antigravity movements, and respiratory effort.
- Excessive tone usually manifests in the flexor or extensor muscles of the extremities, although in certain conditions truncal tone is also increased. In severe circumstances, there may be neck stiffness or 'posturing'.

Possible reasons for abnormal tone include the following:

- Neonatal encephalopathy
- Sepsis
- Hypoglycemia
- Hypermagnesemia, due to administration of magnesium sulfate to the mother
- Intracranial hemorrhage
- Spinal cord injury

- Drugs/anesthesia
- Neonatal abstinence syndrome (NAS) or neonatal opiate withdrawal (NOW)
- Chromosomal abnormality
- Congenital CNS disorders
- Inborn errors of metabolism
- Neuromuscular disorders

Abnormalities of tone are important to identify because they may:

- Relate to conditions that require urgent specific therapy
- Require early intervention within a specific time frame
- Indicate a pre-existing brain injury or problem with development.

In acute conditions (e.g., early in the course of HIE), an infant's tone may be normal, increased, or decreased at birth. Later, however, the infant may become hypotonic and develop other neurologic signs, including seizures. In other conditions, such as trisomy 21 or neuromuscular disorders, the infant is hypotonic at birth and this condition does not change over time.

Abnormalities in tone and activity for gestational age are often subtle but important indicators of neurologic conditions requiring urgent/timely assessment, monitoring, and intervention.

Abnormal level of alertness*

The level of alertness in a well term neonate will vary depending on a number of factors, including time from last feed, environmental stimuli, and GA.

A preterm neonate's level of alertness is difficult to assess reliably before 28 weeks GA, but infants this age and younger should rouse, for brief periods, in response to persistent stimuli. After 28 weeks of age, a well infant should be more easily rousable with gentle stimuli and remain alert for longer periods of time. Spontaneous periods of alertness should also be present in newborns beyond 28 weeks GA. After 32 weeks GA, neonates should show frequent, spontaneous arousal and roving eye movements. Sleep–wake cycles, meaning regular periods of sleep followed by periods of wakefulness, should become evident.

Term and late preterm infants have sleep–wake cycles after 36 weeks of age. When awake, they are visually attentive and respond to external stimuli (e.g., the human voice and other sounds, touch, light, and pain). Infants who are sleeping can be roused into a fully awake state, and those who are crying can be soothed. Motor and feeding behaviours are well organized. They respond to hunger and exhibit well developed primitive reflexes, such as rooting, suck, grasp, and the Moro reflex. When the palms or soles are 'tickled', they withdraw the stimulated limb.

The recognition of abnormal levels of alertness is important because they are the most common neurologic abnormalities observed in the neonatal period. Hyperalert infants are easily roused and may be difficult to settle. These infants are often described as 'irritable' and demonstrate exaggerated responses to normal stimuli, such as sound and touch. Hyperalertness may be an early sign of CNS irritability.

The presentation of an infant with decreased level of alertness is more worrisome. Terms such as 'stupor' and 'coma' are often used to describe infants with decreased levels of alertness. These terms are imprecise and poorly defined because the progression of decreasing level of alertness is a continuum. When assessing an infant's state, care providers need to consider appearance (awake or asleep), response to attempts to rouse with a gentle stimulus, light, or sound, and the quality and quantity of motor response to noxious stimuli (i.e., a pinch or pinprick). 'Stupor' generally refers to an infant who appears to be sleepy or asleep and has a lower response to attempts at arousal, but retains largely intact, purposeful motor responses to noxious stimuli. The comatose infant appears to be asleep, with no arousal responses. These infants have markedly lower (or absent) motor responses to noxious stimuli.

When assessing alertness, it is important to note the presence or absence of all or some of the behaviours described.

Infants with encephalopathy may appear to be alert or hyperalert but on closer inspection are found to lack other behaviours expected with normal wakefulness. Absence of these behaviours should raise concern about an abnormal level of alertness and the possibility of neonatal encephalopathy.

Abnormal movements*

Movement patterns in a well term infant are rarely, if ever, purposeful, but they are highly variable and predominantly symmetric.

Abnormal movements in a newborn include frequent, repetitive or stereotypical movement patterns, such as lip-smacking, repetitive sucking or chewing, and 'bicycling' of the legs. Movement may also be classified as abnormal due to an overall decrease in the amount of activity normally expected for age.

The term 'jitteriness' or 'tremors' describes the presence of involuntary, rhythmic, oscillatory movements of equal amplitude. They are further classified as being 'fine' high frequency (greater than 6 cycles per sec) and low amplitude (less than 3 cm), or 'coarse', low frequency (fewer than 6 cycles per sec) and high amplitude (greater than 3 cm).

Two-thirds of healthy newborns exhibit physiologic fine jitteriness during the first few days of life. This typically disappears by day 3. About one-half of these infants are jittery only when startled, crying, or upset, while the other half are jittery during periods of alertness or other behavioural states. Less commonly, jitteriness is present beyond the neonatal period and can extend to a mean age of 7.2 months without long-term complications, possibly indicating the role of maturational events (Table 5.1).

Jitteriness can often be elicited by a particular stimulus, diminishes with passive flexion or containment of an extremity, and is not associated with abnormal gaze or eye movements, or with autonomic signs, such as hypertension or apnea. Physiological jitters can be confirmed in an infant who has a normal serum glucose level by a positive response to the suckling stimulation test. This response is elicited by placing an infant in the supine position with head straight and both hands free. When the examiner places a middle finger in the infant's mouth, the jitteriness ceases, and returns upon removal of the examiner's finger.

Mild jitteriness in the absence of an underlying etiology is a benign finding.

Infants who have fine jitters while quiet or sleeping or whose jitteriness initially presents beyond day 3 post-birth require a limited evaluation, at least. Coarse jitters should always be considered pathological and warrant a more comprehensive evaluation (Table 5.2). Jittery newborns are more likely than nonjittery newborns to develop seizures and to have abnormal electroencephalograms (EEGs) with epileptiform transients. Jittery newborns with a history of perinatal complications are more likely to have an adverse neurodevelopmental outcome.

> Differentiating jitteriness from seizures is clinically important Table 5.2. Jitteriness can be so severe that it is confused with a clonic seizure. Jitteriness can be normal or abnormal. Seizures in the newborn almost always arise from a pathological cause.

Table 5.1.
Common causes of jitteriness

Hypoglycemia	Discussed in ACoRN Chapter 7, Fluid and Glucose
Hypocalcemia	Low serum calcium (ionized calcium ≤ 1.0 mmol/L or total serum calcium ≤ 2.25 mmol/L) as a result of poor intake, induced alkalosis, prematurity, or a metabolic disorder
Neonatal abstinence syndrome/Neonatal opioid withdrawal	Opioids (heroin, methadone, morphine, and related drugs) used during pregnancy. Intrauterine exposure to CNS stimulants, CNS depressants, hallucinogens, antidepressants (SSRIs and SNRIs), and other licit (e.g., nicotine) or illicit drugs, can also cause neurologic symptoms and abnormal behaviours in the neonatal period
CNS irritability	Due to brain malformation, hemorrhage, encephalopathy, or CNS stimulants

CNS: central nervous system; SSRIs: selective serotonin reuptake inhibitors; SNRIs: serotonin–norepinephrine reuptake inhibitors

Table 5.2.
Distinguishing jitteriness from seizure activity

Observation	Jitteriness	Seizures
Alert	Yes	Impaired
Abnormal gaze or eye movement	No	Yes
Movements exquisitely sensitive to stimuli	Yes	No
Predominant movement	Oscillatory tremor	Clonic jerking
Movements cease with passive flexion	Yes	No
Autonomic changes (e.g., tachycardia, increase in blood pressure, or apnea)	No	Yes
Often migrates from one body area to another	No	Yes

Adapted from Volpe JJ. Neurology of the Newborn, 5th ed. Philadelphia, PA: WB Saunders, 2008.

Seizures in newborns usually present as subtle changes in activity, clonic movements, or tonic posturing. These movements do not stop when the limb is held or flexed. Seizures may also present with changes in autonomic function, such as heart rate (HR), blood pressure (BP), saturations and apnea. Due to immaturity of the newborn's neural pathways, classic tonic-clonic seizures are not seen in the neonate.

Recurrent apnea in the late preterm or term infant may be considered a manifestation of seizures.

Seizures are important to identify (Tables 5.3, 5.4) because they may:

- Relate to a condition that requires urgent, specific therapy (e.g., hypoglycemia) or early intervention within a specific time frame (e.g., therapeutic hypothermia for HIE).
- Interfere with important physiological functions, such as breathing or swallowing.
- Signal and/or aggravate a pre-existing brain injury.

Four types of seizures can occur in newborns (Table 5.3).

Table 5.3.
Newborn seizure types and characteristics

Type (% Frequency)	Characteristics
Subtle (30%)	• Horizontal tonic deviation of the eyes, with or without jerking movements • Repetitive blinking or staring episodes • Chewing, lip-smacking, or drooling • 'Bicycling' of the legs and other rhythmic-appearing, purposeless movements • Apnea • Sudden tachycardia at rest, *or* increase in blood pressure, *or* decrease in SpO2 • Posturing

Clonic (25%)	• Rhythmic, slow movements (1 to 3 jerks/sec) involving the face and/or the upper and/or lower extremities on one side of the body (therefore called focal)
	  ○ The infant is usually conscious during focal seizures.
	• Course, jerking movements of one or two limbs that migrate to the contralateral part of the body (therefore called multifocal) in a nonorderly fashion
	  ○ When movements generalize to involve both sides of the body, loss of consciousness usually occurs.

Tonic (20%)	• Sustained, rigid posturing of a limb or asymmetric posturing of the trunk or neck (focal), with or without tonic eye deviation • Premature infants may develop generalized tonic seizures that include flexion or extension of the neck, trunk, and upper extremities, and extension of the lower extremities (similar to decorticate or decerebrate posturing), with or without autonomic phenomena.
Myoclonic (25%)	• Rapid contractions of flexor muscles in one limb (focal), several parts of the body (multifocal), or the whole body (generalized) ○ In 'benign sleep myoclonus', which usually disappears by 6 months of age with no sequelae, any of the three forms can be present. This condition is characterized by immediate cessation of abnormal movements with arousal.

The infant's age is a clue to the cause of seizures (Table 5.4).

Table 5.4.
Common causes of seizures in the newborn period

Age	Cause
At birth	• Acute drug withdrawal caused by naloxone administration to the infant of a narcotic-using mother • Local anesthetic injected into fetal scalp during pudendal block
Day 1	• HIE seizures usually present in the first 6 to 24 h • Hypoglycemia • Metabolic abnormalities (e.g., hypocalcemia) • Trauma, including subdural hemorrhage
Day 2 to 3	• NAS/NOW • Neonatal stroke • Metabolic disturbances • Inborn errors of metabolism—may present with seizures, hypotonia, and altered consciousness, often with other abnormalities such as hypoglycemia, metabolic acidosis, and hyperammonemia • Meningitis/encephalitis • Subarachnoid hemorrhage
Day 3 to 7	• Neonatal stroke • Hypocalcemia • Brain malformation • Meningitis/encephalitis • NAS/NOW due to methadone withdrawal
Day 7	• Meningitis/encephalitis

NAS: neonatal abstinence syndrome; NOW: neonatal opiate withdrawal

Newborns at risk for HIE

Newborns that experience a significant perinatal hypoxic ischemic event usually have a recognizable sentinel event during labour. A perinatal sentinel event may include:

• Fetal HR monitoring abnormalities, such as late decelerations, complicated variable decelerations, minimal or absent variability, and bradycardia.
• Evidence or suspicion of bleeding from placental abruption, fetal hemorrhage, cord occlusion or cord prolapse.

These infants are often depressed at birth and require more prolonged resuscitation. They are further identified using the following signs:

• An Apgar score of 0 to 3 for 5 min or longer *or* of 0 to 5 for 10 min or longer.
• An umbilical cord arterial pH less than 7.15.
• Umbilical cord arterial base deficit of 10 mmol/L or higher, or lactate greater than 5 mmol/L.

Risk factors for HIE identify newborns who require close observation and assessment because they are at higher risk for developing HIE. They may be candidates for therapeutic hypothermia, provided they meet the necessary criteria for treatment. Early consultation with your regional referral centre is recommended.

Clinical signs of end-organ perfusion problems indicate a higher risk of long-term sequelae from moderate to severe HIE. These signs include:

- Clinical encephalopathy (hypotonia, seizures, coma, abnormal activity).
- Evidence of multisystem organ dysfunction in the immediate neonatal period, usually of the renal, hepatic, cardiovascular, respiratory, and gastrointestinal systems.
  - Kidney damage is indicated by decreased urine output, microscopic hematuria, elevation of serum creatinine, and low serum sodium.
  - Hepatic injury manifests as elevated liver enzymes, abnormal clotting factors and other abnormalities in synthetic function, such as albumin production and glucose control.
  - Thrombocytopenia may accompany abnormal clotting factors.
  - Signs of cardiac injury include poor contractility, low BP, reduced peripheral perfusion, and (occasionally) heart failure and arrhythmias.
  - Significant acidosis may result in persistent pulmonary hypertension of the newborn (PPHN), causing cyanosis.
  - Gastrointestinal injury can manifest as ileus or necrotizing enterocolitis.
- Early imaging studies showing evidence of acute, non-focal cerebral abnormality.

In infants greater than 35 weeks GA with moderate to severe HIE, neurodevelopmental outcome can be improved by initiating therapeutic hypothermia within 6 hours of birth.

Core Steps

The essential Core Step in the ACoRN Neurology Sequence is to determine the presence and degree of neonatal encephalopathy using the Encephalopathy Assessment Table (Table 5.5).

Table 5.5.
Encephalopathy Assessment

Category	Normal	Mild	Moderate	Severe
Level of alertness	☐ Alert, normal sleep–wake cycles	☐ Hyperalert	☐ Lethargy	☐ Stupor or coma
Spontaneous activity	☐ Normal	☐ Normal	☐ Decreased activity	☐ No activity
Posture	☐ Flexed	☐ Mild distal flexion	☐ Arms flexed, legs extended (decorticate)	☐ Arms and legs extended (decerebrate)
Tone	☐ Normal	☐ Normal to mild hypotonia	☐ Hypotonic	☐ Flaccid
Primitive reflexes	☐ Normal suck and Moro	☐ Weak suck, strong Moro	☐ Weak suck, incomplete Moro	☐ Absent suck, absent Moro
Autonomic (one of)				
Pupils	☐ Reactive	☐ Dilated reactive	☐ Constricted	☐ Dilated or nonreactive
Heart rate	☐ Normal	☐ Tachycardia	☐ Bradycardia	☐ Variable heart rate
Respirations	☐ Normal	☐ Normal	☐ Periodic breathing	☐ Apnea
Seizures	☐ None	☐ None	☐ Common	☐ Uncommon

Adapted from Sarnat HB, Sarnat MS. Neonatal encephalopathy following fetal distress: A clinical and electroencephalographic study. Arch Neurol 1976 33(10):696–705. For more information on reflexes, see Table 5.7, page 166.

Well infants present with findings only in the 'normal' column of the Encephalopathy Assessment Table. Infants with mild encephalopathy present with no findings in the 'severe' column and do not meet criteria for moderate to severe encephalopathy.

The Encephalopathy Assessment Table helps the ACoRN provider to document changes in neurologic status during the first days of life.

> Criteria for moderate or severe encephalopathy are met when infants present with at least one 'moderate' or 'severe' finding in three or more categories, *or* if they present with seizures.

Organization of Care

In the ACoRN Neurology Sequence, Organization of Care is first determined by glucose levels in the presence of one or more of the ACoRN Alerting Signs. The immediate course of action depends on:

- Blood glucose level and, subsequently,
- Whether the infant presents with a seizure-like event or other ACoRN Neurology Alerting Signs.

Infants presenting with symptomatic hypoglycemia, hypoglycemia in the presence of additional risks for neurologic injury (HIE), or seizure-like events, require rapid assessment and intervention to optimize outcomes.

Response

Symptomatic hypoglycemia

Symptomatic hypoglycemia in the Neurology Sequence may present with nonspecific signs, such as:

- Jitteriness, tremor, seizure-like activity, or coma
- Irritability, lethargy, or stupor
- Hypotonia or limpness
- Exaggerated Moro reflex
- Apnea or cyanotic spells
- Poor feeding, poor sucking reflex
- Hypothermia
- High-pitched crying

Symptomatic hypoglycemia is assumed when blood glucose is less than 2.6 mmol in the first 72 h post-birth or less than 3.3 after 72 h, together with an Alerting Sign in the ACoRN Neurology Sequence *or* any of the previously listed nonspecific signs. Symptomatic hypoglycemia is an emergency because it is associated with an increased risk for neurodevelopmental sequelae.

Infants with symptomatic hypoglycemia require emergent treatment with IV dextrose solution. A bolus of 2 mL/kg of D10W, delivered over 15 min, should be given immediately. When starting an IV proves difficult, the ACoRN provider may consider administering 40% dextrose gel to the oral mucosa, at a dose of 0.5 mL/kg, *while establishing parenteral access*. Dextrose boluses must be followed by a continuous D10W infusion at 4 mL/kg/h to provide a constant glucose infusion rate.

> Establishing a continuous infusion of D10W is essential because a D10W bolus or dextrose gel only remains in the circulation for about 15 to 30 min, depending on the infant's rate of glucose utilization.

Successfully managing an infant with symptomatic hypoglycemia involves initial administration of a D10W infusion at 4 mL/kg/h, with ongoing monitoring and glucose infusion rate adjustments as detailed in the ACoRN Fluid and Glucose Sequence. The goal of treatment is to normalize blood glucose as soon as possible. Therefore, blood glucose level must be retested 30 min after the bolus of D10W is completed and actively managed until the level is above 2.6 mmol/L. Details for ongoing management are discussed in Chapter 7, Fluid and Glucose.

Seizure-like movements

Seizure-like movements must also be interpreted in the context of glucose levels. When associated with hypoglycemia, they are presumed to indicate symptomatic hypoglycemia and the infant is treated immediately as previously directed.

If hypoglycemia is *not* present or has been corrected, seizure-like movements may relate to another underlying pathology, such as HIE, CNS infection, metabolic abnormalities, intracranial bleeding, stroke, or malformation.

Prolonged or persistent seizures can lead to physiological compromise, neurologic injury, and long-term sequelae, and require immediate intervention. If hypoglycemia is *not* present, seizure-like movements require treatment with an anticonvulsant medication.

In most centres, phenobarbital is the first-line therapy for an infant believed to be having seizures.

- Start phenobarbital. The usual loading dose of phenobarbital is 20 mg/kg IV, given slowly over 20 min.

When seizure control is not achieved by this initial dose, infants may need an escalating load of phenobarbital (the initial 20 mg/kg dose, followed by up to two 10 mg/kg doses, 30 to 60 min apart), to a maximum 40 mg/kg, before considering the administration of a second anticonvulsant drug.

- Careful observation for onset of respiratory depression and hypotension is needed when high doses of anticonvulsants are used.
- Adding a second anticonvulsant may be necessary when seizures are refractory. The choice of anticonvulsant should be discussed with the referral centre (see also Appendix C, Medications).

Descriptive documentation of abnormal movements (Table 5.6) is important because the clinical diagnosis of seizures is unreliable in newborns. Electroclinical dissociation—defined as abnormal movements without epileptiform discharges on EEG, and epileptiform EEG without abnormal movements—is common in newborns and increases after anticonvulsants have been administered.

When available, continuous amplitude-integrated electroencephalography (aEEG) monitoring can help with diagnosis and prognostication for newborns with seizure-like activity.

No hypoglycemia, no seizure-like movements

Infants entering the Neurology Sequence as **At risk for HIE**, or those with an abnormal neurologic exam but no seizures, require careful investigation, further assessment, and possible management.

Infants at risk for HIE who develop abnormal tone, activity, or level of alertness within 6 h of birth, with or without seizure-like activity, may be eligible for therapeutic hypothermia (see Appendix A). Early identification of these infants is critically important.

Table 5.6.
Documenting abnormal movements

Time/Duration	At what time did the seizure occur and how long did it last?
Suppression	Were the movements suppressed by grasping the extremity or if the infant is wakened?
Origin/Spread	Where did the seizure originate (e.g., arm, leg, or face)? Did the seizure spread to other parts of the body? If so, where?
Eye movements	Were there accompanying eye movements such as horizontal deviation of the eyes, jerking, or staring?
Mouth movements	Was there lip-smacking, chewing, tongue movements, or drooling?
Level of alertness	Was the infant awake or asleep? Did the infant, • Respond to visual and auditory stimuli? • Rouse from sleep with tactile stimulation? • Cry periodically while awake?
Autonomic changes	Were there changes in heart rate, saturations, respirations and/or blood pressure before, during, or after the seizure?
Other signs	Was there a change in the infant's colour? Were there signs of regurgitation or choking? Did the infant have difficulty breathing? Did the infant have apnea?

Abnormal tone, activity, or level of alertness may also present in infants with CNS infection or in-born errors of metabolism. These conditions also require emergent care.

Neurologic symptoms in the presence of critical hyperbilirubinemia may indicate acute bilirubin encephalopathy. Bilirubin encephalopathy is a medical emergency (see Chapter 8, Jaundice).

Further information and assessment are needed to determine the underlying pathology in other conditions, including neonatal stroke, CNS injury, neuromuscular disorder, or CNS malformation.

Next Steps

ACoRN Next Steps are to obtain a focused history, conduct a physical examination, order diagnostic tests, and establish a working diagnosis.

Focused history

Essential information to gather during the focused neurology history includes the following:

Antepartum

- Maternal health before and during pregnancy, including nutrition and specific illnesses related to, or complicated by, pregnancy
- Dosage and duration of medications taken during pregnancy
- Substance use (illicit drugs, prescription drugs, alcohol and tobacco)
- Congenital or inherited disorders
- Family history of sleep myoclonus
- Perception of fetal movements

Intrapartum

- Nature of labour, analgesia used, type of delivery, including degree of difficulty and any complications (including sentinel events, such as cord prolapse, abruption, shoulder dystocia)
- Indicators of fetal compromise, such as atypical or abnormal electronic fetal monitor tracing or acidosis noted on a fetal scalp sampling

Neonatal

- Umbilical cord blood gas (arterial and venous) obtained at birth
  - Arterial cord gases reflect the degree of acidosis in the fetus, while venous blood gases reflect the degree of acidosis in the blood coming from the placenta.
  - With a malfunctioning placenta, acidosis is present in both arterial and venous gases and the arteriovenous difference tends to be small.
  - With an acute interruption of umbilical circulation, acidosis is worse in the arterial cord blood and the arteriovenous difference is large.
- Condition at birth and time of onset of respiration
- Need for resuscitation at birth and extent of the resuscitative efforts
- Apgar scores (including extended scores at 10 and 20 min)
- GA
- Feeding history

Focused physical examination

In addition to the examination conducted during the ACoRN Primary Survey, a focused neurologic examination should include the following:

Observation

- Level of alertness and activity
- Posture
- Spontaneous movements
- Any skin changes (e.g., rashes suggestive of HSV or other infections, or neurocutaneous stigmata, jaundice, pallor)

Assessment of vital signs: respiratory rate (RR), HR, temperature, BP, and pulse oximetry.

Examination

Assess for encephalopathy as per Table 5.5, page 161, as well as using the following indicators.

- Head circumference (measure and plot on a chart)
- Evidence of external injury (e.g., a skull fracture or cephalohematoma)
- Posture and tone (popliteal angle, pull-to-sit manoeuvre, ventral suspension)
- Fullness/tension of fontanels and measurement of suture separation
- Primitive reflexes (e.g., suck–swallow, Moro, palmar and plantar grasps, response to traction)
- Brain stem reflexes (e.g., gag, corneal, pupillary size and reaction to light, oculovestibular)
- Deep tendon reflexes (biceps and patellar)
- Spontaneous extraocular movements
- Funduscopic appearance (e.g., retinal hemorrhage or chorioretinitis)

Assessing brain stem activity and primitive reflexes

Checking essential cranial nerve functions and primitive reflexes is key to neurologic examination in the newborn because the brain stem is an important site of injury in acute neonatal encephalopathy. The essential reflexes to assess are shown in Table 5.7.

Table 5.7.
Assessing brain stem activity and primitive reflexes

Reflex	Description
Sucking	Should be strong and rhythmic beyond 36 weeks GA and is tested using a gloved finger inserted into the infant's mouth.
Gag	Should be strong, with contraction of the pharynx and is tested by touching the infant's soft palate with a gloved finger or catheter.
Moro or 'startle'	Has three phases: Abduction of the upper extremities with splaying of the hands, followed by adduction back to midline and, finally, an audible cry. The Moro reflex is elicited by a variety of stimuli, including loud noise or, most commonly, a downward drop of the infant's head relative to the body. In extremely preterm infants, splaying of the hands may be noted with abduction of the upper extremities, becoming more prevalent by 32 weeks GA. The adduction phase is generally seen by 37 weeks. A weak Moro reflex may be seen with any CNS depression, while an asymmetric Moro suggests peripheral (especially brachial plexus) nerve injury.
Rooting	Results in head-turning to the side of stimulation, opening of the mouth, and sucking, and is elicited by stimulating the perioral skin. Weak responses are common but non-specific features of cortical or brain stem dysfunction. Rooting persists until 3 to 4 months of age and may be present longer in infants with CNS dysfunction.
Grasp	Strength increases with increasing GA and is elicited by stimulating the palm or sole. The grasp reflex appears by 26 to 27 weeks GA and generally begins to regress as voluntary grasp starts to develop, at around 2 months of age.
Pupillary response to light	Normal constriction reaction is present starting from 28 to 30 weeks GA.
Corneal	The eyes should close when the cornea is gently touched with the tip of a cotton swab.
Oculocephalic, or 'doll's eyes'	The eyes should deviate in the opposite direction when the head is turned from one side to the other in a supine infant.

CNS: central nervous system; GA: gestational age

Diagnostic tests

Many of the diagnostic tests used to differentiate neurologic disorders are specialized, but a few simple blood tests can assist in reaching a working diagnosis:

1. Complete blood count and differential
   - Assists in the diagnosis of acute anemia from blood loss, polycythemia presenting with hyper viscosity syndrome, or sepsis
2. Blood gas
   - To rule out metabolic acidosis

3. Blood culture
   - This test will not affect immediate management, but the specimen must be drawn before antibiotics are administered.
   - In the presence of significant neurologic findings, a lumbar puncture (LP) should be considered as soon as the infant is stable. Consider drawing an extra tube of CSF for HSV and enterovirus.
4. Blood chemistry
   - To rule out electrolyte abnormalities (sodium, calcium, potassium, and magnesium levels)
   - Serum bilirubin. Although rare, bilirubin encephalopathy should be considered in infants:
     - presenting after 24 h with altered neurologic status, or
     - earlier, with risk factors for hyperbilirubinemia (blood type incompatibilities or metabolic/genetic conditions resulting in hemolysis).

Specific Diagnosis and Management

Diagnosing neurologic conditions in newborns usually requires specialized investigations, and the etiology may remain obscure. However, a working diagnosis based on groups of symptoms can guide care planning, ongoing investigation, and management.

It is critical to identify infants presenting with abnormal neurologic Alerting Signs who are also at risk for HIE.

Hypoxic ischemic encephalopathy

Most newborns exposed to a perinatal hypoxic ischemic event are asymptomatic and have a normal neurologic examination and normal long-term outcomes. These infants do not develop permanent neurologic impairment. Others, however, are symptomatic at birth and develop a form of neonatal encephalopathy called HIE.

- Most infants with mild HIE have normal outcomes.
- In moderate HIE, death is uncommon but long-term sequelae develop in approximately 25% to 30% of survivors.
- Most infants with severe HIE will die or live with significant long-term sequelae.

The signs and symptoms of HIE develop in the early postnatal period but can vary depending on the severity and timing of injury. The systemic effects seen in some cases of HIE occur when oxygen levels and/or blood supply are inadequate to meet the metabolic needs of tissues. The organs affected develop hypoxia and lactic acidosis which, if left uncorrected, can result in further cellular injury and organ dysfunction. In infants with HIE, the neurologic insult results from cell necrosis in the areas most affected and from delayed neuronal death through apoptosis in neighbouring areas. Discovery of the importance of delayed cell death as a contributor to neurologic outcomes in HIE has established the 'therapeutic window' for hypothermia to decrease the incidence of permanent damage.

In HIE, insult to the brain is global, with symmetrical distribution of dysfunction and injury apparent both on clinical and on neuroradiological examinations. The pattern and duration of insult determines which areas of the brain are most affected. Specifically, the areas of highest energy requirement (basal ganglia and brain stem) are damaged when the insult is acute and total, and the areas with the most fragile blood supply (watershed regions of the cortex and subcortex) become impaired when the insult is partial but prolonged.

Possible long-term neurologic sequelae of HIE include motor disorders, seizures, cognitive impairment, sensorineural deficits, and feeding difficulties. Cerebral palsy subsequent to an intrapartum hypoxic-ischemic injury may develop in newborn infants who present with signs of neonatal encephalopathy.

Risk factors for developing long-term sequelae include:

- Persistent abnormalities on EEG,
- Seizures that persist or are difficult to control,
- An abnormal neurologic examination beyond 1 week post-birth or at time of discharge, and/or
- An inability to feed by mouth that requires prolonged gavage feeding.

> Initiating therapeutic hypothermia within 6 h of birth reduces infant mortality and often prevents or minimizes morbidity in the longer term.

All newborns who are identified as being at risk for HIE should be closely monitored during the first 6 h post-birth to determine whether they meet criteria for initiating therapeutic hypothermia. Strict normothermia should be initiated while decisions about therapeutic hypothermia are pending. To maximize identification of eligible candidates for this treatment, the criteria listed to identify newborns as **At Risk for HIE** are more inclusive than the criteria for determining eligibility for therapeutic hypothermia.

To qualify for therapeutic hypothermia, the newborn should be 35 weeks GA or greater and meet *either* treatment criteria A *or* B and *also* meet criteria C:

Criteria A: Cord pH less than or equal to 7.0 or base deficit greater than or equal to 16, **or**

Criteria B: pH 7.01 to 7.15 or base deficit 10 to 15.9 on cord gas or blood gas within 1 h of age, **and**

History of acute perinatal event (e.g., cord prolapse, placental abruption, or uterine rupture) **and**

Apgar score less than or equal to 5 at 10 min, or at least 10 min of positive-pressure ventilation

and

Criteria C: Evidence of moderate or severe encephalopathy, as demonstrated either by the presence of seizures or by observing at least one sign in three or more of the 'moderate' or 'severe' columns of the Encephalopathy Assessment Table 5.5, page 161.

The goal of therapeutic hypothermia is neuroprotection. The mechanism of action is multifactorial and thought to include reduction in cellular apoptosis, reduced cellular energy loss and oxygen consumption in recovering cells, reduced release of cytotoxic mediators, and the induction of genes that reduce neuronal death.

Therapeutic hypothermia can be achieved safely using either selective head cooling or total body cooling. Total body cooling is preferred for ease of use and set-up as well as better access to aEEG or EEG monitoring. The target core body temperature for therapeutic effect in total body cooling is 33°C to 34°C. Hypothermia is maintained for 72 h, and rewarming is done slowly over an average of 6 to 12 h.

Neonates for whom therapeutic hypothermia is contraindicated include those with:

- Unstable pulmonary hypertension,
- Unstable coagulopathy or significant active hemorrhage, and/or
- Palliative care as the treatment goal.

Therapeutic hypothermia should *only* be considered after:

- Neonatal resuscitation, the ACoRN Primary Survey, and the appropriate ACoRN Sequences have been completed;
- The tertiary care referral centre has been consulted; and
- Following a strict protocol (see Appendix A).

Therapeutic hypothermia decreases metabolic activity and alters metabolism by the liver. Therefore, pharmacokinetics may be significantly altered during the cooling process.

For infants who do not meet criteria for therapeutic hypothermia, who are more than 6 h old, or for whom this treatment is contraindicated:

- Initiate strict normothermia (i.e., active thermal management to avoid hyperthermia). The goal is to maintain the infant's axillary temperature between 36.5°C and 37.0°C and avoid overheating (see Chapter 9, Thermoregulation).

Neuroimaging, such as a magnetic resonance imaging scan, is useful for diagnostic and prognostic assessment. Such studies are done later in the treatment course, after rewarming.

When managing any infant with abnormal neurologic status or suspected neonatal encephalopathy, consider these essential steps:

- Carefully observe the infant to ensure that ventilation and oxygenation are within the normal range (refer to the Resuscitation and ACoRN Respiratory Sequences).
  - Assisted ventilation may be required.
  - Hyperoxia must be avoided.
  - Hypocarbia and alkalosis must be avoided.
- Assess for clinical signs of poor perfusion, low pulse, or low BP (refer to the Cardiovascular Sequence), and maintenance of adequate circulation.
  - An echocardiogram may be helpful for infants with signs of poor circulation or persistent pulmonary hypertension of the newborn (PPHN).
  - Volume expanders or inotropes may be required.
  - Monitor for signs of PPHN.
- Carefully manage the infant's fluids and glucose, to avoid hypoglycemia, fluid overload, and hyponatremia (refer to Chapter 7, Fluid and Glucose).
  - Restrict initial fluid intake to 2 to 3 mL/kg/h (approximately 50 to 75 mL/kg/day) of D10W. Most newborns are initially oliguric or anuric and may require less fluid.
  - Monitor blood glucose every 2 to 4 h until stable. Restricted fluid intake may not meet glucose requirements and more concentrated dextrose solutions may require central line insertion.
  - Monitor serum electrolytes every 6 to 12 h. Excessive fluid intake and abnormal renal function may lead to hyponatremia (serum Na less than 135 mmol/L) and/or hyperkalemia (serum K greater than 4.5 mmol/L).
  - Monitor and correct any other metabolic disturbances, such as hypocalcemia or hypomagnesemia.
- Maintain body temperature within the desired target range: strict normothermia is 36.5°C to 37.0°C, and therapeutic hypothermia is 33.5°C ± 0.5°C. (Refer to Chapter 9, Thermoregulation, and Appendix A for further guidance).
- Consult early and refer as needed.

Hyperthermia must be avoided because it increases the risk for, and severity of, neurodevelopmental morbidity.

Other diagnoses

Effects of intrauterine exposures

Neonatal abstinence syndrome (NAS) / neonatal opiate withdrawal syndrome (NOWS)

A positive and supportive relationship between the mother and care providers is essential. Asking about prescription medication and illicit drug use in a sensitive, nonjudgemental way is a routine part of perinatal care and should not be reserved for cases when drug use is suspected.

- Find out which drugs have been used, their timing in relation to pregnancy and delivery, and the frequency and routes of administration.
- Explain the need to screen for infection to mothers with a history of intravenous drug use.
- Implement protocols to prevent or treat perinatal transmission of infections, when indicated.

Toxicology tests in mothers and infants have limited therapeutic value because treatment decisions are based on severity of symptoms. Other concerns regarding such testing include:

- False-negative results, particularly when a drug is not used just before birth or a sample is not obtained shortly after birth.
- False-positive results, sometimes caused by interacting with other medications or food.
- The potential for use of the results outside of a health care context.
- Issues of informed consent. Toxicology testing in mothers or infants requires the mother's informed consent and cannot be performed under general consent for care protocols. Such testing is not considered best practice in Canada.

The clinical presentation of NAS/NOWS varies with the drug or medication being used, the quantity, frequency, and duration of intrauterine exposure, and timing (i.e., when the drug was last used before delivery). When signs present within the first 24 h post-birth, consideration should be given to other fetal exposures, such as nicotine, caffeine, or polysubstance use.

With maternal heroin or methadone use, a newborn appears physically and behaviourally normal at birth. Signs of withdrawal from methadone tend to appear later—in the first week or two—than from heroin—in 2 to 3 days—because of methadone's long half-life. Signs and symptoms found in infants with NAS/NOWS include:

W	**w**akefulness
I	**i**rritability, increased tone, increased Moro reflex
T	**t**remulousness (jittery), temperature instability, tachypnea
H	**h**yperactivity, high-pitched cry, hiccups, hypersensitivity to sound, hyperreflexia
D	**d**iarrhea (explosive), diaphoresis, disorganized suck
R	**r**unny nose, regurgitation, respiratory distress, rub marks

A	**a**pnea, autonomic dysfunction (change in HR and RR)
W	**w**eight loss
A	**a**lkalosis (respiratory)
L	**l**acrimation (tearing of eyes) and lethargy
S	**s**nuffles, sneezing, seizures

Monitoring temperature to avoid hyperthermia is essential for infants at risk for, or experiencing, signs of NAS/NOWS. These infants should also be:

- Loosely swaddled.
- Handled gently.
- Cared for skin-to-skin with parents.
- Placed in a quiet, dimly lit environment.
- Fed frequently to ensure adequate fluid and caloric intake.
- Encouraged to breastfeed, unless the mother is HIV-positive or there is documented polydrug use.
- Observed for seizures.

A recognized scoring system should be used to assess the severity of withdrawal symptoms and help determine the need for additional monitoring, nursing, and medical or pharmacologic therapies. Finnegan's Neonatal Abstinence Scoring System is one scoring system commonly used to observe and manage infants with opiate/opioid withdrawal. Other scoring systems include the Lipsitz, Neonatal Narcotic Withdrawal Index, the Neonatal Withdrawal Inventory, and the Eat, Sleep, Console Assessment.

Pharmacological intervention is usually considered after ruling out other medical conditions in infants who show the following signs despite receiving supportive environmental measures:

- Inconsolable crying
- Poor sleep
- Persistent tremors or jitteriness when undisturbed
- Poor weight gain or excessive weight loss (> 10%).

For infants experiencing increasing severity of symptoms of opioid withdrawal, the drug of choice is oral morphine. Start morphine in accordance with your regional protocol. The initial dose is titrated up or down based on the infant's response. Some infants require treatment for 4 weeks or longer.

Pharmacotherapy should be titrated based on an accepted assessment tool. Response to treatment is inferred by an improving score or assessment.

Infants less than 32 weeks GA may not show typical withdrawal symptoms, and the decision to evaluate using a particular scoring system should be made on a case-by-case basis.

Infants requiring pharmacologic treatment may require admission to a special care nursery or NICU for observation and cardiorespiratory monitoring while therapy is initiated.

Naloxone should **not** be administered to an infant whose mother has a history of chronic illicit or prescription narcotic use because it can precipitate seizures.

SSRI/SNRI neonatal behavioural syndrome

SSRI/SNRI neonatal behavioural syndrome (SNBS) is associated with maternal use of specific antidepressants during pregnancy, typically an SSRI, such as paroxetine (Paxil), sertraline (Zoloft), and fluoxetine (Prozac), or an SNRI, such as venlafaxine (Effexor).

An estimated 10% to 30% of infants exposed to antidepressants during the third trimester of pregnancy show signs of SNBS. It is not clear whether they signal withdrawal from antidepressants, drug toxicity in the developing brain, or both. Signs usually present within hours of delivery and can be identified during the ACoRN Primary Survey. They include:

- Tachypnea, respiratory distress, cyanosis
- Jitteriness, tremors, seizures
- Increased muscle tone
- Irritability

- Eating or sleeping difficulties
- Vomiting
- Hypoglycemia
- Hypothermia

These signs are typically mild and usually resolve within 2 weeks. PPHN is a rare complication of SNBS. Infants with SNBS should be clinically observed for respiratory and neurobehavioural symptoms for at least 48 h.

Neonatal stroke

Neonatal stroke occurs in approximately 1:4000 births, usually around time of delivery and often without a recognized hypoxic insult. Stroke is caused by interruption of blood flow and often affects the middle cerebral artery. Risk factors for neonatal stroke include congenital heart disease and hereditary or acquired thrombophilias. In many cases, risk factors are never identified. Infants may present with focal seizures in the first days of life or be asymptomatic and only recognized at a later age as having had a stroke. Unless the stroke is severe, neurocognitive sequelae tend to be mild.

Intracranial hemorrhage

Subarachnoid hemorrhage usually occurs in the absence of hypoxic insult or trauma.

- Small subarachnoid hemorrhages are common, present with minimal symptoms, and usually have a good prognosis.
- If seizures occur, they often appear on day 2 or 3, and the infant appears well between seizures.

Periventricular hemorrhage (PVH) or intraventricular hemorrhage (IVH) originates in the germinal matrix, a fragile, loosely supported capillary network in the external wall of the lateral ventricles. PVH/IVH is more common in sick, ventilated preterm infants but can occur in otherwise healthy preterm newborns. PVH/IVH is uncommon in term infants.

- Infants with PVH/IVH are usually asymptomatic.
- In severe cases, PVH/IVH may be accompanied by subtle seizures, decerebrate posturing, and/or generalized tonic seizures.

Subdural hemorrhage is sometimes associated with head trauma (e.g., due to difficult delivery). It is a space-occupying lesion that may exert pressure on brain tissue, causing focal seizures.

CNS infections

Bacterial meningitis or viral encephalitis can cause altered level of alertness, abnormal tone, or seizures. Diagnostic guidance and recommendations for management are provided in Chapter 10, Infection.

- Obtain blood for culture, white cell and differential count, platelet count and glucose, and cerebral spinal fluid for cell count, bacterial and viral cultures, polymerase chain reaction, protein and glucose.
- Start antibiotics ± antiviral promptly, pending test results.

Performing an LP is beyond the scope of practice for some clinicians. When bacterial meningitis is suspected, obtaining a cerebral spinal fluid sample is less important than initiating antibiotics. Before performing an LP, make sure there are no contraindications to this procedure, such as thrombocytopenia or a significant family history of bleeding disorders.

Brain malformations

Conditions associated with abnormal brain growth or anatomy include single-gene disorders, chromosomal or other genetic anomalies, and exposure in utero to a chemical or infectious agent. Diagnosis and management of brain malformations involve specialized investigations and subspecialty care that are usually only available at tertiary care referral centres. Timely identification, consultation, and referrals are required.

Metabolic, genetic, or neuromuscular disorders

Hypoglycemia, hypocalcemia, hypomagnesemia, hyponatremia, and hypernatremia can lead to generalized seizure activity. Persistent hypoglycemia is also associated with neurodevelopmental impairment in the longer term. Initial management is directed by Chapter 7, Fluid and Glucose.

Hyperbilirubinemia is a rare cause of neonatal encephalopathy in the era of maternal and newborn screening, but should be considered in any unwell neonate presenting with Alerting Signs in the Neurology Sequence. Early recognition and prompt treatment of hyperbilirubinemia can prevent neurologic sequelae such as bilirubin-induced neurologic dysfunction and chronic bilirubin encephalopathy. Investigation and management of hyperbilirubinemia is discussed in Chapter 8, Jaundice.

Inborn errors of metabolism are rare. Reduced levels of alertness—from depression to coma— seizures, metabolic acidosis, and/or hyperammonemia are more common presentations of metabolic conditions.

Neuromuscular disorders are rare. They present with hypotonia and weakness. There is often a prenatal history of decreased fetal movement and polyhydramnios.

Diagnosis and management of symptomatic newborns with metabolic, genetic, and neuromuscular disorders are medical emergencies requiring specialized investigations and subspecialty care. Consultation with a level 3 referral centre is required.

Level of Risk: Neurology
In the ACoRN Neurology Sequence, level of risk is based on abnormal findings on the Encephalopathy Assessment Table, the presence of seizure-like movements, and risk for developing hypoxic ischemic encephalopathy (HIE).

 Green:
- Normal findings on Encephalopathy Assessment Table
- No risk factors for HIE

 Yellow:
- Mild abnormalities based on Encephalopathy Assessment Table
- Risk factors for HIE

Infants at a Yellow Level of Risk require increased levels of attention and consultation. Transfer is required if needs exceed site capabilities.

 Red:
- Moderate to severe findings based on Encephalopathy Assessment Table
- Seizure-like movements
- Infant meets criteria for active HIE management

Infants at a Red Level of Risk require level 3 care. Transfer is required if needs exceed site capabilities.

Neurology: Case 1—The floppy baby

You have just been informed that your patient, a mother in her second pregnancy, has delivered a baby by urgent Caesarean section at 37 weeks GA, following a head-on collision in a motor vehicle. The mother has wakened from her anesthetic and is doing well. She has no injuries related to the accident, but her baby required resuscitation. You know from your prenatal care of the mother that she is healthy. You arrive when the baby is 1 h old. She is on a radiant warmer in the observation nursery area. She is breathing regularly and without difficulty, her vital signs (RR, HR, BP, SpO2) are normal, and she is pink in room air.

You determine that the baby shows none of the Resuscitation Alerting Signs.

Skin colour, perfusion, and peripheral pulses are normal. The nurse tells you the baby's tone appears low. You observe her lying with arms and legs extended. The temperature probe on the radiant heater reads 36.7°C, and an axillary temperature is being taken.

1. **Complete the ACoRN Primary Survey and Consolidated Core Steps, and generate a Problem List.**

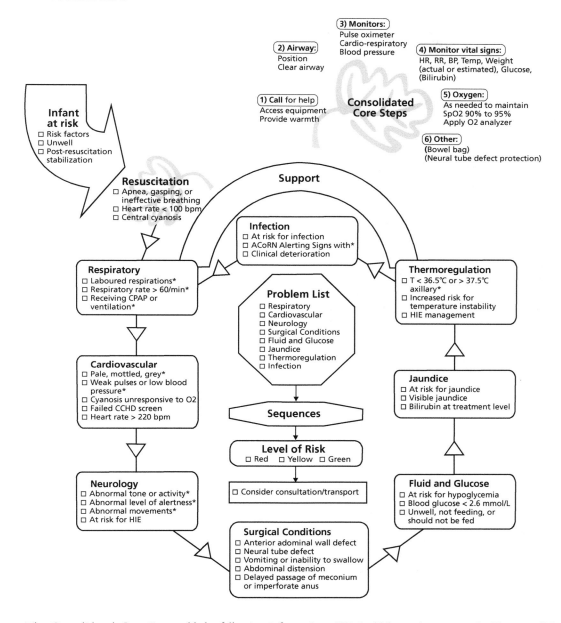

The Consolidated Core Steps add the following information: HR is 130, respiratory rate is 40, mean BP is 48, and axillary temperature 36.8°C. Her weight is 3500 g. Her blood glucose is 3.5 mmol/L.

Neurology, Fluid and Glucose, Thermoregulation, and Infection are prioritized on your Problem List.

2. **Neurology is the first sequence identified. Which Alerting Signs would you mark? Why?**

> **Neurology**
> ☐ Abnormal tone or activity*
> ☐ Abnormal level of alertness*
> ☐ Abnormal movements*
> ☐ At risk for HIE

The baby appears visually attentive, is responsive to stimuli, and is easily roused. Rooting is absent but suck, grasp, and Moro reflexes are present.

She is lying on the warmer with minimal flexion of her extremities. You see no abnormal movement suggestive of seizures, and the baby is not jittery at this time. You agree with the nurse's assessment of mildly decreased tone.

The anterior fontanel is flat. The baby's pupils are equal and reactive to light. The corneal, oculocephalic, and gag reflexes are present.

3. As the Core Step in the Neurology Sequence, you complete the Encephalopathy Assessment Table.

Category	Normal	Mild	Moderate	Severe
Level of alertness	☐ Alert, normal sleep–wake cycles	☐ Hyperalert	☐ Lethargy	☐ Stupor or coma
Spontaneous activity	☐ Normal	☐ Normal	☐ Decreased activity	☐ No activity
Posture	☐ Flexed	☐ Mild distal flexion	☐ Arms flexed, legs extended (decorticate)	☐ Arms and legs extended (decerebrate)
Tone	☐ Normal	☐ Normal to mild hypotonia	☐ Hypotonic	☐ Flaccid
Primitive reflexes	☐ Normal suck and Moro	☐ Weak suck, strong Moro	☐ Weak suck, incomplete Moro	☐ Absent suck, absent Moro
Autonomic (one of) Pupils Heart rate Respirations	☐ Reactive ☐ Normal ☐ Normal	☐ Dilated reactive ☐ Tachycardia ☐ Normal	☐ Constricted ☐ Bradycardia ☐ Periodic breathing	☐ Dilated or nonreactive ☐ Variable heart rate ☐ Apnea
Seizures	☐ None	☐ None	☐ Common	☐ Uncommon

Your assessment is that she does not show signs of moderate or severe encephalopathy.

4. How do you Organize Care for this infant?

While considering your working diagnosis and what blood work to order, the nurse tells you she noted contractions on the mother's arrival to the ER. The initial fetal HR tracing showed late decelerations and minimal variability.

A scalp pH was unobtainable because the cervix was closed, and the presenting part had not yet descended. The obstetrician opted to proceed with Caesarean section. A cord blood gas was obtained at time of birth.

Apgar scores were 1 at 1 min, 3 at 5 min, and 5 at 10 min. The baby required bag-and-mask ventilation for 11 min, after which she began to breathe spontaneously.

You perform a focused physical examination.

The baby's appearance, growth parameters, and head circumference are normal. You note that she is becoming sleepier yet rousable. Suck, grasp, and Moro reflexes are all present. You see no abnormal movement suggestive of seizures and the baby is not jittery at this time.

While checking for abnormal tone, you note that the baby's popliteal angle is 130°. Also, the pull-to-sit manoeuvre shows her head has a moderate lag in extension. On ventral suspension, her head is raised but not to the body axis, and her back is slightly curved.

5. What could these signs indicate?

_____

_____

The baby continues to breathe regularly at 54 breaths/min. HR is 160 bpm, the pulses are easy to palpate over the femoral arteries, and BP is normal.

You learn that the cord arterial pH was 6.98, with a base deficit of 18 mmol/L.

6. How would you describe these blood gas results? Is there need for immediate intervention?

☐ Respiratory acidosis   ☐ Respiratory alkalosis

☐ Metabolic acidosis   ☐ Metabolic alkalosis

7. What do you suspect the working diagnosis to be?

You exit the Neurology Sequence to complete the other sequences in your Problem List in order of priority. A 'to-do' list of investigations is identified and being worked on by your team. You reassess this baby using the Primary Survey and Consolidated Core Steps, and re-enter the Neurology Sequence to consider Specific Diagnosis and Management.

The only positive findings so far are low tone and some lethargy. You feel this baby has mild encephalopathy and is at risk for progressing to moderate to severe HIE.

You decide to observe her closely and actively manage her temperature to maintain strict normothermia. An aEEG is not available at your site. You place a call to your referral centre for advice.

8. What five key pieces of information obtained from your focused history assist with a provisional diagnosis?

1)

2)

3)

4)

5)

One of the questions raised as you completed the ACoRN Primary Survey was whether this baby with Alerting Signs on the Neurology Sequence should be orally fed.

9. How do you determine whether this baby should be orally fed?

_____

_____

In consultation with the transport coordinating physician, you decide to keep the baby NPO and start IV fluids.

Continue to use the ACoRN Primary Survey and Sequences, rechecking blood glucose and the Encephalopathy Assessment Table on an hourly basis.

Neurology: Case 2—A 2-h-old baby with seizures (*continued from Case 1*)

The baby is now 2 h old. An intravenous with D10W at 3 mL/kg/h is infusing. She is lying quietly in her incubator, breathing easily, and remains pink in room air.

You take a BP reading (normal) and auscultate heart and lungs. The HR is 120 bpm and regular. Blood glucose has remained > 3.3 mmol/L.

You notice the baby's left arm starting to twitch rhythmically. Observing her movements carefully, you see rhythmic, coarse, jerky movements in all extremities which do not stop when held. Also, her eyes deviate to the left, and she has a glazed look. The episode lasts 20 seconds.

1. Is this baby having a seizure?

☐ Yes ☐ No

2. Which of the following signs are associated with seizures?

☐ A glazed look.
☐ Eye deviation.
☐ Abnormal movements precipitated by doing BP.
☐ Fine oscillatory tremors.
☐ Inability to suppress movements with flexion.
☐ Generalization of abnormal movements to all extremities.

You determine the baby shows none of the Alerting Signs for Resuscitation and quickly repeat the Primary Survey and the Consolidated Core Steps.

Now her SpO2 is 92% in room air, the airway is clear, and there are no abnormalities on auscultation of the chest. The blood glucose done at the bedside is 3.9 mmol/L.

There are no Alerting Signs from the ACoRN Respiratory or Cardiovascular Sequences. You re-enter the ACoRN Neurology Sequence, reviewing the Alerting Signs and completing the Core Steps.

On focused neurologic assessment, the baby is lethargic and hypotonic, and spontaneous activity has decreased. Her posture is in mild distal flexion. She has a weak suck and incomplete Moro reflex. Her pupils are small but reactive to light. Respiration is regular and airway secretions minimal.

You redo the Encephalopathy Assessment Table using the new information.

3. How would you complete the Encephalopathy Assessment Table now?

Category	Normal	Mild	Moderate	Severe
Level of alertness	☐ Alert, normal sleep–wake cycles	☐ Hyperalert	☐ Lethargy	☐ Stupor or coma
Spontaneous activity	☐ Normal	☐ Normal	☐ Decreased activity	☐ No activity
Posture	☐ Flexed	☐ Mild distal flexion	☐ Arms flexed, legs extended (decorticate)	☐ Arms and legs extended (decerebrate)
Tone	☐ Normal	☐ Normal to mild hypotonia	☐ Hypotonic	☐ Flaccid
Primitive reflexes	☐ Normal suck and Moro	☐ Weak suck, strong Moro	☐ Weak suck, incomplete Moro	☐ Absent suck, absent Moro
Autonomic (one of)				
Pupils	☐ Reactive	☐ Dilated reactive	☐ Constricted	☐ Dilated or nonreactive
Heart rate	☐ Normal	☐ Tachycardia	☐ Bradycardia	☐ Variable heart rate
Respirations	☐ Normal	☐ Normal	☐ Periodic breathing	☐ Apnea
Seizures	☐ None	☐ None	☐ Common	☐ Uncommon

The table now indicates the baby has several signs of moderate encephalopathy, including seizures.

You approach Organization of Care for this baby based on her blood glucose being in the normal range and the presence of seizures. This baby is not hypoglycemic, but seizure-like activity is present, and she has risks for HIE. You decide to order phenobarbital.

4. How much phenobarbital will you give and how will you direct your staff to give it?

_____

_____

You administer the phenobarbital and continue documenting the seizure activity of this baby.

5. Based on the information collected so far, how would you describe the seizure this baby is having?

Time/ duration	Suppress by holding	Origin/ spread	Eye/ mouth movements	Level of alertness	Autonomic changes	Other signs

With the presence of seizures in the setting of risk factors for HIE, the categorization of moderate encephalopathy can now be made.

You place a second call to the referral centre, and they agree with the diagnosis of HIE. The baby qualifies for therapeutic hypothermia: there is moderate encephalopathy, her gestational age is 37 weeks, and she is 2 h old. Discussion ensues as to whether passive cooling for therapeutic hypothermia should be initiated before arrival of the transport team. Review your regional hypothermia protocol and ACoRN Appendix A.

The parents ask, 'How can we tell if our baby will be okay?'

6. What information would you convey to parents at this point?

_____

_____

On arrival, the transport team assumes care of the infant and prepares to continue therapeutic hypothermia during transport.

Neurology: Case 3—A newborn whose mother has reported using an illicit substance

A 20-h-old baby boy is currently rooming in with his mother. His nurse reports he has been jittery and irritable. You find, from the birth record, that he was born at 39 weeks GA to a 21-yo primigravida and weighs 3000 g. The mother had no documented prenatal care, and no concerns were identified during labour and birth.

In the observation area of the nursery, the nurse is rocking the baby, trying to console him because he has been crying constantly.

1. **Complete the ACoRN Primary Survey and Consolidated Core Steps, and generate a Problem List with the infant in the nurse's arms.**

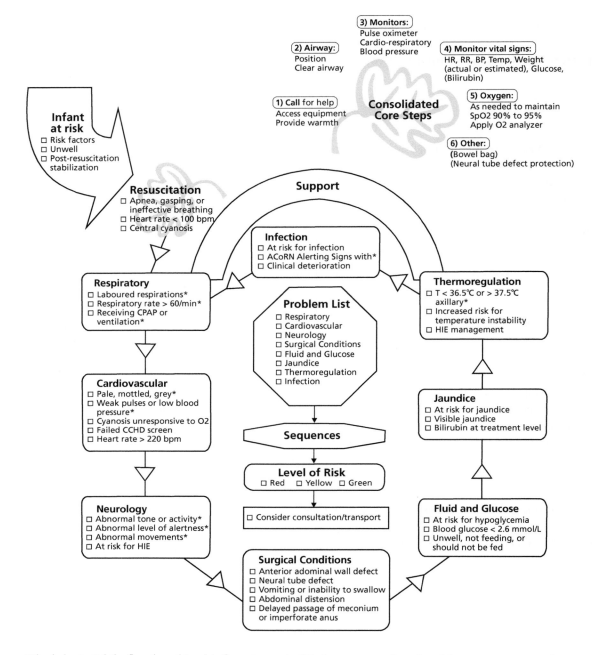

The baby is tightly flexed, sucking his fists vigorously. His legs are tremulous, but this movement stops when you hold his feet. Vital signs are stable and within normal limits. He has been bottle-fed 4 times since birth, and his mother has declined to breastfeed. The nurses have noticed his suck is not well coordinated.

The baby has no Alerting Signs in the Respiratory or Cardiovascular Sequences. Abnormal movements are witnessed, and you are concerned that his tone is increased. The Consolidated Core Steps add the following information: point of care glucose is 4.5 mmol/L and temperature is 37°C.

The Neurology Sequence is the first sequence identified in your prioritized Problem List.

As indicated in the Core Steps, you complete the Encephalopathy Assessment Table and determine he has no signs to indicate an encephalopathy.

You continue down the Neurology Sequence.

2. How do you Organize Care for this infant?

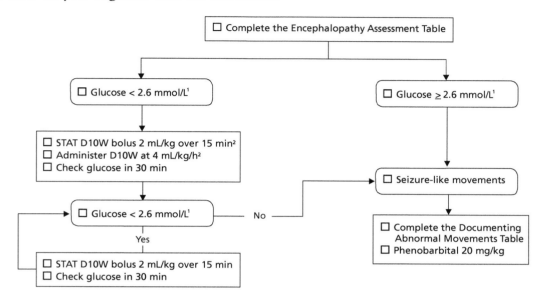

3. Is this baby having seizures? Why or why not?

_____

_____

You Organize Care based on these findings and proceed to Next Steps.

The mother says she used heroin during her pregnancy, including on the day of delivery. She has no co-existing medical conditions. She came to hospital fully dilated and delivered quickly. Membranes ruptured at the time of delivery. No paternal history is available. The baby was vigorous at birth. Apgar scores were 8 at 1 min and 9 at 5 min. No resuscitation was required.

On examination, the baby is irritable and yawns and sneezes frequently. He has a shrill cry and is difficult to console. He wakes crying approximately 30 min after each feed. Tone is high and he startles easily. There are no other positive physical findings.

You order a complete blood count and differential but feel that no other blood work is indicated at this time. Your index of suspicion for infection is made lower by the identification of a likely explanation for this infant's presentation. Your working diagnosis is NAS. The baby remains with mother in couplet care, supported by the nursing staff. She maintains oral feeding with a normal glucose, so there is no need to enter the Fluid and Glucose or Thermoregulation Sequences. The possibility of infection remains on your differential, but there are no additional risk factors. You elect to observe this infant closely and await the results of your complete blood count and differential before ordering a blood culture and starting antibiotics.

You place a call to the attending paediatrician to review your findings and plan management. Your Level of Risk assignment for this baby will depend on the infant's response to environmental and nonpharmacologic supportive measures and the level of care available at your facility.

Nonpharmacological comfort measures are initiated by the nursing staff.

You ensure the baby will be nursed in a quiet setting, with lights dimmed and lower noise levels. Nonnutritive sucking, swaddling, and kangaroo care may help to settle this baby.

Scoring is initiated using your nursery's standard protocol.

4. Determine the infant's NAS score by completing the following table.

Neonatal abstinence syndrome score

System	Signs and symptoms	Score	Time					Comments
Central nervous system	Excessive high-pitched cry	2						
	Continuous high-pitched cry	3						
	Sleeps < 1 h after feeding	3						
	Sleeps < 2 h after feeding	2						
	Sleeps < 3 h after feeding	1						
	Hyperactive Moro reflex	2						
	Markedly hyperactive Moro reflex	3						
	Tremors disturbed	2						
	Mild tremors undisturbed	3						
	Moderate-to-severe tremors undisturbed	4						
	Increased muscle tone	2						
	Excoriation (specify area)	1						
	Myoclonic jerks	3						
	Generalized convulsions	5						
Metabolic Vasomotor Respiratory	Sweating	1						
	Fever 37.5°C to 38.3°C	1						
	Fever >38.4°C	2						
	Frequent yawning > 4 sec/interval	1						
	Mottling	1						
	Nasal stuffiness	1						
	Frequent sneezing > 4×/interval	1						
	Nasal flaring	2						
	Respiratory rate > 60/min	1						
	Respiratory rate > 60/min + retractions	2						
GI	Excessive sucking	1						
	Poor feeding	1						
	Regurgitation	2						
	Projectile vomiting	3						
	Loose stools	2						
	Watery stools	3						
Total Score								
Scorer's initials								

Adapted from Finnegan L, Connaughton JF Jr, Kron RE, Emich JP. Neonatal abstinence syndrome: Assessment and management. Addict Dis 1975;2(1–2):141–58.

Despite nonpharmacological measures, the baby has increasing severity of symptoms that do not appear to be influenced by environment.

5. What are your next steps?

_____

_____

_____

_____

Bibliography

American Academy of Pediatrics, Committee on Drugs. Neonatal drug withdrawal. Pediatrics 2012;129(2):e540–60.

Armentrout DC, Caple J. The jittery newborn. J Pediatr Health Care 2001;15(3):147–9.

Blume HK, Li CI, Loch CM, Koepsell TD. Intrapartum fever and chorioamnionitis as risks for encephalopathy in term newborns: A case-control study. Dev Med Child Neurol 2008;50(1):19–24.

de Vries LS, Toet MC. Amplitude integrated electroencephalography in the full-term newborn. Clin Perinatol 2006;33(3):619–32.

Finnegan L, Connaughton JF Jr., Kron RE, Emich JP. Neonatal abstinence syndrome: Assessment and management. Addict Dis 1975;2(1–2):141–58.

Grossman MR, Lipshaw M, Osborn RR, Berkwitt AK. A novel approach to assessing infants with neonatal abstinence syndrome. Hosp Pediatr 2018;8(1):1–8.

Gunn AJ, Bennet L. Timing of injury in the fetus and neonate. Curr Opin Obstet Gynecol 2008;20(2):175–81.

Hendson L, Shah V, Trkulja S; Canadian Paediatric Society, Fetus and Newborn Committee. Selective serotonin reuptake inhibitors or serotonin-norepinephrine reuptake inhibitors in pregnancy: Infant and childhood outcomes. In press: www.cps.ca/en/documents/position/SSRI-infant-outcomes.

Hill A. Development of tone and reflexes in the fetus and newborn. In: Polin RA, Fox WW, eds. Fetal and Neonatal Physiology, 2nd edn. Philadelphia, PA: W. B. Saunders; 1998.

Huntsman RJ, Lowery NJ, Sankaran K. Nonepileptic motor phenomena in the neonate. Paaediatr Child Health 2008;13(8):680–4.

Jacobs SE, Morely CJ, Inder TE, et al. Whole-body hypothermia for term and near-term newborns with hypoxic ischemic encephalopathy. Arch Pediatr Adolesc Med 2011;165(8):692–700.

Lacaze-Masmonteil T, O'Flaherty P, CPS Fetus and Newborn Committee. Managing infants born to mothers who have used opioids during pregnancy. Updated June 28, 2018: www.cps.ca/en/documents/position/opioids-during-pregnancy.

Laptook AR. Use of therapeutic hypothermia for term infants with hypoxic-ischemic encephalopathy. Pediatr Clin North Am 2009;56(3):601–16.

Laptook A, Tyson J, Shankaran S, et al. National Institute of Child Health and Human Development Neonatal Research Network. Elevated temperature after hypoxic-ischemic encephalopathy: Risk factor for adverse outcomes. Pediatrics 2008;122(3):491–9.

Lemyre B, Chau V, Canadian Paediatric Society; Fetus and Newborn Committee. Hypothermia for newborns with hypoxic ischemic encephalopathy. Paediatr Child Health 2018;23(4):285–91.

Minnesota Hospital Association. Neonatal Abstinence Syndrome (NAS) Toolkit: www.mnhospitals.org/Portals/0/Documents/patientsafety/Perinatal/Neonatal%20Abstinence%20Syndrome%20Toolkit.pdf

Mizrahi EM. Neonatal seizures and neonatal epileptic syndromes. Neurol Clinics 2001;19(2):427–63.

Moulsdale W, Hermann S. In utero exposure to selective serotonin reuptake inhibitors: Evidence for poor neonatal adaptation. Newborn Infant Nurs Rev 2008;8(3):123–30.

O'Grady MJ, Hopewell J, White MJ. Management of neonatal abstinence syndrome: A national survey and review of practice. Arch Dis Child Fetal Neonatal Ed 2009;94(4):F249–52.

Osborn DA, Jeffery HE, Cole MJ. Opiate treatment for opiate withdrawal in newborn infants. Cochrane Database Syst Rev 2010 Oct 6: https://doi.org/10.1002/14651858.CD002059.pub3

Osborn DA, Jeffery HE, Cole MJ. Sedatives for opiate withdrawal in newborn infants. Cochrane Database Syst Rev 2010 Oct 6: https://doi.org/10.1002/14651858.CD002053.pub3

Pellock JM. Other nonepileptic paroxysmal disorders. In: Wyllie E, Cascino GD, Gidal BE, Goodkin HP, eds. Wyllie's Treatment of Epilepsy: Principles and Practice, 5th ed. Philidelphia, PA: Wolters Kluwer, Lippincott Williams & Wilkins; 2011.

Ringer SA, Aziz K. Neonatal stabilization and postresuscitative care. Clin Perinatol 2012;39(4):901–18.

Sarnat HB, Sarnat MS. Neonatal encephalopathy following fetal distress: A clinical and electroencephalographic study. Arch Neurol 1976;33(10):696–705.

Shankaran S, Laptook A, Ehrenkranz RA, et al. Whole-body hypothermia for neonates with hypoxic-ischemic encephalopathy. N Engl J Med 2005;353(15):1574–84.

Society of Obstetricians and Gynecologists of Canada. Fetal health surveillance: Antepartum and intrapartum consensus guideline. SOGC CPG No. 197, September 2007. https://sogc.org/wp-content/uploads/2013/01/gui197CPG0709r.pdf (Accessed April 1, 2017)

Task Force on Neonatal Encephalopathy and Cerebral Palsy. Neonatal encephalopathy and cerebral palsy: Defining the pathogenesis and pathophysiology. Washington, DC: American College of Obstetricians and Gynecologists and American Academy of Pediatrics; 2003.

Thibeault-Eybalin MP, Lortie A, Carmant L. Neonatal seizures: Do they damage the brain? Pediatr Neurol 2009;40(3):175–80.

Volpe JJ. Neurology of the Newborn, 5th ed. Philadelphia, PA: W. B. Saunders; 2008.

Wirrell EC. Neonatal seizures: To treat or not to treat? Semin Pediatr Neurol 2005;12(2):97–105.

Young TE, Mangum B. Neofax 2008. Raleigh, NC: Thomson Reuters; 2008.

Answer key: Neurology Case 1—The floppy baby

1. **Complete the ACoRN Primary Survey and Consolidated Core Steps, and generate a Problem List.**

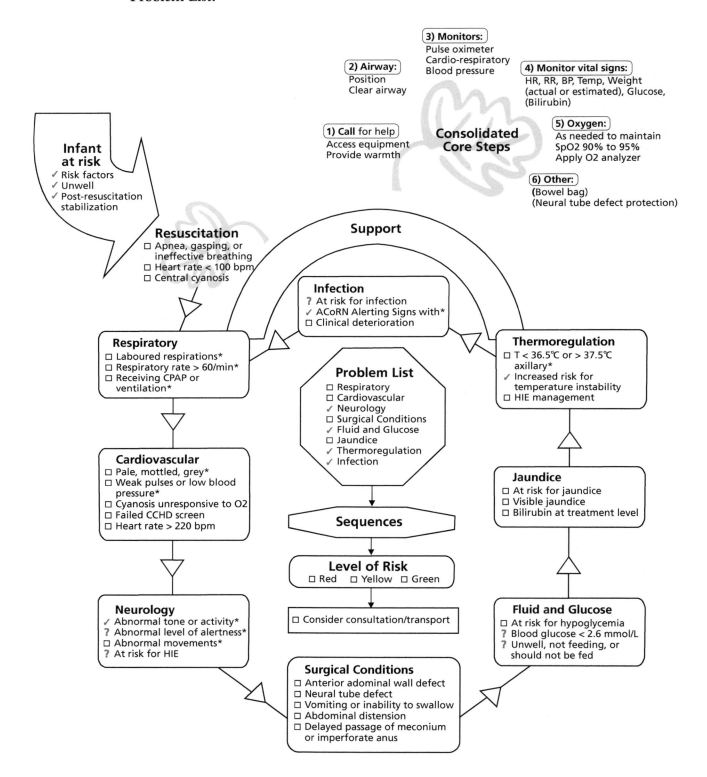

3) Monitors:
Pulse oximeter
Cardio-respiratory
Blood pressure

2) Airway:
Position
Clear airway

4) Monitor vital signs:
HR, RR, BP, Temp, Weight
(actual or estimated), Glucose,
(Bilirubin)

1) Call for help
Access equipment
Provide warmth

Consolidated Core Steps

5) Oxygen:
As needed to maintain
SpO2 90% to 95%
Apply O2 analyzer

6) Other:
(Bowel bag)
(Neural tube defect protection)

Infant at risk
✓ Risk factors
✓ Unwell
✓ Post-resuscitation stabilization

Resuscitation
☐ Apnea, gasping, or ineffective breathing
☐ Heart rate < 100 bpm
☐ Central cyanosis

Support

Infection
? At risk for infection
✓ ACoRN Alerting Signs with*
☐ Clinical deterioration

Respiratory
☐ Laboured respirations*
☐ Respiratory rate > 60/min*
☐ Receiving CPAP or ventilation*

Thermoregulation
☐ T < 36.5℃ or > 37.5℃ axillary*
✓ Increased risk for temperature instability
☐ HIE management

Problem List
☐ Respiratory
☐ Cardiovascular
✓ Neurology
☐ Surgical Conditions
✓ Fluid and Glucose
☐ Jaundice
✓ Thermoregulation
✓ Infection

Cardiovascular
☐ Pale, mottled, grey*
☐ Weak pulses or low blood pressure*
☐ Cyanosis unresponsive to O2
☐ Failed CCHD screen
☐ Heart rate > 220 bpm

Jaundice
☐ At risk for jaundice
☐ Visible jaundice
☐ Bilirubin at treatment level

Sequences

Level of Risk
☐ Red   ☐ Yellow   ☐ Green

Neurology
✓ Abnormal tone or activity*
? Abnormal level of alertness*
☐ Abnormal movements*
? At risk for HIE

☐ Consider consultation/transport

Fluid and Glucose
☐ At risk for hypoglycemia
? Blood glucose < 2.6 mmol/L
? Unwell, not feeding, or should not be fed

Surgical Conditions
☐ Anterior adominal wall defect
☐ Neural tube defect
☐ Vomiting or inability to swallow
☐ Abdominal distension
☐ Delayed passage of meconium or imperforate anus

The Primary Survey identifies no Alerting Signs in the Respiratory or Cardiovascular Sequences.

More information is needed about this baby's risk for HIE and level of alertness (?'s), but she has abnormal tone, requiring further stabilization (✓) in the Neurology Sequence.

Under Fluid and Glucose, we do not yet know her blood glucose (?), and we are not sure whether her neurologic status is appropriate for feeding (?).

She is at increased risk for thermoregulatory issues (✓) because she is on a radiant warmer.

The baby has Alerting Signs with an asterisk (*), indicating the need to consider infection.

2. Neurology is the first sequence identified. Which Alerting Signs would you mark? Why?

Neurology
✓ Abnormal tone or activity*
? Abnormal level of alertness*
  Abnormal movements*
? At risk for HIE

The nurse reported that this baby had low tone and you witnessed her positioned on the radiant warmer with arms and legs extended—at 37 weeks GA you would expect a healthy newborn to display a flexed position.

The history does not provide you with enough information to confirm or comment on her level of alertness or risk for HIE. You need to gather additional information, so you place a **?** beside both of these Alerting Signs.

No abnormal movements have been observed, so this Alerting Sign is left blank.

3. As the Core Step in the Neurology Sequence, you complete the Encephalopathy Assessment Table.

Category	Normal	Mild	Moderate	Severe
Level of alertness	✓ Alert, normal sleep–wake cycles	☐ Hyperalert	☐ Lethargy	☐ Stupor or coma
Spontaneous activity	✓ Normal	☐ Normal	☐ Decreased activity	☐ No activity
Posture	☐ Flexed	✓ Mild distal flexion	☐ Arms flexed, legs extended (decorticate)	☐ Arms and legs extended (decerebrate)
Tone	☐ Normal	✓ Normal to mild hypotonia	☐ Hypotonic	☐ Flaccid
Primitive reflexes	✓ Normal suck and Moro	☐ Weak suck, strong Moro	☐ Weak suck, incomplete Moro	☐ Absent suck, absent Moro
Autonomic (one of) Pupils Heart rate Respirations	✓ Reactive ✓ Normal ✓ Normal	☐ Dilated reactive ☐ Tachycardia ☐ Normal	☐ Constricted ☐ Bradycardia ☐ Periodic breathing	☐ Dilated or nonreactive ☐ Variable heart rate ☐ Apnea
Seizures	✓ None	☐ None	☐ Common	☐ Uncommon

This baby does not have findings in the 'moderate' or 'severe' column in three or more categories, and there have been no concerns about seizures. She does not meet the criteria for moderate or severe encephalopathy.

4. How do you Organize Care for this infant?

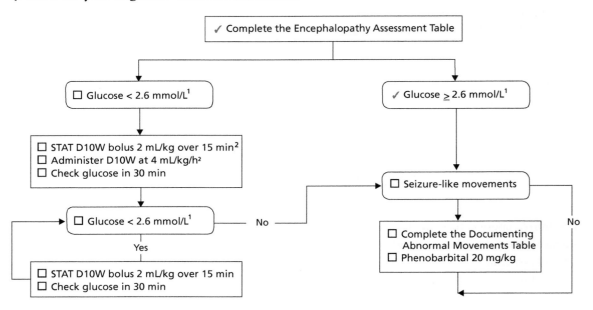

The baby presented with abnormal tone and blood glucose of 3.5 mmol/L. Organization of Care is based on normal blood glucose levels and absence of seizure-like movements, and you proceed to Next Steps.

5. What could these signs indicate?

These signs (popliteal angle is 130°, moderate head lag in extension and, on ventral suspension, her head is raised but not to body axis and back is slightly curved) all suggest decreased tone (hypotonia).

6. How would you describe these blood gas results? Is there need for immediate intervention?

☐ Respiratory acidosis   ☐ Respiratory alkalosis
✓ Metabolic acidosis   ☐ Metabolic alkalosis

These results are consistent with a metabolic acidosis. This baby has no Alerting Signs from the ACoRN Resuscitation, Respiratory, or Cardiovascular Sequences. Therefore, there is no need at this time to consider treating the metabolic acidosis indicated by the base deficit of 18 mmol/L.

With adequate cardiorespiratory function, you anticipate that metabolic acidosis will gradually resolve on its own.

7. What do you suspect the working diagnosis to be?

You suspect a working diagnosis of early-stage neonatal encephalopathy, based on intrapartum findings (e.g., poor variability and late decelerations), an urgent Caesarean section, placental abruption, the baby's condition at birth (i.e., Apgar scores 1, 3, and 5 at 1, 5, and 10 min; bag-and-mask ventilation × 11 min;

spontaneous respirations thereafter), cord blood gas results (i.e., metabolic acidosis), and the current physical findings (i.e., stable vital signs, mild hypotonia).

8. What five key pieces of information obtained from your focused history assist with a provisional diagnosis?

1) Late decelerations and minimal variability on the electronic fetal monitoring tracing.
2) Apgar scores of 1 at 1 min, 3 at 5 min, and 5 at 10 min.
3) Requirement for bag and mask ventilation for 11 minutes.
4) Persistent hypotonia.
5) Cord gases—acidosis and increased base deficit.

9. How do you determine whether this baby should be orally fed?

An infant should not be fed unless level of alertness is normal, the airway protective reflexes (gag and cough) are present, and the suck–swallow mechanism is mature. The suck–swallow mechanism involves rooting and coordinated sucking and swallowing.

In a baby that is just born, it is reasonable to give some time to see if the situation resolves and feeding is deemed safe. It is recommended that the decision to feed orally be made within 1 h from birth for an asymptomatic newborn, and earlier for preterm or symptomatic babies. If not feeding, blood glucose should be monitored closely.

Answer key: Neurology Case 2—A 2-h-old baby with seizures (*continued from Case 1*)

1. Is this baby having a seizure?

✓ Yes   ☐ No

2. Which of the following signs are associated with seizures?

✓ A glazed look.
✓ Eye deviation.
☐ Abnormal movements precipitated by doing BP.
☐ Fine oscillatory tremors.
✓ Inability to suppress movements with flexion.
✓ Generalization of abnormal movements to all extremities.

3. How would you complete the Encephalopathy Assessment Table now?

Category	Normal	Mild	Moderate	Severe
Level of alertness	☐ Alert, normal sleep wake cycles	☐ Hyperalert	✓ Lethargy	☐ Stupor or coma
Spontaneous activity	☐ Normal	☐ Normal	✓ Decreased activity	☐ No activity
Posture	☐ Flexed	✓ Mild distal flexion	☐ Arms flexed, legs extended (decorticate)	☐ Arms and legs extended (decerebrate)

Tone	☐ Normal	☐ Normal to mild hypotonia	✓ Hypotonic	☐ Flaccid
Primitive reflexes	☐ Normal suck and Moro	☐ Weak suck, strong Moro	✓ Weak suck, incomplete Moro	☐ Absent suck, absent Moro
Autonomic (one of)				
Pupils	☐ Reactive	☐ Dilated reactive	✓ Constricted	☐ Dilated or nonreactive
Heart rate	✓ Normal	☐ Tachycardia	☐ Bradycardia	☐ Variable heart rate
Respirations	✓ Normal	☐ Normal	☐ Periodic breathing	☐ Apnea
Seizures	☐ None	☐ None	✓ Common	☐ Uncommon

The table now indicates the baby has several signs of moderate encephalopathy, including seizures in a clinical setting consistent with HIE.

4. How much phenobarbital will you give and how will you direct your staff to give it?

20 mg/kg intravenously, 20 mg/kg × 3.5 kg = 70 mg, IV over 20 min (maximum rate = 1 mg/kg/min).

5. Based on the information collected so far, how would you describe the seizure this baby is having?

Time/ duration	Suppress by holding	Origin/ spread	Eye/ mouth movements	Level of alertness	Autonomic changes	Other signs
09:00 at 2 h of age Lasted 20 sec	No	Left arm, then all extremities	Eyes deviated to left	Glazed look	No	No

In combination with Table 5.6, you document the seizure as clonic, multifocal, and subtle and note the time and duration of seizure activity.

6. What information would you convey to parents at this point?
- Their question cannot be answered immediately with certainty.
- Not all babies with seizures/encephalopathy develop long-term sequelae.
- Further tests and observation of her condition in hospital will help determine the degree of CNS injury and level of risk for long-term sequelae.
- Long-term outcome will only be certain as development is observed over time.

Answer key: Neurology Case 3—Baby born to a mother who reported using an illicit substance

1. Complete the ACoRN Primary Survey and Consolidated Core Steps, and generate a Problem List with the infant in the nurse's arms.

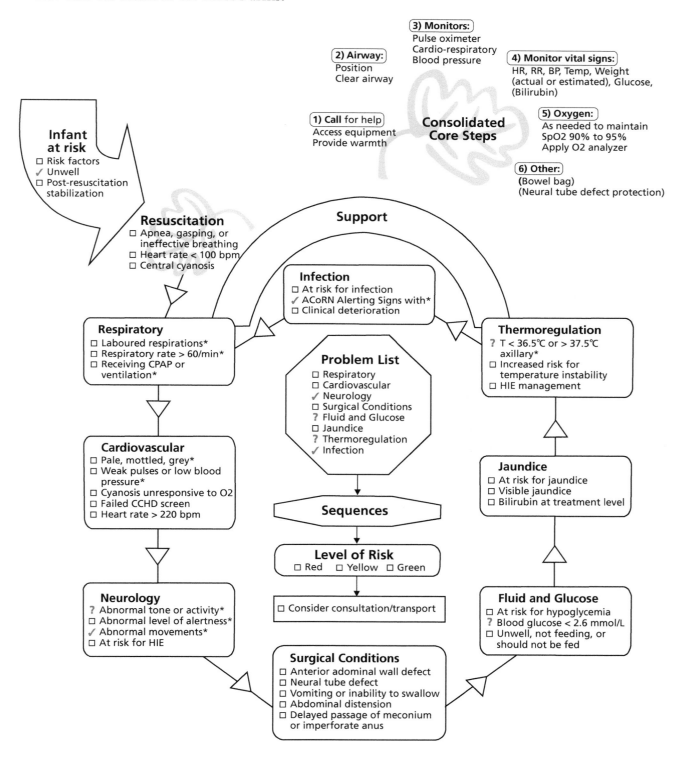

3) Monitors:
Pulse oximeter
Cardio-respiratory
Blood pressure

2) Airway:
Position
Clear airway

4) Monitor vital signs:
HR, RR, BP, Temp, Weight
(actual or estimated), Glucose,
(Bilirubin)

1) Call for help
Access equipment
Provide warmth

**Consolidated
Core Steps**

5) Oxygen:
As needed to maintain
SpO2 90% to 95%
Apply O2 analyzer

6) Other:
(Bowel bag)
(Neural tube defect protection)

**Infant
at risk**
☐ Risk factors
✓ Unwell
☐ Post-resuscitation
stabilization

Support

Resuscitation
☐ Apnea, gasping, or
ineffective breathing
☐ Heart rate < 100 bpm
☐ Central cyanosis

Infection
☐ At risk for infection
✓ ACoRN Alerting Signs with*
☐ Clinical deterioration

Respiratory
☐ Laboured respirations*
☐ Respiratory rate > 60/min*
☐ Receiving CPAP or
ventilation*

Problem List
☐ Respiratory
☐ Cardiovascular
✓ Neurology
☐ Surgical Conditions
? Fluid and Glucose
☐ Jaundice
? Thermoregulation
✓ Infection

Thermoregulation
? T < 36.5℃ or > 37.5℃
axillary*
☐ Increased risk for
temperature instability
☐ HIE management

Cardiovascular
☐ Pale, mottled, grey*
☐ Weak pulses or low blood
pressure*
☐ Cyanosis unresponsive to O2
☐ Failed CCHD screen
☐ Heart rate > 220 bpm

Sequences

Jaundice
☐ At risk for jaundice
☐ Visible jaundice
☐ Bilirubin at treatment level

Level of Risk
☐ Red   ☐ Yellow   ☐ Green

Neurology
? Abnormal tone or activity*
☐ Abnormal level of alertness*
✓ Abnormal movements*
☐ At risk for HIE

☐ Consider consultation/transport

Fluid and Glucose
☐ At risk for hypoglycemia
? Blood glucose < 2.6 mmol/L
☐ Unwell, not feeding, or
should not be fed

Surgical Conditions
☐ Anterior adominal wall defect
☐ Neural tube defect
☐ Vomiting or inability to swallow
☐ Abdominal distension
☐ Delayed passage of meconium
or imperforate anus

The baby has no Alerting Signs in the Respiratory or Cardiovascular Sequences. Abnormal movements have been observed and you are concerned about increased tone. However, while his tone may appear to be increased, this determination requires more assessment than just observation and should be present centrally as well as peripherally. It is not wrong to place a **?** here if you are uncertain. It will remind you to reassess this Alerting Sign as you proceed. This baby has no obvious risk factors for HIE. The Consolidated Core Steps established that glucose and temperature are normal. You can remove the **?** marks from the Fluid and Glucose and Thermoregulation Sequences. They are also removed from your Problem List, and you do not need to enter these sequences at present. This baby has been feeding and, although he has been reported as poorly coordinated, he is maintaining a stable blood glucose. He has one ACoRN Alerting Sign with *****, so infection is being considered.

2. How do you Organize Care for this infant?

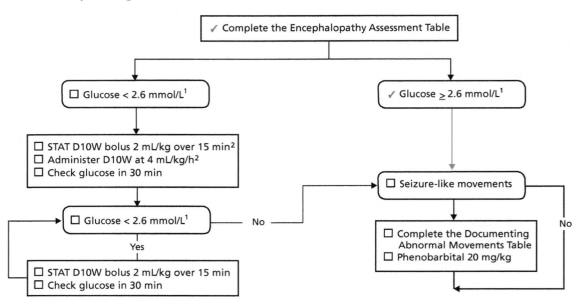

This infant's glucose is 4.6 mmol/L. At this point in the Organization of Care, you need to determine whether this infant's abnormal movements are consistent with seizures.

3. Is this baby having seizures? Why or why not?

No, the baby is not having seizures because movements stop when extremities are held. You organize care based on the normal glucose reading and absence of seizures, and proceed to Next Steps.

4. Determine the infant's NAS score by completing the following table.

Neonatal abstinence syndrome score

System	Signs and symptoms	Score	Time					Comments
			10:15					
Central nervous system	Excessive high-pitched cry	2	2					
	Continuous high-pitched cry	3						
	Sleeps < 1 h after feeding	3	3					
	Sleeps < 2 h after feeding	2						
	Sleeps < 3 h after feeding	1						
	Hyperactive Moro reflex	2	2					
	Markedly hyperactive Moro reflex	3						
	Tremors disturbed	2	3					
	Mild tremors undisturbed	3						
	Moderate-to-severe tremors undisturbed	4						
	Increased muscle tone	2						
	Excoriation (specify area)	1						
	Myoclonic jerks	3						
	Generalized convulsions	5						
Metabolic Vasomotor Respiratory	Sweating	1						
	Fever 37.5°C to 38.3°C	1						
	Fever > 38.4°C	2						
	Frequent yawning > 4 sec/ interval	1	1					
	Mottling	1						
	Nasal stuffiness	1	1					
	Frequent sneezing > 4 × /interval	1	1					
	Nasal flaring	2						
	Respiratory rate > 60/min	1						
	Respiratory rate > 60/min + retractions	2						
GI	Excessive sucking	1						
	Poor feeding	1	1					
	Regurgitation	2						
	Projectile vomiting	3						
	Loose stools	2						
	Watery stools	3						
Total Score			14					
Scorer's initials			*AS*					

The baby's scores are elevated, and the history and physical exam are consistent with NAS. Nonpharmacologic measures are initiated but are not successful in controlling the baby's symptoms.

5. What are your next steps?

You counsel the mother about how to assess her baby's level of comfort and what additional calming measures she can use.

- The initial score, at around 2 h of age, reflects baseline behaviour. Subsequent scores are performed at 4-h intervals.
- If a score is 8 or greater, scoring is completed every 2 h, until 24 h from the last score of 8.
- A higher score implies greater severity.
- If scores consistently remain under 8 until an infant is 48 h of age, continue observation every 8 h for 5 to 7 days to help detect late withdrawal.

You administer morphine in accordance with your regional protocol to treat the ongoing symptoms. Scoring is continued to help titrate the morphine dose. You counsel the mother about how to assess her baby's level of comfort and what additional calming measures she can use.

Surgical Conditions

Educational objectives

Upon completion of this chapter, you will be able to:

- Identify infants needing stabilization for a surgical condition.
- Apply the Acute Care of at-Risk Newborns (ACoRN) Surgical Conditions Sequence.
- Provide immediate management for infants with anterior abdominal wall defects.
- Provide immediate management for infants with neural tube defects.
- Identify and provide immediate management for infants suspected of having a gastrointestinal (GI) obstruction, including imperforate anus.
- Recognize the importance of delayed passage of meconium and provide management to these infants.
- Prepare and stabilize a newborn prior to surgical care.
- Recognize when to exit the Surgical Conditions Sequence to other ACoRN sequences.

Key concepts

1. Infants with major surgical conditions require care by a specialized medical-surgical team in a regional facility.
2. Early recognition, preferably in utero, improves quality of care and outcomes.
3. Infants who show one or more of the ACoRN Alerting Signs for surgical conditions should be investigated promptly to identify or exclude pertinent associated conditions and causes.
4. Medical stabilization precedes surgery in all infants presenting with major surgical conditions.
5. The timing of surgical intervention varies based on the condition and degree of medical stabilization. In most cases, surgical intervention can be delayed until optimal medical stabilization is achieved.

Skills

- Bowel bag application (see Appendix A)
- Application of a sterile dressing for neural tube defects
- Nasal gastric tube or Replogle tube insertion
- Gastric suctioning (continuous versus intermittent)
- Basic chest and abdominal radiograph interpretation (see Appendix B)

A number of conditions that may require surgery soon after birth first require stabilization. This chapter focuses on neonatal care and management before surgery for anterior abdominal wall defects, neural tube defects, and GI obstructions. Surgical conditions of the respiratory or cardiovascular system are discussed in their respective ACoRN chapters, and other surgical conditions fall outside the scope of ACoRN.

Most serious surgical anomalies are now detected antenatally. Planning for care at the time of birth can significantly improve the infant's quality of care and outcome. Prenatal diagnosis allows the care team to:

- Identify or exclude associated conditions and causes, such as chromosomal anomalies or genetic syndromes.
- Optimize counselling for parents on potential outcomes, intervention options, and the most appropriate timing, location, and mode of delivery.
- Plan special care requirements. Collaborative care planning will involve the family, the mother's antenatal care provider, maternal–fetal medicine specialists, neonatologists, paediatric surgeons, and geneticists.
- Arrange a family visit to the facility where the mother and infant will be cared for, and a meeting with members of the care team.
- Determine need and timing for prenatal transport or family relocation.

Some surgical conditions, however, are not detected during routine maternal ultrasound examination, or parents may have opted not to receive imaging during pregnancy. Sometimes, too, an infant with a known surgical condition is born early, before the mother travels to a level 3 centre. Newborns with surgical conditions can present at any time, in any facility. Their subsequent care and outcomes depend on:

- Prompt recognition,
- Medical stabilization, and
- Urgent transport to a tertiary facility.

Alerting Signs

An infant who shows one or more of the following Alerting Signs enters the ACoRN Surgical Conditions Sequence.

> **Surgical Conditions**
> ☐ Anterior adominal wall defect
> ☐ Neural tube defect
> ☐ Vomiting or inability to swallow
> ☐ Abdominal distension
> ☐ Delayed passage of meconium or imperforate anus

ACoRN Surgical Conditions Sequence

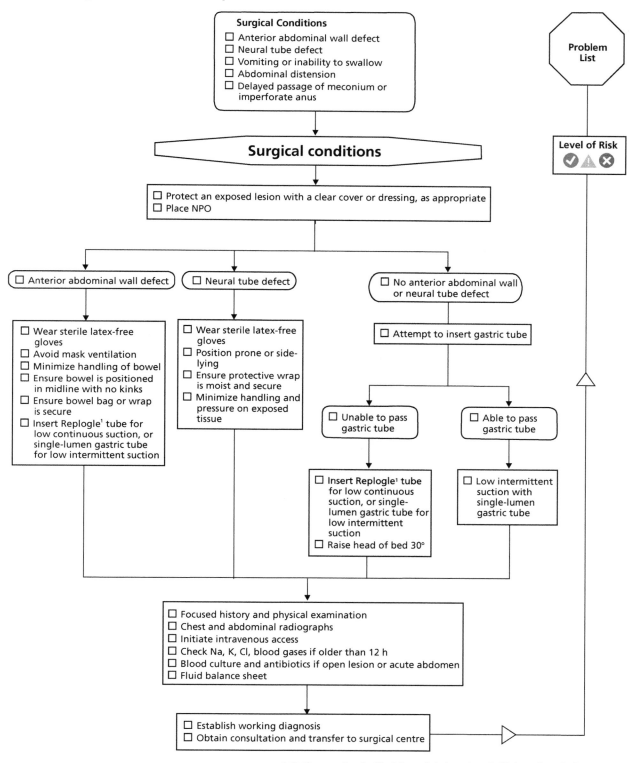

Surgical Conditions
- ☐ Anterior abdominal wall defect
- ☐ Neural tube defect
- ☐ Vomiting or inability to swallow
- ☐ Abdominal distension
- ☐ Delayed passage of meconium or imperforate anus

Problem List

Surgical conditions

Level of Risk ✓ ⚠ ✗

- ☐ Protect an exposed lesion with a clear cover or dressing, as appropriate
- ☐ Place NPO

☐ Anterior abdominal wall defect

☐ Neural tube defect

☐ No anterior abdominal wall or neural tube defect

Anterior abdominal wall defect:
- ☐ Wear sterile latex-free gloves
- ☐ Avoid mask ventilation
- ☐ Minimize handling of bowel
- ☐ Ensure bowel is positioned in midline with no kinks
- ☐ Ensure bowel bag or wrap is secure
- ☐ Insert Replogle[1] tube for low continuous suction, or single-lumen gastric tube for low intermittent suction

Neural tube defect:
- ☐ Wear sterile latex-free gloves
- ☐ Position prone or side-lying
- ☐ Ensure protective wrap is moist and secure
- ☐ Minimize handling and pressure on exposed tissue

☐ Attempt to insert gastric tube

☐ Unable to pass gastric tube

☐ Able to pass gastric tube

- ☐ Insert Replogle[1] tube for low continuous suction, or single-lumen gastric tube for low intermittent suction
- ☐ Raise head of bed 30°

- ☐ Low intermittent suction with single-lumen gastric tube

- ☐ Focused history and physical examination
- ☐ Chest and abdominal radiographs
- ☐ Initiate intravenous access
- ☐ Check Na, K, Cl, blood gases if older than 12 h
- ☐ Blood culture and antibiotics if open lesion or acute abdomen
- ☐ Fluid balance sheet

- ☐ Establish working diagnosis
- ☐ Obtain consultation and transfer to surgical centre

1. Continuous suction should only be applied when using a double-lumen "sump" tube (e.g., Replogle). If a double-lumen tube is not available, intermittent suction should be used.

Abbreviations: Cl - chloride, h - hours, K - potassium, Na - sodium, NPO - nothing by mouth

Anterior abdominal wall defect

Gastroschisis and omphalocele are the two most common abdominal wall defects, with varying etiologies and a wide spectrum of prognosis.

Gastroschisis

The small intestine and, sometimes, other organs (stomach, large bowel, spleen) protrude through a small opening in the abdominal wall to the right of the umbilicus (Figure 6.1). The umbilical cord is not involved and is anatomically normal. The exposed intestine is not covered by a peritoneal membrane and often appears thick, foreshortened, and matted. The intestine is usually anatomically normal, but all infants with gastroschisis have abnormal rotation and fixation of the intestines. Some infants may have other GI anomalies, including volvulus, intestinal atresia, intestinal stenosis, or intestinal perforation. Coexisting chromosomal anomalies are unusual in infants with gastroschisis.

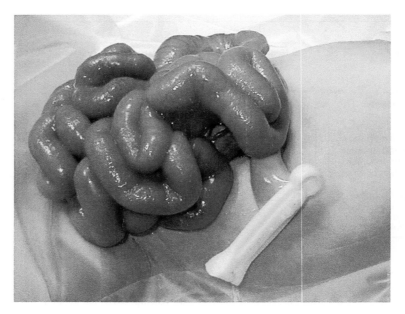

Figure 6.1. Infant with gastroschisis.

Source: Christison-Lagay ER, Kelleher CM, Langer JC. Neonatal abdominal wall defects. Seminars in Fetal and Neonatal Medicine. 2011;16(3):162–72. Used with permission from Dr. Jacob C. Langer.

Omphalocele

Characteristically a midline defect, an omphalocele occurs at the insertion point of the umbilical cord, with a translucent sac composed of amnion, Wharton's jelly, and peritoneum covering the herniated abdominal contents. The umbilical cord inserts into the membrane rather than the abdominal wall. In most cases, only the small intestine is visible, but when the omphalocele is large (sometimes called a 'giant omphalocele'), the liver and other organs may be seen. A giant omphalocele (Figure 6.2) is difficult to repair because there may not be enough space in the abdominal cavity to replace exposed organs.

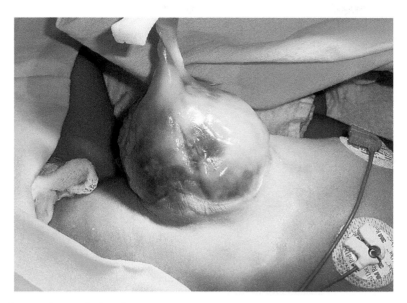

Figure 6.2. Infant with omphalocele.

Source: Christison-Lagay ER, Kelleher CM, Langer JC. Neonatal abdominal wall defects. Seminars in Fetal and Neonatal Medicine. 2011;16(3):162–72. Used with permission from Dr. Jacob C. Langer.

All infants with omphalocele have malrotation of the intestines, but unlike gastroschisis, it is rare to have other intestinal anomalies. There is a high incidence of associated conditions (30% to 40%) and chromosomal abnormalities in infants with omphalocele that may impact prognosis, including survival. Infants with a giant omphalocele have a higher incidence of respiratory failure due to a combination of chest deformity, pulmonary hypoplasia, and diaphragmatic dysfunction. It is important to assess whether the sac is intact or ruptured at the time of birth and throughout stabilization.

Neural tube defect

Neural tube defects can occur in the spinal column (spina bifida) or head (encephalocele). Spina bifida can range from small lesions in the distal spine (Figure 6.3) to more extensive lesions in the thoracic and lumbar regions. An encephalocele is a sac-like protrusion of meninges and brain tissue through a defect in the skull. The effects of a neural tube defect can range from minor impairment to total paralysis, depending on the level and extent of the defect.

Infants with neural tube defects may also have an associated central nervous system (CNS) malformation, such as agenesis of the corpus callosum and Arnold–Chiari malformation.

Spina bifida includes four main types of defects (Figure 6.4):

1. Spina bifida occulta is the mildest form of this condition, and it is often discovered coincidentally during an imaging test done for unrelated reasons. Spina bifida occulta is a small separation in one or more of the vertebrae without spinal cord or meningeal herniation.
2. Meningocele is an opening in the vertebrae, through which a sac containing meninges and cerebrospinal fluid protrudes.

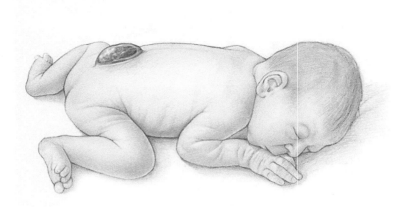

Figure 6.3. Infant with spina bifida (myelomeningocele).

3. Myelomeningocele is the most common form of spina bifida. In addition to meningocele, nerve tissue protrudes through the vertebral opening. It is covered by a sac and may be partially or completely covered by skin.

4. Myeloschisis is an open defect of the spine that may involve exposure of the entire spinal cord. It is the most severe type of spina bifida.

Vomiting or inability to swallow

An infant presenting with vomiting or the inability to swallow secretions raises concern for a GI tract obstruction or dysfunction. The presence of bile, degree of abdominal distention, or associated airway findings may give a clue as to the location of the problem.

Vomiting

Infants with obstruction of the proximal intestinal tract (e.g., gastric, duodenal, or jejunal) usually present with vomiting. Vomiting due to a GI obstruction can be clear or bilious (green), depending on where the obstruction is located.

Nonbilious vomiting can be caused by an obstruction proximal to the point where the common bile duct enters the duodenum:

- Pyloric stenosis can present as early as the first week to months after birth, with nonbilious, forceful vomiting, and dehydration.
- Proximal duodenal webs or atresia will present within hours of birth.

Bilious vomiting in the newborn should be considered evidence of mechanical intestinal obstruction, until proven otherwise. Causes include:

- Duodenal atresia, stenosis, or web, with obstruction distal to the entry of the common bile duct into the duodenum;

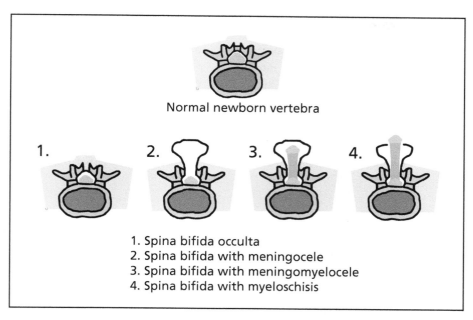

Normal newborn vertebra

1.
2.
3.
4.

1. Spina bifida occulta
2. Spina bifida with meningocele
3. Spina bifida with meningomyelocele
4. Spina bifida with myeloschisis

Figure 6.4. Types of neural tube defect.

- Jejunal–ileal atresia; and
- Malrotation with volvulus.

Volvulus is a surgical emergency. If the condition is unrecognized or surgery is delayed, necrosis of the entire intestine, shock, and death can ensue.

Infants with more distal obstruction due to meconium ileus or colonic atresia will also exhibit bilious vomiting, usually preceded by abdominal distension. Other possible causes of bilious vomiting include duodeno-gastric reflux (which is more common in preterm infants), functional intestinal obstruction (e.g., Hirschsprung's disease), metabolic disturbances, or sepsis.

Bilious vomiting is not always due to a GI obstruction, but obstruction must be ruled out urgently.

Inability to swallow (or handle secretions)

Esophageal atresia (EA)/tracheoesophageal fistula (TEF) can present with difficulty feeding, noisy and laboured breathing (especially during attempted feeds), and inability to handle oral secretions (excessive drooling). There may also be periods of cyanosis and apnea during attempted feeds, as the infant aspirates milk or oral secretions into the lungs. When a tracheoesophageal fistula is present, infants may experience increasing abdominal distension, especially during noninvasive respiratory support or mechanical ventilation.

Abdominal distension

The differential for abdominal distension is broad and can include each of the diagnoses described for vomiting. Infants with an obstruction of the intestinal tract distal to the junction between the jejunum and ileum (e.g., ileal atresia) usually present initially with abdominal distension. Abdominal distension may also be caused by an abdominal mass, peritonitis, or ascites.

> When the infant's abdomen is tender as well as distended, it is important to exclude causes of acute abdomen, such as necrotizing enterocolitis (NEC), volvulus, or GI perforation (ruptured bowel).

1. **NEC** is a condition of multifactorial pathogenesis and is more common in preterm infants. NEC commonly occurs in the terminal ileum and proximal colon. Manifestations vary widely, from abdominal distension with fresh blood in the stool to fulminant sepsis, intestinal perforation, and necrosis of the entire intestinal tract. Age of onset can be days in term or late preterm infants but can be delayed by weeks in infants born more preterm. NEC without peritonitis or perforation will generally be managed medically with bowel rest, antibiotics, and close monitoring.
2. **Volvulus** occurs when the bowel twists on itself, leading to intestinal ischemia. Infants with volvulus may present with abdominal distension, bilious emesis, bloody stools, and hemodynamic instability. Volvulus can be secondary to malrotation or the bowel can twist on a lead point, such as in congenital Meckel's diverticulum or enteric duplication.
3. **Spontaneous gastric or intestinal perforations** are focal and occur more commonly in preterm infants.

Delayed passage of meconium or imperforate anus

Infants with functional or anatomic obstruction of the distal intestinal tract present with failure or delay in the passage of meconium. An infant who has not passed meconium by 48 h (or 72 h in a preterm infant) should be identified early, preferably before the infant's abdomen becomes distended, to avoid complications such as colitis due to bacterial overgrowth. Passage of meconium may be delayed by:

- Imperforate anus, with or without a perineal or genitourinary fistula,
- Microcolon,
- Colonic atresia,
- Meconium ileus, or
- Hirschsprung's disease (congenital absence of the myenteric plexus).

> In all newborns, ensure that the anus is patent. A presumed anal opening may in fact be a blind pouch. There may be seepage of meconium through the urethra, vagina, or perineal fissure in infants with imperforate anus.

Core Steps

The essential Core Steps in the ACoRN Surgical Conditions Sequence are to:

- Protect an exposed lesion with a clear cover or dressing, as appropriate (see Appendix A),
- Place NPO

Congenital lesions that are not covered with skin must be addressed immediately to reduce the risk for breakdown, infection, or thermal, fluid, and electrolyte loss. Positioning the infant with a gastroschisis or omphalocele in a bowel bag is preferable to a moist gauze dressing, which impedes visualization, has a rough surface, can absorb fluid from the lesion, and may leave residual particles behind.

When an infant has a neural tube defect, the lesion should be covered with a sterile, moist dressing.

Organization of Care

Care in the ACoRN Surgical Conditions Sequence is organized initially based on whether the infant has:

- An anterior abdominal wall defect,
- A neural tube defect,
- No anterior wall defect but signs of GI obstruction (i.e., vomiting, inability to swallow, abdominal distension, delayed passage of meconium, or an imperforate anus), *and* whether a gastric tube can be inserted.

Response

When stabilizing newborns with a surgical condition, response aims to optimize the infant's condition and minimize complications before surgery.

For the infant who has an anterior abdominal wall defect, optimal care includes the following:

- Manage the infant on an overhead warmer or in an incubator, to prevent heat loss.
- Maintain sterile technique when manipulating the bowel (wear a mask and latex-free sterile gloves).
- Place the infant in a sterile bowel bag (Figure 6.5) and secure at the level of the nipples or apply a transparent occlusive covering to the bowel to minimize heat and fluid losses.
- Avoid mask ventilation, continuous positive airway pressure (CPAP), and noninvasive positive pressure ventilation (NiPPV) to minimize gaseous distension of the intestines. Intubate early if the infant is in respiratory distress and needs ventilatory support.
- Minimize handling of the exposed bowel or viscera to prevent secondary damage and infection. For infants with an omphalocele, take care not to tear the sac.
- Avoid pressure on the mesentery and potential kinking of the bowel by using rolls to support the bowel midline in either a supine or side-lying position.
- Decompress the GI tract by inserting a #10 Fr double-lumen Replogle 'sump' tube for continuous suction or a #8 Fr or #10 Fr single-lumen gastric tube, on low, intermittent suction.

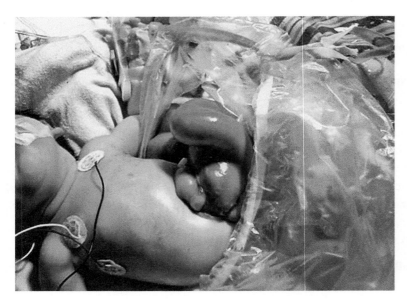

Figure 6.5. Applying a protective bowel bag.

Used with permission from Dr. Joseph J. Tepas.

○ A double-lumen Replogle tube allows continuous suction through one lumen with the other vented to air, to prevent the catheter from generating a vacuum against the mucosa. Start suction at 40 mmHg to 60 mmHg and maintain pressure in the low range, never exceeding 80 mmHg.

○ If a single-lumen gastric tube is inserted to decompress the GI tract, use intermittent suction only. Continuous suction using this device can collapse the stomach, creating a vacuum pressure on the mucosa, which can cause ulceration, hemorrhage, or perforation. Use a regulator that has an intermittent suction setting, with preset on-and-off cycles. Start suction at 40 mmHg to 60 mmHg and maintain pressure in the low range, never exceeding 80 mmHg.

For the infant who has a neural tube defect, optimal care includes the following:

• Manage the infant on an overhead warmer or in an incubator to prevent heat loss.
• Maintain sterile technique when examining or dressing the lesion (wear a mask and latex-free sterile gloves to minimize risk for developing latex sensitivity).
• Ensure the defect is covered with a sterile moist protective wrap.
• Position prone or side-lying.
• Create or use a pre-packaged 'donut' dressing on skin surrounding the lesion to prevent pressure on the protruding sac.
• Keep the sac intact to prevent cerebrospinal fluid leakage or damage to the nerve tissue.

For the infant with no abdominal wall or neural tube defect but signs of gastrointestinal obstruction, attempt to insert a gastric tube to a premeasured depth.

Able to pass gastric tube

• To decompress the gastrointestinal tract, insert a #8 Fr or #10 Fr single-lumen gastric tube and apply low intermittent suction.

Unable to pass gastric tube

The tube may 'bounce' and not advance or come back out through the infant's mouth. Do not apply force, but leave the tube inserted to the point of resistance until an X-ray is performed. Suspect esophageal atresia with or without a tracheoesophageal fistula (EA/TEF), with pooling of secretions within the blind esophageal pouch.

- Raise the head of the infant's bed 30° to minimize aspiration from the esophageal pouch or gastroesophageal reflux through a distal fistula.
- Initiate low continuous suction using a double-lumen Replogle tube placed in the upper esophageal segment, and set the level of suction at 40 mmHg to 60 mmHg.
- If a Replogle tube is not available, insert a single-lumen gastric tube to the point of resistance and apply low intermittent suction at 40 mmHg to 60 mmHg.
- Avoid mask ventilation, CPAP, or NiPPV for infants with EA/TEF to minimize gaseous distension of a blind esophageal pouch or GI tract via a fistula. Intubate early if the infant is in respiratory distress and requires ventilatory support.

Next Steps

Next Steps in the ACoRN Surgical Conditions Sequence are to obtain a focused history, conduct a physical examination, order diagnostic tests, establish IV access, initiate a fluid balance sheet, and establish Level of Risk.

Focused history

Important information to gather during the focused surgical history includes the following:

Antepartum

- Maternal age: risk for gastroschisis increases in mothers younger than 25 years old and is highest in mothers under 20 years old
- Medical, obstetrical, and family history
- Maternal diabetes or hypothyroidism
- Maternal medications during pregnancy, including potential teratogens
- Other risk factors include suboptimal prenatal care, low socio-economic status, smoking during pregnancy, occupational or recreational exposure to solvents, or use of amphetamine-related drugs or cocaine during pregnancy
- Previous fetuses or children with congenital anomalies
- Prenatal genetic screening
- Prenatal ultrasound findings. Most conditions described in this chapter are easily seen on ultrasounds, but others, such as EA/TEF, become suspected in the absence of a fluid-filled stomach or polyhydramnios on ultrasound.

Because many lesions are associated with other congenital anomalies, obtaining a full antenatal record, including any fetal echocardiography results, is important for care planning and infant outcomes.

Intrapartum

- Spontaneous or induced labour
- Meconium or bile-stained amniotic fluid
- Mode of delivery

Neonatal

- Gestational age
- Birth weight: small, appropriate, or large for gestational age
- Need for resuscitation
- Onset of feeding and type of feeds
- Any changes in feeding pattern
- Difficulty feeding: coughing, choking, cyanosis, or apnea
- If vomiting, time of onset and colour of vomitus
- Passage of meconium at or post-delivery
- Colour of stool and presence of blood
- If abdominal distension, time of onset

Focused physical examination

A thorough examination of any infant with a surgical condition is imperative, due to potential for other congenital anomalies in syndromic or chromosomal conditions. Examples include:

- The association of omphalocele with Pentalogy of Cantrell, Beckwith-Wiedemann syndrome, OEIS complex (omphalocele, exstrophy of the cloacae, imperforate anus, and spinal deformity) or with aneuploidies, such as trisomy 13 and 18; and
- EA/TEF or imperforate anus may be components of the VACTERL association (vertebral defects, anal atresia, cardiac defects, tracheoesophageal fistula, renal anomalies, and limb abnormalities).

Abdominal wall defect

- Check for a covering membrane and whether it is intact.
- With gastroschisis, assess the bowel for kinking, cyanosis, or necrosis. Presence of meconium on the bowel surface may indicate a rupture. Positioning to avoid kinking or pressure on the bowel and monitoring the health of the bowel through the bowel bag, before and during transfer to a level 3 centre, is important.

Neural tube defect

- Observe lesion for the level of spine involved and the presence of intact covering.
- Measure head circumference and evaluate anterior fontanelle and cranial sutures. Hydrocephalus can complicate spina bifida cases with coincident Chiari malformation.
- Conduct a thorough neurologic exam for signs of deficit, such as abnormal tone and movement of lower limbs, absence of anal sphincter tone, or dribbling of urine.

- Determine hip stability.
- Check for skin abnormalities such as hemangioma, pigmented nevi, or dermal sinus.

For infants presenting with surgical conditions beyond the first few hours of life, always check for the following.

- Signs of dehydration: dry mucous membranes, sunken anterior fontanel, excessive weight loss since birth (i.e., greater than 10%)
- Colour of fluid in an infant's gastric tube
- Stool colour and texture, and presence of blood
- Abdominal distension, discolouration, or tenderness. Measure the infant's abdominal girth as a baseline
- Bowel sounds

Chest and abdominal radiographs

In many cases, a chest and abdominal radiograph provides enough information to establish the course of action.

- Confirm location of the Replogle or single-lumen gastric tube tip within the stomach.
- With esophageal atresia, the gastric tube typically ends at an air-filled pouch, mid-chest. The pouch can often be seen at the level of the tube. The radiograph may also show air in the stomach, confirming the presence of a distal tracheoesophageal fistula.
- Air pattern in the bowel often indicates the level of obstruction. A classic 'double bubble' (dilation of the stomach and proximal duodenum) with no distal air is seen in duodenal atresia. Lack of distal air in an acute abdomen may signal a life-threatening volvulus. A diffusely dilated small or large bowel suggests a lower obstruction or atresia. Lack of air in the rectum may be seen in Hirschsprung's disease or imperforate anus.
- Bowel wall thickening, an asymmetric bowel gas pattern, bubbly looking or linear lucencies ('string of pearls') in the bowel wall (pneumatosis) or branching lucencies in the liver (portal air), suggest NEC.
- A cross-table lateral radiograph with the infant in a supine position can best identify air-fluid levels within the bowel loops (seen in intestinal obstruction) and free air in the peritoneal cavity.
- Calcifications in the peritoneal cavity suggest intrauterine bowel perforation, sometimes in association with meconium ileus (meconium peritonitis).
- Assessment of the vertebral column is important with neural tube defects but also when other congenital anomalies are present. The presence of hemivertebrae or fused vertebrae may suggest VACTERL association.

Initiate intravenous access

Administer fluids as directed in Chapter 7, Fluid and Glucose.

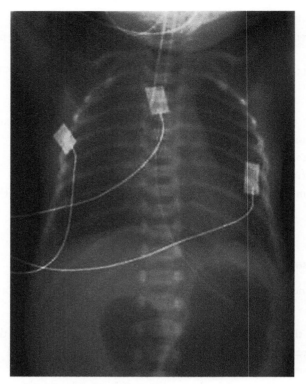

Duodonel obstruction with 'double bubble' sign.

Reprinted from: Obstetric Imaging: Fetal Diagnosis and Care. Braun T, Henrigh W (eds.). Intestinal obstruction, pp. 11–24, 2018. With permission from Elsevier.

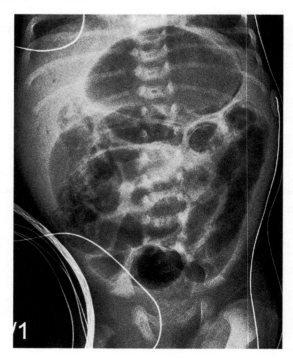

Necrotizing enterocolitis (NEC). Linear lucencies in bowel wall are visible, most notably in the left upper quadrant, as well as bubbly lucencies on the right side of the abdomen (pneumatosis). Branching lucencies are seen within the liver (portal air).

(a)

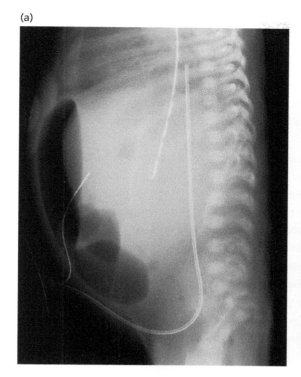

(b)

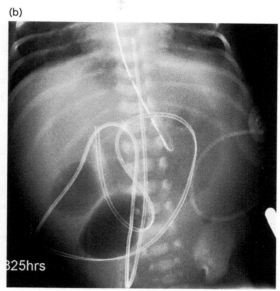

325hrs

Perforation. (a) This cross-table lateral image clearly shows anterior abdominal free air in the peritoneal cavity. (b) The AP image shows a central lucency that is more difficult to discern and may be missed. Both show the presence of a low-lying UVC, a UAC in good position at T-8, and a Replogle tube in the stomach.

Blood tests

Order serum sodium, potassium, and chloride to determine whether there are electrolyte abnormalities resulting from excessive water or electrolyte losses by evaporation (with an abdominal wall defect), or by vomiting, suctioning, or third-spacing (with intestinal obstruction or an acute abdomen). This electrolyte assessment should be routine after 12 h of age because measurements earlier than this usually reflect maternal values.

Blood gases should be performed to assess for metabolic alkalosis (in vomiting), or metabolic acidosis (in dehydration or acute abdomen), or respiratory acidosis with coincident respiratory decompensation.

Blood culture and antibiotics

Blood cultures and antibiotics should be initiated when there is an open lesion or evidence of an acute abdomen.

Fluid balance sheet

Newborns with surgical conditions require a fluid balance sheet to monitor intake and output volumes, including fluid aspirated through a Replogle or single-lumen gastric tube.

In gastroschisis, the exposed bowel may lead to excessive fluid loss by evaporation, intestinal edema, or both. Using a bowel bag and handling the bowel carefully can reduce fluid losses but paying continuous attention to the fluid status of the infant is important. Decisions on IV fluid administration should be made in consultation with the tertiary surgical site while awaiting transport.

Establish a working diagnosis
Obtain a consult and request transfer to a surgical centre as soon as possible

Specific Diagnosis and Management

While a definitive diagnosis and surgical management typically occur at the tertiary care centre and are outside the scope of ACoRN, some considerations follow here:

Gastroschisis should be managed as soon after birth as possible by tertiary paediatric surgeons, to preserve gut viability and minimize risk of infection. Unless the bowel is easily reduced into the abdomen, this will usually involve placing the bowel in a silo, with progressive reduction into the abdomen before surgical closure (Figure 6.6).

The urgency to repair an **omphalocele** depends on whether the sac is ruptured or not. The timing of the surgery also depends on the dimension of the defect, the infant's size, and the presence or absence of other anomalies. In cases of large omphaloceles, the bowel and viscera will not fit within the abdomen and the sac will be allowed to epithelialize rather than making an attempt at surgical closure.

Surgical repair of **neural tube defects** should occur in the first 24 to 48 h of life, to help prevent infection and preserve neurologic function. Magnetic resonance imaging will also determine the presence or absence of hydrocephalus or Chiari malformation.

Surgical repair for **esophageal atresia/tracheoesophageal fistula** depends on the results of initial investigations and type of lesion. Although there are 5 types of **EA/TEF** (Figure 6.7), types A and C are the most common and most easily diagnosed. Type C (EA with distal fistula) is present in 85% of cases and type A (EA without distal fistula) in 8%. They are differentiated by the presence or absence of air in the abdomen, which reflects the presence of a distal fistula. Surgical management of type A consists of primary or delayed anastomosis of the esophageal pouch to the distal esophagus. In type C, in addition to esophageal anastomosis, the distal fistula will be ligated urgently to prevent the abdominal contents from refluxing into the

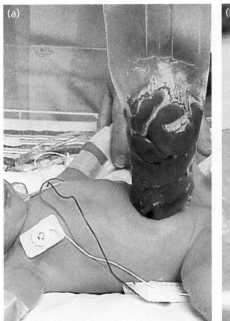
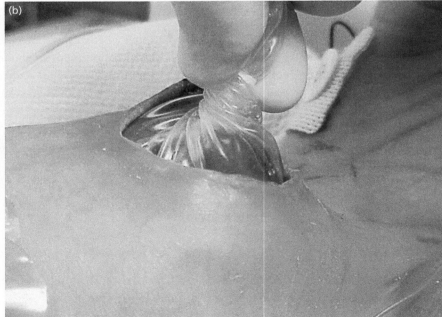

Figure 6.6. Showing the bowel siloed (a), then reduced (b) into an infant's abdomen.

Used with permission from Dr. Jacob C. Langer.

infant's lungs and also decrease risk for overdistension or perforation of the stomach. In both types, timing the esophageal anastomosis depends on the length of the gap between the proximal and distal esophagus.

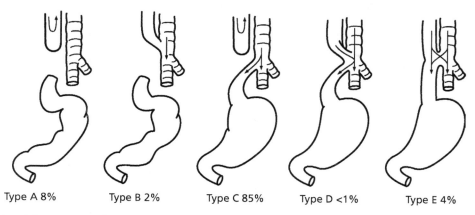

Type A 8%   Type B 2%   Type C 85%   Type D <1%   Type E 4%

Figure 6.7. The 5 types of EA/TEF, with prevalence (%).

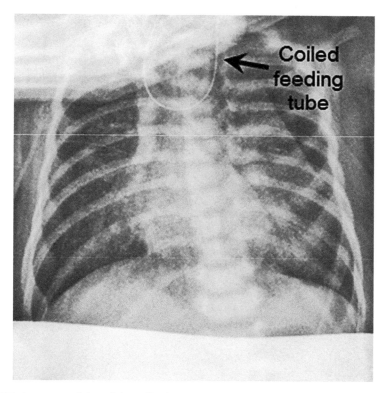

Type C EA/TEF (pre-repair), with coiled gastric tube.

Source: Higano NS, Bates AJ, Tkach JA, et al. Pre- and post-operative visualization of neonatal esophageal atresia/tracheoesophageal fistula via magnetic resonance imaging. J Pediatr Surg Case Rep 2018;29:5–8. Reproduced with permission.

Type E (also known as 'H type-fistula') is difficult to diagnose and may present later in the newborn period, with coughing and choking during feeds or in early childhood and a history of recurrent pneumonia.

Surgical management for **vomiting/abdominal distension/delayed passage of meconium** or **imperforate anus** depends on the lesion and clinical status of the infant.

- *Duodenal/jejunal–ileal atresias:* These obstructions require abdominal decompression and a laparotomy for intestinal reanastomosis.
- *Malrotation/volvulus:* In the presence of an acute abdomen and cardiorespiratory instability, this is a surgical emergency. Emergent consultation and transport are paramount.
- *Meconium ileus:* If uncomplicated, this condition can be treated with specialized enemas. For a complicated meconium ileus with in utero perforation resulting from the initial obstruction, there are two outcomes:
  - When the perforation has sealed and there is no intestinal obstruction, a laparotomy may not be necessary.
  - Laparotomy is required when there is an intestinal obstruction, evidence of persistent peritonitis, or an abdominal mass.
- *NEC:* The absolute indications for surgical intervention include pneumoperitoneum and intestinal gangrene. A laparotomy is performed to inspect the entirety of the GI tract. Necrotic or perforated segments of the bowel are resected, and an ostomy is performed.
- *Imperforate anus:* Surgical management includes a colostomy until the rectum and anus can be reconstructed at a later age.
- *Hirschsprung's disease:* The usual management is a diverting colostomy proximal to the transition zone, with resection of the aganglionic segment of the bowel. The definitive treatment, when the ganglionic bowel is brought down and anastomosed with the anal canal, becomes possible when the infant weighs more than 10 kg.

Level of Risk: Surgical Conditions	
	In the ACoRN Surgical Conditions Sequence, the level of risk is always RED. All infants need consultation and management in a level 3 surgical facility.

Surgical Conditions: Case 1—Abdominal wall defect

You are called to a 37-week GA baby post-delivery. She was born with loops of small bowel extruding from her abdominal wall. She is breathing regularly in room air and appears otherwise appropriate.

You recognize that this is an unwell baby with a visible anomaly and call for assistance as you move the baby to the over-bed warmer for better assessment. As help arrives, you position the baby to open the airway and apply the monitors as part of the Consolidated Core Steps. Your colleague begins the ACoRN Primary Survey.

The baby's breathing is regular and effective at a rate of 48 breaths/min. She is pink in room air, with a heart rate of 145 bpm room air. Her blood pressure is 50/38 with a mean of 42. Her temp is 36.9°C. She has normal tone and activity. The abdominal wall defect has no covering, and you identify the need to protect it as part of the Consolidated Core Steps.

1. **How would you protect the exposed bowel during early stage care of this infant? Tick all that apply.**
   - ☐ Use sterile technique.
   - ☐ Wear sterile, latex-free gloves.
   - ☐ Examine the bowel for areas of stricture or atresia.
   - ☐ Let gravity determine the position of the bowel on the bed.
   - ☐ Cover the defect with a sterile, dry gauze dressing.
   - ☐ Place the baby inside a bowel bag or the bowel inside an occlusive, transparent covering.

The baby is under a radiant warmer.

You carefully place her into a bowel bag to protect the exposed viscera. The bag is secured at nipple level. A colleague uses rolled towels to support the bowel in a midline position. The visible bowel includes several loops of small intestine that look pink and well perfused. Their appearance is carefully noted and monitored, but these loops are not otherwise disturbed or examined.

2. **What does your Problem List look like?**

Problem List
- ☐ Respiratory
- ☐ Cardiovascular
- ☐ Neurology
- ☐ Surgical Conditions
- ☐ Fluid and Glucose
- ☐ Jaundice
- ☐ Thermoregulation
- ☐ Infection

The Surgical Conditions Sequence is the first sequence in your prioritized Problem List. You enter the sequence with the Alerting Sign of an anterior abdominal wall defect, confirm coverage of the exposed bowel, and place the baby NPO.

You continue to monitor the infant's vital signs, including oxygen saturations, as part of the Consolidated Core Steps.

3. How do you Organize Care for this baby?

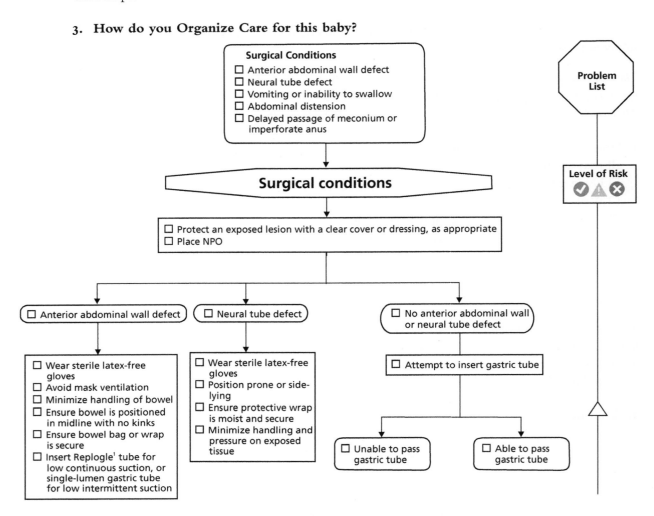

You obtain a focused history and learn that the mother is a 17-yo who had minimal prenatal care.

Except for the abdominal wall defect, the baby's focused physical examination is unremarkable, and she has no apparent dysmorphic features or other anomalies.

Your working diagnosis is gastroschisis, with no obvious associated anomalies. You order chest and abdominal radiographs, and initiate an IV. You request a blood culture be added to the blood work list, with a plan to start antibiotics due to the open abdominal wall defect. You initiate a fluid balance sheet to document IV fluid intake and gastric losses.

4. Based on the Surgical Conditions Sequence, what is this baby's Level of Risk?
☐ Red   ☐ Yellow   ☐ Green

After completing the remaining ACoRN Sequences down to Next Steps, you call your regional surgical centre for consultation and request advice and transport. You inform the specialist that you have ordered a chest and abdominal radiograph to document the position of the gastric tube, that you started a peripheral IV with D10W, and have given antibiotics (ampicillin and gentamicin).

You review this infant's fluid requirements while waiting for transport.

Surgical Conditions: Case 2—Inability to pass a nasogastric tube

A 6-h-old, term baby boy is not tolerating feeding, and you are called to complete an assessment. Breastfeeding was initiated in the delivery room and seemed to be well tolerated at first. While attempting to breastfeed at 3 h of age, however, the baby experienced an apneic episode and colostrum was observed exiting his nose. Subsequent feeding attempts resulted in coughing, and feeding has now been abandoned.

The mother tells you her baby has been drooling and mucousy since birth, and that she has wiped his mouth with a soft cloth several times.

Vital signs and tone are normal. The baby is breathing regularly and looks pink in room air, but his breathing is noisy. He is drooling heavily, and you hear a few crackles when you auscultate his chest.

Because the baby shows none of the Resuscitation Alerting Signs, your team begins the ACoRN Primary Survey and Consolidated Core Steps.

I. **Complete the ACoRN Primary Survey and Consolidated Core Steps, and generate a Problem List.**

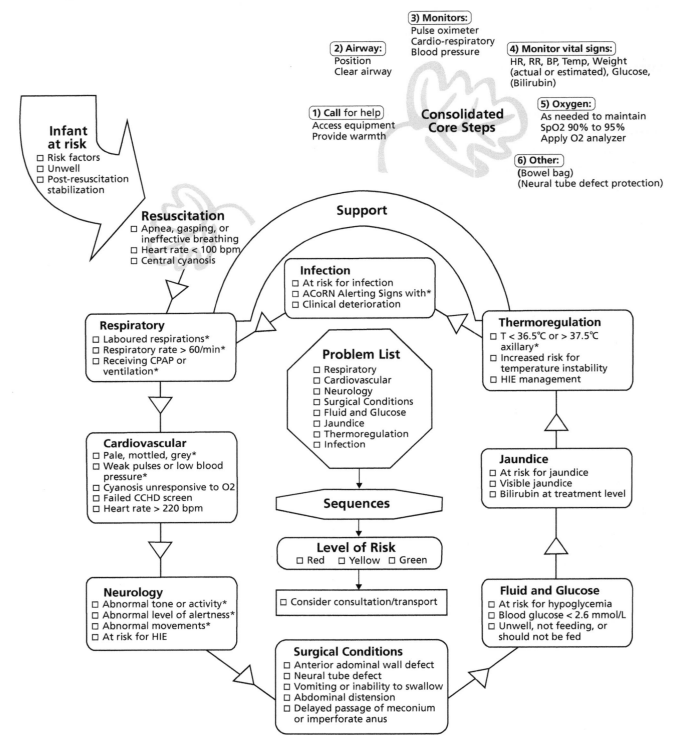

You enter the Surgical Conditions Sequence because of vomiting or inability to swallow.

You talk to the baby's parents and explain why further attempts at feeding should be withheld. The baby needs to be observed and assessed.

You gently examine the baby's mouth, oropharynx and nose, suctioning a small amount of secretions, then attempt to pass a gastric tube to a premeasured depth into the stomach.

2. How do you Organize Care for this baby?

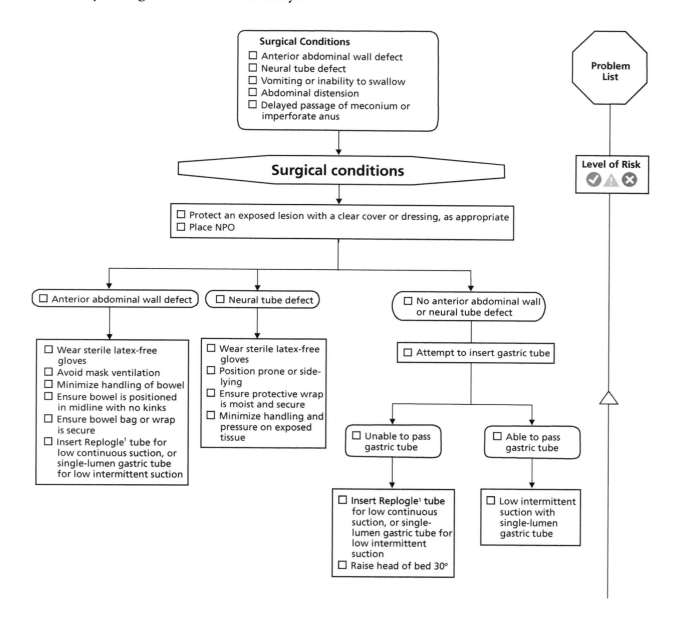

3. Why are you inserting a nasogastric (NG) tube? Tick all that apply.

☐ To feed the baby.

☐ Because this baby has an anterior abdominal wall defect.

☐ Because the baby may vomit and aspirate stomach contents.

☐ Because a GI tract obstruction may be present.

☐ Because positioning the NG tube may help determine whether and, if so, where there is an obstruction.

You gently insert a single-lumen NG tube but meet resistance at about 10 cm and then see the tip of the tube re-emerge from the baby's mouth. You try again. The same thing happens.

4. What do you do now? Tick all that apply.

☐ Re-attempt NG insertion with a smaller gauge catheter.

☐ Secure the tube at the point of resistance.

☐ Leave the tube open to air.

☐ Apply low intermittent suction at 40 mmHg to 60 mmHg, using a regulator with preset on-off cycles.

☐ If a regulator is not available, use a 10 mL or 20 mL syringe to apply suction intermittently.

☐ Raise the head of the bed 30°.

☐ Order a chest and abdo X-ray.

You tell the parents that the baby looks well now, the focused physical examination is normal, and you are awaiting the results of a chest and abdomen radiograph, ordered as part of the Next Steps. You exit the Surgical Sequence and enter the next sequence on the Problem List.

You have completed the Fluid and Glucose Sequence and started a D10W infusion via a peripheral IV, because the baby cannot be fed. He is being cared for in a servo controlled isolette to maintain a thermo neutral environment and so that you can observe for any further episodes of choking or vomiting.

Meanwhile, the x-ray image has arrived.

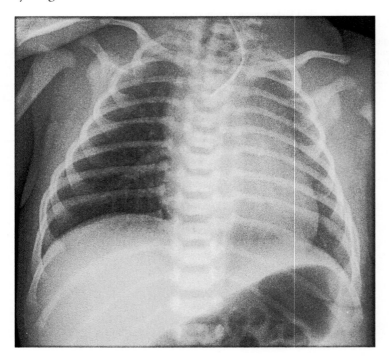

5. What can you see in this radiograph? Tick all that apply.

☐ The gastric tube ends in the upper esophagus.

☐ There is no air in the stomach.

☐ The lung markings appear to be increased.

☐ The cardiac shadow looks normal in size and shape.

☐ There are many abnormal-looking vertebrae.

6. What is your working diagnosis?

☐ Esophageal atresia with fistula.

☐ Esophageal atresia without fistula.

☐ Aspiration of secretions or milk.

☐ Duodenal atresia.

☐ VACTRL association.

7. Based on the Surgical Conditions Sequence, what is this baby's Level of Risk?

☐ Red   ☐ Yellow   ☐ Green

After completing the remaining ACoRN Sequences down to Next Steps, you call your regional centre for consultation and request advice and transport. The specialist asks you to pull the gastric tube out 2 cm to allow it to sit in the bottom of the blind pouch or, if possible, replace it with a double-lumen Replogle sump tube so you can apply low continuous suction for better drainage of secretions.

She also asks your team to institute comfort measures to minimize crying, decrease risk for gastric distension, and prevent reflux or aspiration from the suspected esophageal atresia.

You tell the mother that her baby appears to have an interruption in his esophagus and will need to be transferred to be evaluated more carefully.

The infant is transferred to the nearest neonatal regional surgical centre, where the diagnosis of EA with distal fistula (Type C) is confirmed.

Bibliography

Adzick NS, Thom EA, Spong CY, et al. A randomized trial of prenatal versus postnatal repair of myelomenigocele. N Engl J Med 2011;364(11):993–1004.

Campbell KH, Copel JA. Gastroschisis. In: Copel JA, D'Alton ME, Feltovich H, et al, eds. Obstetric Imaging: Fetal Diagnosis and Care, 2nd ed. Philadelphia, PA: Elsevier; 2018.

Chabra S, Gleason CA. Gastroschisis: Embryology, pathogenesis, epidemiology. Neoreviews 2005;6(11):e493–9.

Danzer E, Hedrick HL, Rintoul NE, Siegle J, Adzick NS, Panitch HB. Assessment of early pulmonary function abnormalities in giant omphalocele survivors. J Pediatr Surg 2012;47(10):1811–20.

Ein SH, Langer JC. Delayed management of giant omphalocele using silver sulfadiazine cream: An 18-year experience. J Pediatr Surg 2012;47(3):494–500.

Fenichel GM. Disorders of cranial volume and shape. In: Clinical Pediatric Neurology: A Signs and Symptoms Approach, 6th ed. Philadelphia, PA: Saunders/Elsevier; 2009.

Freeman NV, Burger DM, Griffiths M, Malone PSJ, eds. Surgery of the Newborn. London, England: Churchill Livingstone; 1994.

Gamba P, Midrio P. Abdominal wall defects: Prenatal diagnosis, newborn management, and long-term outcomes. Semin Pediatr Surg 2014;23(5):283–90.

Januschek E, Röhrig A, Kunze S, Fremerey C, Wiebe B, Messing-Jünger M. Myelomingocele—a single institute analysis of the years 2007–2015. Childs Nerv Syst 2016;32(7):1281–7.

Lockridge T, Caldwell AM, Jason P. Neonatal surgical emergencies: Stabilization and management. J Obstet Gynecol Neonatal Nurs 2002;31(3):328–99.

Mastroiacovo P, Lisi A, Castilla EE. The incidence of gastroschisis: Research urgently needs resources. BMJ 2006;332(7538):423–4.

Neu J, Walker WA. Necrotizing enterocolits. N Engl J Med 2011;364(3):255–64.

Nixon HH, O'Donnell B. The Essentials of Paediatric Surgery. London, England: W. Heinemann, 1961.

Riboh J, Abrajano CT, Garber K, et al. Outcomes of sutureless gastroschisis closure. J Pediatr Surg 2009;44(10):1847–51.

Ringer SA, Aziz K. Stabilization and post-resuscitation care. Clin Perinatol 2012;39(4):901–18.

Sandler AD. Children with spina bifida: Key clinical issues. Pediatr Clin N Am 2010;57(4):879–92.

Sinha CK, Haider N, Marri RR, Rajimwale A, Fisher R, Nour S. Modified prognostic criteria for oesophageal atresia and tracheo-oesophageal fistula. Eur J Pediatr Surg 2007;17(3):153–7.

Wilson RD, Johnson MP. Congenital abdominal wall defects: An update. Fetal Diagn Ther 2004;19(5):385–98.

Answer key: Surgical Conditions Case 1—Abdominal wall defect

1. How would you protect the exposed bowel during early stage care of this infant?

- ✓ Use sterile technique.
- ✓ Wear sterile, latex-free gloves.
- ☐ Examine the bowel for areas of stricture or atresia.
- ☐ Let gravity determine the position of the bowel on the bed.
- ☐ Cover the defect with a sterile, dry gauze dressing.
- ✓ Place the baby inside a bowel bag or the bowel inside an occlusive, transparent covering.

To mitigate risk for infection, using sterile technique when dressing or manipulating the defect is essential. Wearing latex-free gloves is imperative to avoid a latex sensitivity. Although the bowel will need to be assessed for strictures or atresias, this assessment is not a strategy to protect the exposed bowel.

To maintain bowel integrity, placement in a bowel bag or protecting the exposed portion with an occlusive, transparent covering is recommended. A sterile, dry gauze dressing could adhere to the exposed tissue and cause additional trauma. The covered bowel should be supported with rolls to reduce traction on the tissues and maintain bowel perfusion. A bowel bag or clear, occlusive dressing not only protects the exposed bowel from trauma and contamination, it reduces evaporative losses and allows the health care team to visualize the bowel and assess tissue perfusion.

2. What does your Problem List look like?

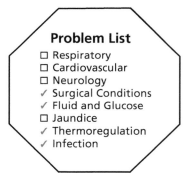

Problem List
- ☐ Respiratory
- ☐ Cardiovascular
- ☐ Neurology
- ✓ Surgical Conditions
- ✓ Fluid and Glucose
- ☐ Jaundice
- ✓ Thermoregulation
- ✓ Infection

The baby has no Alerting Signs in the Respiratory, Cardiovascular, or Neurology Sequences. She has one Alerting Sign from the ACoRN Surgical Conditions Sequence. This is a baby with a surgical condition who should not be fed (Fluid and Glucose Sequence). She is at risk for temperature instability (Thermoregulation Sequence) and infection (Infection Sequence) because of the exposed bowel.

You had also put **?** marks beside Blood glucose < 2.6 mmol/L and T <36.5°C or >37.5°C, to remind yourself to follow up.

3. How do you Organize Care for this baby?

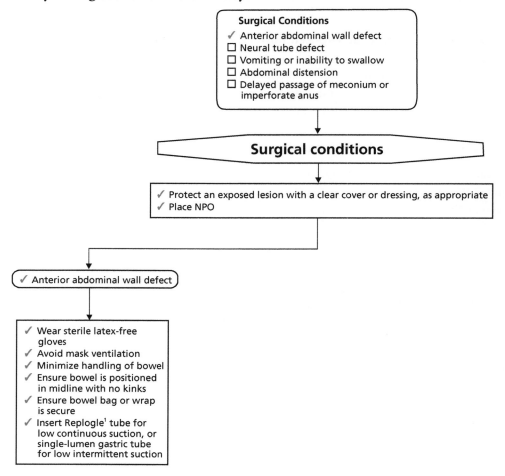

Optimally, a Replogle tube would be inserted into the infant's stomach and connected to continuous suction to provide decompression. When a Replogle is not available, a #8 Fr or #10 Fr gastric tube, connected to low intermittent suction, will also decompress the stomach.

Mask ventilation, CPAP, or NiPPV will increase abdominal distension and should be avoided. Supporting the bowel in the midline position, with the baby in a supine or side-lying position, decreases traction on the tissue and maintains perfusion to the bowel. The head of the bed should remain flat so as not to put additional pressure on the viscera.

4. Based on the Surgical Conditions Sequence, what is this baby's Level of Risk?
✓ Red   ☐ Yellow   ☐ Green

Answer key: Surgical Conditions Case 2—Inability to pass a nasogastric tube

1. Complete the ACoRN Primary Survey and Consolidated Core Steps, and generate a Problem List.

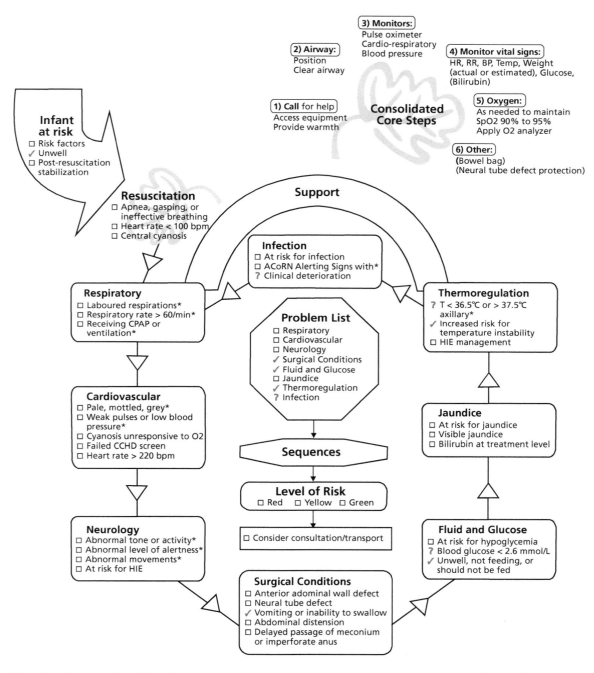

The first Alerting Sign identified on your Primary Survey is the infant's presenting problem of vomiting or inability to swallow secretions. This baby is having difficulty with feeding and should not be fed at this time. He is being assessed on an overbed warmer away from parents, so is at increased risk for temperature instability. You do not yet have a blood glucose or a current temperature, prompting **?** marks beside those Alerting Signs. At present, you are not sure if this was an existing condition or a clinical deterioration, so decide to put a **?** beside this Alerting Sign under Infection to remind you to reassess.

2. How do you Organize Care for this baby?

3. Why are you inserting a nasogastric (NG) tube?

- ☐ To feed the baby.
- ☐ Because this baby has an anterior abdominal wall defect.
- ☐ Because the baby may vomit and aspirate stomach contents.
- ✓ Because a GI tract obstruction may be present.
- ✓ Because positioning the NG tube may help determine whether, and if so, where there is an obstruction.

Inserting an NG tube helps to decompress the GI tract proximal to the obstruction, if one exists. It also helps to confirm the absence or presence of a proximal pouch, on radiograph. Radiologic absence or presence of air in the abdomen further assists in identifying the type of obstruction.

4. What do you do now?

☐ Re-attempt NG insertion with a smaller gauge catheter.

✓ Secure the tube at the point of resistance.

☐ Leave the tube open to air.

✓ Apply low intermittent suction at 40 mmHg to 60 mmHg, using a regulator with pre-set on-off cycles.

✓ If a regulator is not available, use a 10 mL or 20 mL syringe to apply suction intermittently.

✓ Raise the head of the bed 30°.

✓ Order a chest and abdo X-ray.

A smaller gauge catheter will also meet resistance. Once inserted, it is important to note the insertion depth of the gastric tube and secure it in place.

Intermittent suction helps to manage secretions that accumulate in the pouch. Optimally, a Replogle tube is used, or low intermittent suction connected to a regulator. If a regulator is not available in your centre, a 10 mL or 20 mL syringe can be used to manually apply intermittent suction.

Elevating the head of the bed decreases the risk of aspiration by using gravity to manage the secretions.

An X-ray is ordered to determine where the gastric tube is positioned.

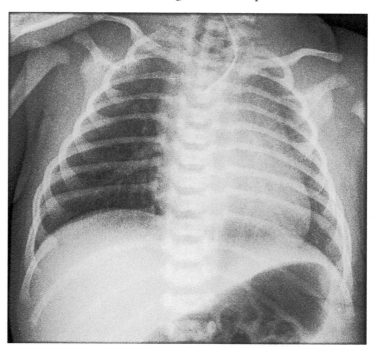

5. What can you see in this radiograph?

✓ The gastric tube ends in the upper esophagus.

☐ There is no air in the stomach.

✓ The lung markings appear to be increased.

✓ The cardiac shadow looks normal in size and shape.

☐ There are many abnormal-looking vertebrae.

The lung markings appear slightly increased, but there is no evidence of pneumonia. The cardiac-thoracic ratio is less than 50%, and therefore within normal limits. The vertebrae appear normal but this does not rule out VACTRL association.

6. What is your working diagnosis?

✓ Esophageal atresia with fistula.

☐ Esophageal atresia without fistula.

☐ Aspiration of secretions or milk.

☐ Duodenal atresia.

☐ VACTRL association.

The presence of a proximal pouch with air in the stomach is consistent with esophageal atresia with a distal fistula. If there were no fistula, the stomach would be gasless.

7. Based on the Surgical Conditions Sequence, what is this baby's Level of Risk?

✓ Red   ☐ Yellow   ☐ Green

Fluid and Glucose

Educational objectives

Upon completion of this chapter, you will be able to:

- Identify infants needing fluid and glucose stabilization.
- Understand the principles of fluid and glucose management in early transition.
- Apply the Acute Care of at-Risk Newborns (ACoRN) Fluid and Glucose Management Sequence.
- Recognize and manage infants with, or at risk for, hypoglycemia.
- Supplement feeds in infants with early transitional hypoglycemia.
- Calculate and manage glucose intake (enterally and/or intravenously) to stabilize hypoglycemia.
- Recognize infants who require intravenous (IV) fluids.
- Recognize infants whose hypoglycemia is unlikely to resolve quickly, who may need consultation and/or transfer to a higher level of care.
- Recognize infants with persistent or refractory hypoglycemia, who need medication to assist counter-regulation or block insulin release.
- Recognize when to exit the Fluid and Glucose Sequence to other ACoRN sequences.

Key concepts

1. Healthy term infants without risk factors for hypoglycemia should breastfeed on cue soon after birth. They do not need fluid supplements, investigation, or screening for hypoglycemia.
2. Well term and late preterm infants with risk factors for hypoglycemia who can be fed, should breastfeed on cue as soon as possible after birth and before the first glucose check at 2 h of age.
3. Unwell infants and those who cannot feed require IV fluids and glucose to maintain normal water balance and energy supply.
4. Water and electrolyte balance should be carefully monitored in infants receiving IV fluids.
5. Reliable and accurate blood glucose screening is essential in all institutions caring for infants. If point-of-care devices are used, appropriate quality control measures should be in place.
6. Glucose infusion rates (GIRs) greater than 8 mg/kg/min indicate need for higher level care. More invasive or intensive management may be required.
7. Hypoglycemia, dehydration, and overhydration can cause short- and long-term complications.

Skills

- Calculation of GIR

Well term infants receive all the fluids, glucose, nutrients, and electrolytes they need from feeding. Breastfeeding is initiated as soon as possible after birth, together with the observation and support of maternal–infant interactions. Well term infants do not need glucose or electrolyte monitoring, supplementation, or fluid management. These procedures can interfere with well-baby care, adaptation, bonding, and the establishment of breastfeeding. The best indicators of well-being in infants are behavioural: normal alertness and activity, latching, and sucking. Urine output is a key indicator of adequate fluid intake after day 1 of age. Meconium should be passed within 48 h of birth. The total postnatal weight loss should not exceed 10% of birth weight.

Term infants at risk for hypoglycemia and late-preterm infants who are well require special attention and glucose monitoring. They should be breastfed as early as possible; ideally within 30 min of birth. Monitoring is crucial but should be minimally intrusive. Perform first blood glucose screen at 2 h of age.

Unwell infants require IV fluids. They either cannot be fed, should not be fed, have symptomatic hypoglycemia, or have hypoglycemia despite managed oral intake. For these infants, the first blood glucose screen should occur as soon as they are determined to be unwell.

Fluid requirements in infants

In assessing fluid status, consider the following types of fluid requirements:

- Maintenance fluids,
- Intravascular volume expanders (to replace deficit), and
- Replacement of excessive or ongoing losses.

Maintenance fluids

A newborn's fluid intake must be sufficient to replace normal losses (from passing urine or stool) and insensible water losses (from evaporation through skin and lungs) and to achieve the calories required for normal growth. The fluid requirement for most infants on day 1 of life is approximately 3 mL/kg/ h but may be as high as 4 mL/kg/h in an extremely premature infant being cared for under a radiant warmer, due to insensible water loss.

Because free water excretion is limited during the normal prediuretic phase of neonatal transition, fluid volumes exceeding 4 mL/kg/h should not be administered before an infant is 24 to 48 h old. For infants with respiratory distress syndrome (RDS) or who are otherwise unwell, this prediuretic phase is more prolonged. Infants with renal dysfunction resulting in lower urine output may not be able to tolerate intake rates over 2 mL/kg/h.

For these reasons, maintenance fluids should not exceed maximum daily tolerance levels during stabilization (Table 7.1, page 236). If they do, however, hyponatremia is the first sign of overhydration in infants receiving solutions with low sodium concentrations. This type of overhydration shifts water into interstitial and intracellular spaces and is also called 'hyposmotic' or 'hypotonic' overhydration. For infants with oliguria (defined as urine output less than 1 mL/kg/h after 24 h of age) the glucose in fluid infusions may need to be concentrated such that the hourly rate of fluid administered will not exceed the maximum tolerance for day of age and condition.

As renal transition proceeds, fluids can be gradually increased. When the infant's diuretic phase is established, a fluid intake of 6 mL/kg/h is both tolerated and needed to deliver nutrients and meet growth demands. In infants with renal dysfunction, oliguria may be followed by a polyuric phase, with urine output exceeding the usual fluid administration rate. These infants should be monitored for dehydration.

Dehydration due to water deficits caused by decreased intake or excessive loss is usually hyperosmotic and hypernatremic. Hypovolemia due to hemorrhage, third-spacing, or gastrointestinal fluid loss is isosmotic.

Think about fluid administration in hourly units

ACoRN measures continuous infusion rates in units of hourly volume/kg (mL/kg/h) rather than daily volume/kg (mL/kg/day) because:

- Infusions are generally ordered in hourly rates,
- Calculations are easy and avoid the step of dividing the total daily volume by 24,
- Calculating the GIR is simpler, and
- It is sometimes necessary to change infusion rates within a 24-h period.

For infants receiving IV fluids, electrolytes are added on or after day 2 of age, when urine output has become established and electrolyte status has been assessed.

For infants with hypoxic ischemic encephalopathy (HIE) and/or oliguria, initial volumes should not exceed 2 mL/kg/h. A lower fluid administration rate may limit glucose delivery, thus increasing the need for blood glucose screening and, potentially, more concentrated glucose solutions.

Intravascular volume expanders

Unwell infants with intravascular volume contraction present with hypotension, hypoperfusion, or shock. They need an isotonic intravascular volume expander to replace deficit. The solution of choice is 0.9% NaCl (normal saline).

Fluid loss volumes can be difficult to estimate but are best assessed by the infant's response to a bolus of 10 mL/kg, administered over 10 to 20 min. A volume expander's effect is judged clinically, by observing an improvement in the infant's condition and vital signs. To track specific indicators of effectiveness, refer to the Clinical Assessment of Circulation Table, in Chapter 4, Cardiovascular.

Replacement of excessive or ongoing losses

Unwell infants may need volume replacement for excessive or ongoing losses. Examples include evaporative loss from an open lesion (e.g., gastroschisis), gastric or enteric fluid loss, or excessive diuresis.

Excess or ongoing fluid losses should be replaced using an IV solution that is similar in electrolyte content to the fluid lost, usually 0.9% NaCl or 0.45% NaCl, with or without potassium chloride. Replacement of excessive or ongoing losses should be in addition to routine maintenance fluids or volume expanders.

Volume expansion, replacement of ongoing losses, and maintenance fluid requirements must each be charted separately on a fluid balance sheet, along with urine output and other measurable losses (in mL/kg/h units).

Glucose requirements and homeostasis

Glucose is the main source of energy for brain cells. Maintaining an adequate blood glucose concentration is essential, because neurologic compromise can occur if the brain is deprived of glucose. Blood glucose concentration is determined by the rate of endogenous glucose production plus the rate of exogenous (external) glucose administration, minus the rate of glucose utilization (Figure 7.1).

The counter-regulation of glucose and energy homeostasis includes the following processes:

- Making new glucose from internal sources (glycogenolysis and gluconeogenesis),
- Using alternative fuels as substrates for brain metabolism (lactate, ketones, amino acids, and fatty acids), and
- Lowering the body's glucose use when availability is limited.

Knowing the glucose content and rate of administration from exogenous sources allows calculation of the minimal GIR needed to meet the infant's utilization. Calculating the GIR allows care providers to estimate the endogenous production deficit. A normal glucose utilization rate is 4 to 6 mg/kg/min. For calculation of GIR, see Next Steps, page 240.

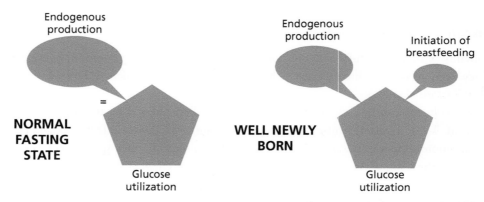

Figure 7.1. Glucose homeostasis in fasting states and normal newborn transition. During the normal fasting state, blood glucose utilization needs are met exclusively by endogenous (internal) production due to counter-regulation. As breastfeeding is established in the normal newborn, endogenous production slowly decreases until intake matches the newborn's utilization rate. Counter-regulation synchronizes with the feed–fast cycle to buffer rising and falling energy intake.

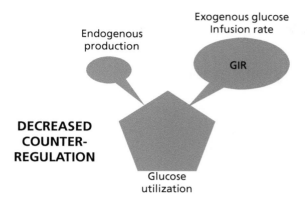

Figure 7.2. Glucose production and intake when counter-regulation is impaired. Counter-regulation may be impaired in infants with at-risk conditions (e.g., infants of diabetic mothers) and is impaired when glycogen stores are insufficient or depleted (e.g., by hyperinsulinism or certain metabolic disorders). When counter-regulation is impaired, the infant's glucose utilization needs must be met from exogenous sources.

Well term infants who are breastfeeding during transition have a glucose intake of approximately 1 to 2 mg/kg/min, derived from lactose. Their intake is well below their baseline glucose utilization rate of 4 to 6 mg/kg/min.

This low glucose intake does not lead to hypoglycemia when glycogen stores are adequate and counter-regulation is normal. As milk volume increases, so does carbohydrate intake. Milk fat also becomes an additional energy substrate.

Premature infants have bigger brains relative to their body size. Both premature and stressed infants have higher metabolic rates. Their baseline glucose utilization rate is slightly higher, at 5 to 7 mg/kg/min.

Infants who are preterm, or have intrauterine growth restriction (IUGR) or HIE, or who are otherwise unwell, have decreased glycogen reserves and may have decreased intake (Figure 7.2).

Large for gestational age (LGA) infants and infants of mothers with diabetes (IDMs), especially those with significant hyperinsulinism, have higher rates of glucose utilization and are less able to mobilize reserves. Insulin drives their metabolic pathways to make glycogen, even when they are hypoglycemic.

Hypoglycemia

Clinically significant hypoglycemia occurs when glucose production and intake cannot meet the rate of glucose utilization, and counter-regulation is underdeveloped or impaired.

Hypoglycemia can be asymptomatic or symptomatic. Infants who are symptomatic enter the ACoRN Neurology Sequence first and receive immediate IV dextrose.

Signs of hypoglycemia in the neonate include:

- Intermittent apneic spells or tachypnea
- Episodes of cyanosis
- Cardiac failure
- Sudden pallor
- Abnormal tone (limpness)
- Abnormal level of alertness (lethargy)

- Abnormal movements (jitteriness or tremors)
- Seizure-like movements
- Weak or high-pitched crying
- Difficulty feeding
- Sweating
- Hypothermia

While other conditions may share these clinical manifestations, it is critical to document glucose levels in the presence of any of these symptoms. Hypoglycemia is more likely to cause long-term neurologic complications when it is symptomatic, persistent, or when it occurs in an infant with other risk factors, such as prematurity, low birth weight, sepsis, or a history of HIE.

Symptomatic or persistent hypoglycemia is a medical emergency and requires immediate treatment with an IV dextrose solution. Follow-up of subsequent blood glucose samples and further clinical investigation are imperative.

Alerting Signs

An infant who shows one or more of the following Alerting Signs enters the ACoRN Fluid and Glucose Sequence.

Fluid and Glucose
☐ At risk for hypoglycemia[1]
☐ Blood glucose < 2.6 mmol/L[2]
☐ Unwell, not feeding, or should not be fed[3]

ACoRN Fluid and Glucose Sequence

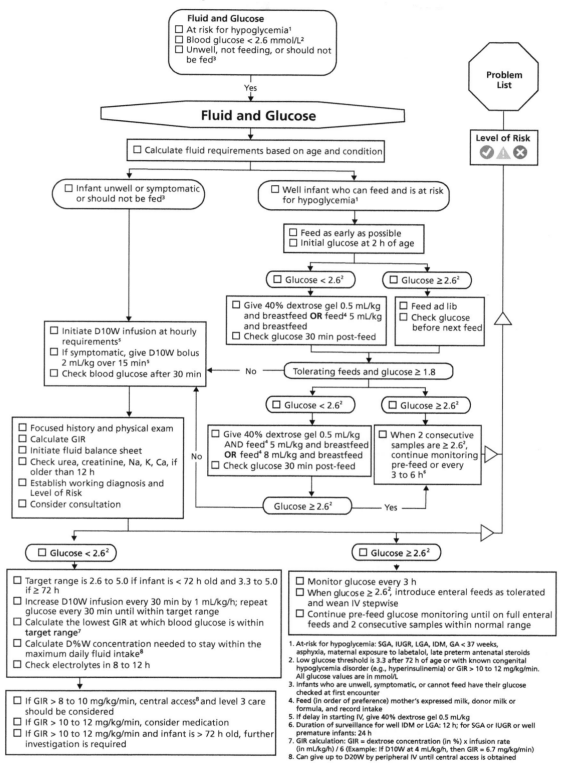

Fluid and Glucose
- ☐ At risk for hypoglycemia[1]
- ☐ Blood glucose < 2.6 mmol/L[2]
- ☐ Unwell, not feeding, or should not be fed[3]

Yes

Fluid and Glucose

- ☐ Calculate fluid requirements based on age and condition

Problem List

Level of Risk

☐ Infant unwell or symptomatic or should not be fed[3]

☐ Well infant who can feed and is at risk for hypoglycemia[1]

- ☐ Feed as early as possible
- ☐ Initial glucose at 2 h of age

☐ Glucose < 2.6[2]   ☐ Glucose ≥ 2.6[2]

- ☐ Give 40% dextrose gel 0.5 mL/kg and breastfeed **OR** feed[4] 5 mL/kg and breastfeed
- ☐ Check glucose 30 min post-feed

- ☐ Feed ad lib
- ☐ Check glucose before next feed

- ☐ Initiate D10W infusion at hourly requirements[5]
- ☐ If symptomatic, give D10W bolus 2 mL/kg over 15 min[5]
- ☐ Check blood glucose after 30 min

No ← Tolerating feeds and glucose ≥ 1.8

☐ Glucose < 2.6[2]   ☐ Glucose ≥ 2.6[2]

- ☐ Focused history and physical exam
- ☐ Calculate GIR
- ☐ Initiate fluid balance sheet
- ☐ Check urea, creatinine, Na, K, Ca, if older than 12 h
- ☐ Establish working diagnosis and Level of Risk
- ☐ Consider consultation

No ←

- ☐ Give 40% dextrose gel 0.5 mL/kg AND feed[4] 5 mL/kg and breastfeed **OR** feed[4] 8 mL/kg and breastfeed
- ☐ Check glucose 30 min post-feed

- ☐ When 2 consecutive samples are ≥ 2.6[2], continue monitoring pre-feed or every 3 to 6 h[6]

Glucose ≥ 2.6[2] ─── Yes ───

☐ Glucose < 2.6[2]

☐ Glucose ≥ 2.6[2]

- ☐ Target range is 2.6 to 5.0 if infant is < 72 h old and 3.3 to 5.0 if ≥ 72 h
- ☐ Increase D10W infusion every 30 min by 1 mL/kg/h; repeat glucose every 30 min until within target range
- ☐ Calculate the lowest GIR at which blood glucose is within **target range**[7]
- ☐ Calculate D%W concentration needed to stay within the maximum daily fluid intake[8]
- ☐ Check electrolytes in 8 to 12 h

- ☐ Monitor glucose every 3 h
- ☐ When glucose ≥ 2.6[2], introduce enteral feeds as tolerated and wean IV stepwise
- ☐ Continue pre-feed glucose monitoring until on full enteral feeds and 2 consecutive samples within normal range

1. At-risk for hypoglycemia: SGA, IUGR, LGA, IDM, GA < 37 weeks, asphyxia, maternal exposure to labetalol, late preterm antenatal steroids
2. Low glucose threshold is 3.3 after 72 h of age or with known congenital hypoglycemia disorder (e.g., hyperinsulinemia) or GIR > 10 to 12 mg/kg/min. All glucose values are in mmol/L
3. Infants who are unwell, symptomatic, or cannot feed have their glucose checked at first encounter
4. Feed (in order of preference) mother's expressed milk, donor milk or formula, and record intake
5. If delay in starting IV, give 40% dextrose gel 0.5 mL/kg
6. Duration of surveillance for well IDM or LGA: 12 h; for SGA or IUGR or well premature infants: 24 h
7. GIR calculation: GIR = dextrose concentration (in %) x infusion rate (in mL/kg/h) / 6 (Example: If D10W at 4 mL/kg/h, then GIR = 6.7 mg/kg/min)
8. Can give up to D20W by peripheral IV until central access is obtained

- ☐ If GIR > 8 to 10 mg/kg/min, central access[8] and level 3 care should be considered
- ☐ If GIR > 10 to 12 mg/kg/min, consider medication
- ☐ If GIR > 10 to 12 mg/kg/min and infant is > 72 h old, further investigation is required

Abbreviations: Ca - calcium, D%W - %age dextrose in water (e.g., D10W = dextrose 10% in water), GA - gestational age, GIR - glucose infusion rate, h - hours, IDM - infants of diabetic mothers, IUGR - intrauterine growth restriction, IV - intravenous, K - potassium, LGA - large for gestational age, min - minutes, Na - sodium, SGA - small for gestational age

At risk for hypoglycemia

Impaired gluconeogenesis is the most common cause of hypoglycemia in newborns. Specific etiologies include excessive insulin production, altered counter-regulatory hormone production, or inadequate substrate supply. These states can occur transiently in infants who:

- Are small for gestational age (SGA; weigh less than 10th percentile),
- Have IUGR,
- Are LGA (weigh greater than 90th percentile),
- Are IDMs born to mothers with gestational or insulin-dependent diabetes,
- Are premature (including late preterm), or
- Experience perinatal stress or hypoxemia,

The risk of neonatal transitional hypoglycemia increases with maternal conditions such as pre-eclampsia or eclampsia, with maternal use of medications such as beta blockers (e.g., labetalol), antenatal steroids, or oral hypoglycemics.

Maternal glucose infusions greater than 100 mL/h of D10W during labour may stimulate increased fetal insulin secretion and result in transitional hypoglycemia in the newborn.

More rarely, infants with congenital syndromes (such as Beckwith–Wiedemann), abnormal physical features (such as midline facial malformations), or certain metabolic and endocrine disorders, may develop transitional or persistent neonatal hypoglycemia.

Screen for hypoglycemia with the following risk factors in mind:

- SGA infants, and especially those who also have IUGR, are at high risk for developing new or recurrent hypoglycemia, with onset up to 24 h post-birth.
- About 8% of LGA infants experience transient hypoglycemia, with onset in the first 12 h.
- IDMs may have transient hyperinsulinism, a condition which is present at birth and usually resolves within 3 to 7 days. Transient hyperinsulinism can limit a newborn's ability to initiate gluconeogenesis and make ketones. Blood glucose levels decline more abruptly in IDMs than in typical infants, with the lowest point occurring at 1 to 2 h of age. Onset of hypoglycemia is unlikely to occur beyond 12 h post-birth. IDMs who are also LGA have an even higher risk for developing hypoglycemia.
- While also at risk for transient hypoglycemia, late preterm infants who are feeding well are unlikely to develop the condition beyond 12 h post-birth.

Screening recommendations:

- Glucose screening at 2 h of age is indicated for well term and late preterm infants at risk for hypoglycemia. These infants should be breastfed or fed on cue as early as possible after birth and before their first glucose check.
- Glucose screening on admission is indicated for preterm infants (less than 35 weeks GA) and all infants who are unwell, cannot feed, or should not be fed for clinical reasons.

Blood glucose less than 2.6 mmol/L

It is difficult to define neonatal hypoglycemia by a single value. The ability of neonates to respond to hypoglycemia and their risk of developing clinical signs or sequelae depend on size and GA at birth, previous occurrence of hypoglycemia, clinical condition, the availability of energy stores, and ongoing energy demands. What is clear is that both persistent (i.e., repeated or prolonged) and symptomatic hypoglycemia are more strongly associated with adverse neurologic outcomes than one brief hypoglycemic event.

> In at-risk or unwell infants, a blood glucose level less than 2.6 mmol/L in the first 72 h postbirth (the transitional period) indicates need for active management and ongoing surveillance. The threshold for treatment of blood glucose beyond 72 h of age is a level less than 3.3 mmol/L.

Unwell, not feeding, or should not be fed

Well term infants tend to feed irregularly on the first day of life, then with increasing frequency until maternal milk supply becomes established by day 2 to 4. After 12 h of age, the term infant that does not wake, display feeding cues, or has to 'work' at feeding requires clinical evaluation, including the ACoRN Primary Survey.

Infants who are not feeding, or should not be fed because they are unwell, require IV fluids and glucose. These include infants with:

- Moderate to severe respiratory distress,
- Cardiovascular instability (shock, cyanosis, or tachyarrhythmia),
- Symptomatic hypoglycemia,
- Neonatal encephalopathy or an Apgar score of 3 or less at 5 min,
- Poor airway protection, seizures, and/or abnormal tone,
- Surgical conditions (e.g., gastroschisis, omphalocele, tracheoesophageal fistula),
- Abdominal distension, vomiting, gross blood in stool (except when due to swallowed maternal blood), or
- Sepsis.

In addition to being at risk for hypoglycemia, infants born less than 34 weeks GA or whose birth weight is less than 1800 g are unable to tolerate full enteral intake from birth. They may develop feeding intolerance or be predisposed to necrotizing enterocolitis (NEC). For these infants, consider administering IV fluids for the first 24 to 48 h of age, along with expressed breast milk feeds that increase slowly over the next several days.

Core Steps

The essential Core Step in the ACoRN Fluid and Glucose Sequence is to calculate fluid requirements based on the infant's age and clinical condition. In most cases, fluid requirements can be calculated based on age alone.

When appropriate, enteral feeding is always preferred over IV fluids, and breastfeeding on cue should be supported over artificial feeding. When feeding measured volumes is required, the feed should be, in order of preference, the mother's expressed milk, human donor milk, or formula. With measured volume feeds, smaller, more frequent feeds are better tolerated than larger, less frequent feeds. The volume and frequency of feedings should be recorded on a fluid balance sheet.

Infants with normal renal function

Intake volumes for infants during normal renal transition increase during the first week post-birth and are outlined in Table 7.1.

Table 7.1.
Guidelines for intake by age in infants requiring measured feeds or IV fluids

Age	Measured feeds (if not breastfeeding on cue)	IV fluids
Day 1	Up to 6 mL/kg q 2 h or 9 mL/kg q 3 h	3 mL/kg/h
Day 2	Up to 8 mL/kg q 2 h or 12 mL/kg q 3 h	4 mL/kg/h
Day 3	Up to 10 mL/kg q 2 h or 15 mL/kg q 3 h	5 mL/kg/h
≥ Day 4	Up to 12 mL/kg q 2 h or 18 mL/kg q 3 h	6 mL/kg/h

Because free water excretion is limited during the normal pre-diuretic phase of neonatal transition, fluid volumes exceeding 4 mL/kg/h should not be administered before an infant is 24 to 48 h old.

q: every; h: hour(s)

For infants receiving IV fluids, electrolytes are added on day 2 to compensate for renal excretion.

Oliguria

Infants at risk for oliguria, including those with or at risk for HIE, should initially receive a restricted hourly fluid volume of 2 mL/kg/h to avoid overload and dilutional hyponatremia. Fluid balance, electrolytes, and glucose should be monitored closely and carefully documented.

Organization of Care

Care in the ACoRN Fluid and Glucose Sequence is organized initially based on whether the infant is:

- A well infant who can feed, and is at risk for hypoglycemia, or
- Unwell or symptomatic or should not be fed.

The well infant who can feed and is at risk for hypoglycemia should be breastfed or fed on cue as early as possible after birth to stimulate milk production, and before their first glucose check. Care in these infants is further organized based on their response to enteral feeds. Those whose hypoglycemia persists and those who cannot tolerate enteral feeding require IV fluid management.

The infant who is unwell or symptomatic or should not be fed requires IV fluid management.

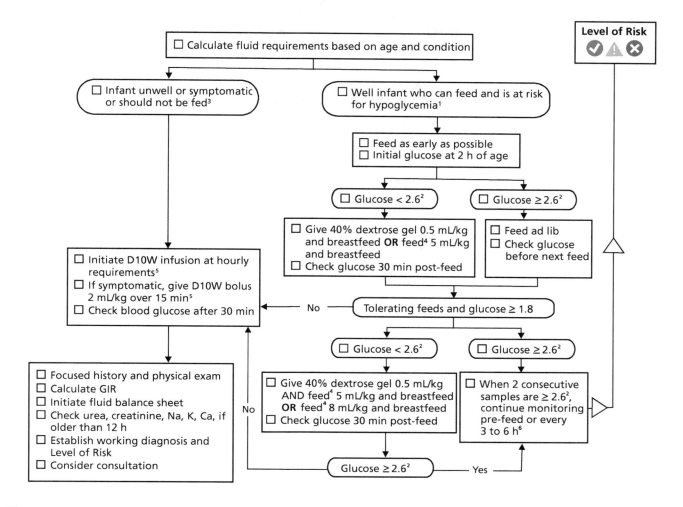

Level of Risk

Response

For the well infant who can feed and is at risk for hypoglycemia, feed as early as possible and check blood glucose at 2 h of age.

- **When the first screen indicates that blood glucose is 2.6 mmol/L or greater,** feeding should continue on cue and be supported. Repeat the glucose before the next feed. Pre-feed monitoring should continue until at least two consecutive samples are 2.6 mmol/L or greater, and the following conditions have been met:
    1. IDMs and LGA infants should be screened until 12 h of age.
    2. SGA, IUGR, and preterm infants should be screened until 24 h of age.
- **When the first glucose screen at 2 h of age is less than 2.6 mmol/L,** it is likely that glycogen stores are inadequate or that counter-regulation is impaired, most commonly by high insulin levels. In either situation, additional carbohydrate intake can be achieved by supplementing a breastfeed with an intrabuccal dose of 0.5 mL/kg 40% dextrose gel or a measured feed of 5 mL/kg. The blood glucose should be rechecked 30 min post-feed.

Supplements to stabilize blood glucose

Assuming a 2-h interval between feeds, 0.5 mL/kg of 40% dextrose gel provides an additional glucose intake of 1.6 mg/kg/min. A measured feed of 5 mL/kg provides an additional glucose intake of 3 mg/kg/min. Most mothers cannot provide a full 5 mL/kg of breast milk during transition, and an alternate milk source (e.g., human donor milk or formula) may be required.

Depending on an infant's glucose utilization rate, supplementing intake may (or may not) stabilize blood glucose at 2.6 mmol/L or greater. For infants with a normal counter-regulation but depleted glycogen stores, or with mild hyperinsulinemia, supplementing early breastfeeds with dextrose gel or a measured feed usually suffices to restore blood glucose levels.

Despite initial management, however, up to one-half of infants who receive enteral supplementation as described still need to be admitted to a specialized nursery for care.

- **If an infant's second blood glucose is 2.6 mmol/L or greater with supplementation**, this approach should be continued until the mother's milk supply increases. There is no available evidence to guide the use of dextrose gel beyond 2 doses.
- **If the infant's second glucose remains less than 2.6 mmol/L but greater than 1.8 mmol/L**, supplementation should be repeated with dextrose gel *and* a measured feed of 5 mL/kg, which provides a glucose intake of 4.6 mg/kg/min. An alternative to dextrose gel is to feed 8 mL/kg, providing a glucose intake of approximately 4.7 mg/kg/min. The infant should continue to receive breast feeds as tolerated. The blood glucose should be rechecked again 30 min post-feed. If the blood glucose remains less than 2.6 mmol/L after this second supplementation attempt, IV dextrose is required.
- If the infant does not tolerate feeding (refuses or vomits) *or* **if the second glucose is less than 1.8 mmol/L**, IV dextrose is required.

For the infant who is unwell or symptomatic or should not be fed, administer IV dextrose. The solution of choice is D10W, administered via peripheral vein, at an initial infusion rate based on age and condition, as indicated in Core Steps.

- **If an infant's blood glucose is less than 2.6 mmol/L and there is a delay in obtaining IV access**, consider administering an intrabuccal dose of 0.5 mL/kg of 40% dextrose gel.
- **If blood glucose is less than 2.6 mmol/L and the infant shows signs of symptomatic hypoglycemia**, a 2 mL/kg bolus of D10W should be administered over 15 min, followed by the D10W infusion. If there is a delay in obtaining IV access, urgently administer 0.5 mL/kg of 40% dextrose gel intrabuccally.
- **For infants who require IV dextrose**, blood glucose level should be checked 30 min after initiating the infusion, administering dextrose gel, or 30 min after completing the IV bolus.

Infants who are at risk but do not develop hypoglycemia, and those who respond to supplementation with glucose levels of 2.6 mmol/L or greater, should room in with their mothers, unless medically contraindicated.

Infant feeding patterns are a focus of care and are assessed and documented at regular intervals. Breastfeeding support and education are provided, as needed, while infant glucose levels and any supplementation needs are routinely monitored and recorded on the fluid balance sheet.

Next Steps

ACoRN Next Steps for the Fluid and Glucose Sequence should include obtaining a focused history, conducting a physical exam, calculating the GIR, initiating the fluid balance sheet, checking urea, creatinine and electrolytes if the infant is greater than 12 h old, and assessing Level of Risk.

Focused history

Important information to gather for fluid and glucose management includes the following:

Antepartum

- Maternal diabetes
- Maternal infection
- Maternal medications (e.g., beta blockers, steroids, or oral hypoglycemics)

Intrapartum

- Excessive maternal glucose infusion during labour (greater than 100 mL/h of D10W)
- Abnormal fetal heart rate

Neonatal

- Umbilical cord pH less than 7.0
- Extent of resuscitation efforts at birth
- Apgar score equal to or less than 3 at 5 min
- Prematurity
- Need for intensive or transitional care
- Birth weight and classification as appropriate for gestational age, SGA, or LGA
- Difficulty feeding or unable to feed
- Suspected or proven infection
- Seizures, jitteriness, irritability, or lethargy
- Number of wet diapers/day
- Passage of meconium

Focused physical examination

A focused fluid and glucose management exam includes the following.

Observation

- Current weight compared with birth weight and previously documented weight
- Skin colour for jaundice or plethoric appearance
- Surgical conditions or congenital anomalies
- Respiratory effort
- Measurement of vital signs: temperature, respiratory rate, heart rate, and blood pressure

Examination

- Signs of dehydration—dry mucosa, and/or poor skin turgor with tenting, sunken fontanel
- Neurologic status—level of activity, jitteriness, irritability, or seizures
- Signs of circulatory instability
- Feeding readiness (ability and intensity of suck-swallow and level of energy)
- Abdominal distension, tenderness, or bowel sounds

Calculate the GIR

It is clinically and diagnostically important to determine the GIR needed to achieve target glucose levels in infants with hypoglycemia. The GIR can be an early indicator of the illness trajectory and resolution time. Calculate a GIR for all infants with hypoglycemia requiring IV dextrose. Using the dextrose concentration and the hourly infusion rate, apply this simple formula:

GIR (mg/kg/min) = dextrose concentration (%) × infusion rate (mL/kg/h)/6

GIR: Examples and insights

- The GIR of a 1-day-old infant needing D10W at 3 mL/kg/h for hypoglycemia is:

  $$D10\,W \text{ at } 3 \text{ mL/kg/h} \rightarrow GIR = 10 \times 3 / 6 \rightarrow GIR = 5.0 \text{ mg/kg/min.}$$

  This infant's glucose requirements are within normal limits (4 to 6 mg/kg/min). The need for active glucose management will likely resolve within 24 to 48 h.

- The GIR of a 1-day-old infant requiring D10W at 4 mL/kg/h for hypoglycemia is:

  $$D10\,W \text{ at } 4 \text{ mL/kg/h} \rightarrow GIR = 10 \times 4 / 6 \rightarrow GIR = 6.7 \text{ mg/kg/min.}$$

  This infant's glucose requirement is slightly elevated. The need for active glucose management will likely continue for a few days.

- The GIR of a 1-day-old infant requiring D15W at 4 mL/kg/h for hypoglycemia is:

  $$D15\,W \text{ at } 4 \text{ mL/kg/h} \rightarrow GIR = 15 \times 4 / 6 \rightarrow GIR = 10 \text{ mg/kg/min.}$$

  This infant may need medication in addition to high concentration dextrose, and should be evaluated for persistent hypoglycemia if increased GIR persists past 72 h or if hypoglycemia recurs. Hospital stay is likely to exceed 1 week.

Initiate the fluid balance sheet

It is important to carefully document enteral and IV fluids and all outputs (urine, stool, or vomitus) for all infants admitted to a special care nursery. All types of enteral feeds should be entered, including breast and supplemental feeds, and route given (i.e., orally or by gastric tube). Each IV fluid, including any boluses, should be entered separately, along with hourly totals. The fluid balance sheet will assist in managing the fluid and glucose status of the infant within daily fluid requirements.

Renal function and electrolytes

Monitor the infant's urea, creatinine and serum electrolytes (i.e., sodium, potassium, and calcium) after 12 h of age when actively managing fluid status with IV fluids. These levels are not useful prior to this point as they reflect maternal levels until this time.

- Infants managed by restricting fluids (i.e., cases with oliguria or HIE) also need careful blood glucose monitoring, because glucose delivery is unlikely to meet the normal utilization rate of 4 to 6 mg/kg/min: D10W at 2 mL/kg/h only delivers 3.3 mg/kg/min of glucose, increasing dependence on counter-regulation to maintain glucose 2.6 mmol/L or greater.
- Infants on maintenance fluids at an hourly fluid rate exceeding the guidelines for intake by age (see Table 7.1, page 236) are at risk of dilutional hyponatremia. This risk increases when the 4 mL/kg/h rate is exceeded on day 1 of age.

Hypocalcemia and other electrolyte, nutritional, or metabolic disturbances are addressed after initial stabilization is complete. Specific care for these conditions is outside the scope of ACoRN.

Establish working diagnosis and Level of Risk

Infants entering the Fluid and Glucose Sequence because they are unwell or should not be fed require IV fluid management due to diagnoses identified in other areas of ACoRN.

Infants with a working diagnosis of hypoglycemia will have differing levels of risk based on the interventions necessary to normalize blood glucose (i.e., dextrose gel, supplemental feeding, or IV therapy).

Infants receiving IV dextrose who remain hypoglycemic have higher glucose utilization rates.

- If blood glucose is less than 2.6 mmol/L 30 min after starting the D10W infusion, it means the infant's glucose utilization rate is higher than the normal rate of 4 to 6 mg/kg/min.
- If blood glucose is less than 2.6 mmol/L 30 min after completing the 2 mL/kg bolus of D10W and starting the D10W infusion, it means the infant's glucose utilization rate is higher than 10 mg/kg/min.

Consider consultation

Level 3 consultation and consideration of transport is needed by infants with a GIR 8 mg/kg/min or greater.

Specific Diagnosis and Management

Specific diagnoses related to **fluid management** include the following.

- **Oliguria**, defined as urine output less than 1 mL/kg/h. Urine output in the prediuretic phase of transition is approximately 1 to 2 mL/kg/h. Urine output in the diuretic phase of transition is proportional to fluid intake.

- **Hyponatremia**, defined as a serum sodium (Na) less than 135 mEq/L.
- **Marked hyponatremia**, defined as Na less than 130 mEq/L.
- **Dilutional hyponatremia**, presumed when hourly fluid rate exceeds the Guidelines for intake by age (see Table 7.1, page 236) and Na is less than 135 mEq/L.
- **Hypernatremia**, defined as Na greater than 145 mEq/L.
- **Excessive postnatal weight loss**, defined as exceeding 10% of birth weight in the first week.
- **Hypertonic dehydration**, presumed when postnatal weight loss exceeds 10% of birth weight in the first week and Na is greater than 145 mEq/L.

Electrolytes should be added to maintenance IV fluids on or after day 2 of age, in accordance with regional guidelines. Management of specific electrolyte disturbances is outside the scope of ACoRN. Consultation is required.

The diagnosis of **hypoglycemia** can be categorized as:

- **Transitional**, responding to supplementation with dextrose gel or measured feeding volumes,
- **Transitional**, requiring IV therapy (GIR less than 8) for less than 72 h post-birth,
- **Persistent or recurrent**, requiring active management past 72 h post-birth (GIR greater than 8), or
- **Refractory**, persistent despite escalation of IV dextrose.

Follow this stepwise process to determine the appropriate IV dextrose solution, infusion rate, and type of IV access needed.

1. The blood glucose target range in an infant with symptomatic or persistent hypoglycemia should be 2.6 to 5.0 mmol/L if the infant is less than 72 h of age, and 3.3 to 5.0 mmol/L if 72 h or older. The upper limit of 5.0 mmol/L is recommended because overtreatment may increase insulin secretion and risk for negative neurodevelopmental outcomes.

2. To achieve the blood glucose target, increase D10W infusion in a stepwise manner, by 1 mL/kg/h every 30 min, and recheck blood glucose levels 30 min after each increase.

3. When the blood glucose target is reached, recalculate the GIR:

$$GIR = (10 \times hourly\,rate)/6.$$

4. To avoid dilutional hyponatremia, a concentrated D%W may be needed to deliver the required GIR without exceeding fluid guidelines in Table 7.1 (page 236). The concentrated D%W can be easily calculated:

$$D\%W = (GIR \times 6)/desired\,rate.$$

5. Administer the concentrated D%W by peripheral vein. Central access is recommended if dextrose concentrations greater than D12.5W are needed for prolonged periods. Escalation of D%W concentration should not be delayed while central access is obtained. Concentrations up to D20W can be administered peripherally for short periods if central access is not possible. Frequent assessment of the IV site is necessary.

---

6. Check serum electrolytes in 8 to 12 h for infants on high concentration dextrose infusions.
7. Consultation and higher-level care are needed for any infant who is receiving concentrated dextrose solutions greater than or equal to D12.5W, or when the GIR needed to achieve the blood glucose target exceeds 8 mg/kg/min.
8. Medication such as glucagon or steroids (to assist counter-regulation) should be considered when an infant's GIR exceeds 10 mg/kg/min. Consultation is required.

For infants with hypoglycemia requiring IV dextrose therapy, when the target glucose range is obtained and IV infusion is stable at a rate appropriate for day of life, monitor glucose every 3 h. Enteral feeds can be reintroduced, and IV dextrose weaned in a stepwise fashion when glucose is within the normal range for age (2.6 mmol/L or higher up to 72 h of age and 3.3 mmol/L or higher after 72 h of age). For these infants, pre-feed glucose monitoring should continue until they are on full enteral feeds and two consecutive samples are within the normal range for age.

For infants with persistent or recurrent hypoglycemia past 72 hours or with refractory hypoglycemia, further investigations are necessary to determine etiology, including endocrine and metabolic causes. These investigations are outside the scope of ACoRN and require tertiary consultation and transport.

Level of Risk: Fluid and Glucose
In the ACoRN Fluid and Glucose Sequence, level of risk is based on: whether the infant is well and can feed or unwell and cannot feed, blood glucose levels and their response to management, the treatment intensity required, and the presence or absence of neurological signs associated with hypoglycemia.
Green: • Infant is well and feeding • Blood glucose is within target range for age • Blood glucose is within target range in response to 40% dextrose gel and/or measured feeds
Yellow: • A D10W infusion is needed because the infant is unwell and cannot feed • A D10W infusion is needed to maintain blood glucose within recommended target, with a GIR less than 8 mg/kg/minute **Infants at a Yellow Level of Risk require increased levels of attention and consultation. Transfer is required if needs exceed site capabilities.**
Red: • Minimum GIR required to maintain blood glucose within target is greater than 8 mg/kg/minute • Neurologic signs are present that may be associated with hypoglycemia **Infants at Red Level of Risk require level 3 care. Transfer is required if needs exceed site capabilities.**

Fluid and Glucose: Case 1—The infant of a diabetic mother

A baby girl is born at 37 weeks GA to a mother with juvenile-onset, insulin-dependent diabetes. Maternal blood glucose has been difficult to control during pregnancy. This is her first baby. There was no need for resuscitation at birth.

The baby weighs 4000 g, is LGA and plethoric, and appears well. She is placed skin-to-skin, latches, and sucks on the breast. Mom is aware that her baby is at risk for hypoglycemia and that her blood glucose level will need to be screened.

1. Complete the ACoRN Primary Survey and Consolidated Core Steps, and generate a Problem List.

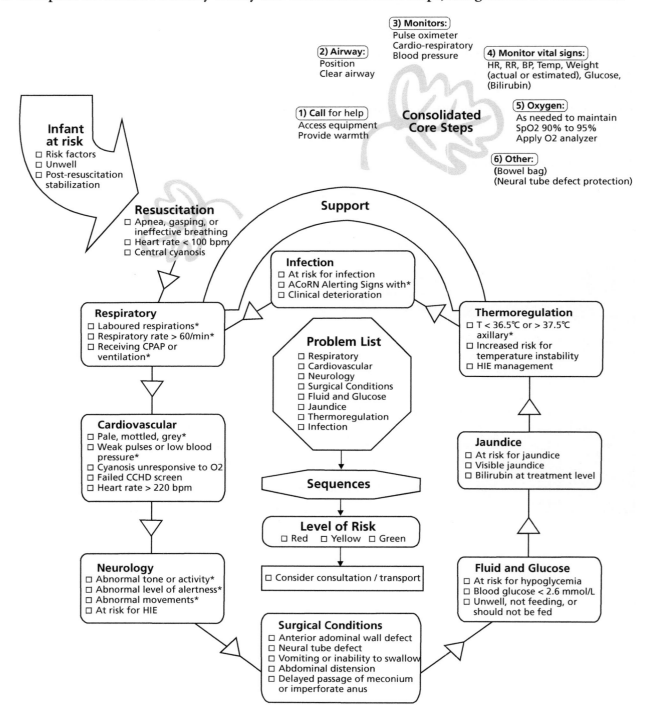

2. **This baby is at risk for hypoglycemia because her mother has diabetes. When should the first glucose screen occur?**
   ☐ At birth, because glucose control during pregnancy was difficult.
   ☐ At birth, as part of the Consolidated Core Steps in the first cycle through the Primary Survey.
   ☐ At 1 h of age, because the baby has breastfed well.
   ☐ At 2 h of age, because that is when blood glucose in infants at risk for hypoglycemia is best assessed.

The baby looks very well. She is now skin-to-skin with mom, who says that she is impressed with how well the baby took to breast. The baby has voided and passed meconium.

You complete an initial set of vital signs as part of your routine care of the well newborn.

The infant has one Alerting Sign in the Fluid and Glucose Sequence, and a question mark beside another.

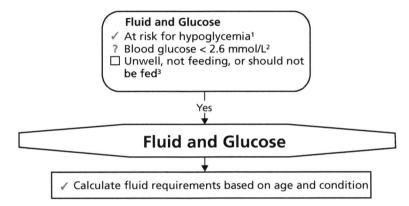

As indicated in the Core Steps of the Fluid and Glucose Sequence, you calculate the baby's fluid requirements based on age and condition.

3. **According to the Guidelines for Intake by Age Table, what are this baby's fluid requirements? (Enter a tick mark.)**

Age	Measured feeds (if not breastfeeding on cue)	IV fluids
☐ Day 1	Up to 6 mL/kg q 2 h or 9 mL/kg q 3 h	3 mL/kg/h
☐ Day 2	Up to 8 mL/kg q 2 h or 12 mL/kg q 3 h	4 mL/kg/h
☐ Day 3	Up to 10 mL/kg q 2 h or 15 mL/kg q 3 h	5 mL/kg/h
☐ ≥ Day 4	Up to 12 mL/kg q 2 h or 18 mL/kg q 3 h	6 mL/kg/h
Because free water excretion is limited during the normal pre-diuretic phase of neonatal transition, fluid volumes exceeding 4 mL/kg/h should not be administered before an infant is 24 to 48 h old.		

4. **Is there an indication to restrict breastfeeding at this time?**
   ☐ Yes   ☐ No

5. **Is there an indication to restrict fluid intake at this time?**
   ☐ Yes   ☐ No

You continue down the Fluid and Glucose Sequence.

6. How do you Organize Care for this infant?

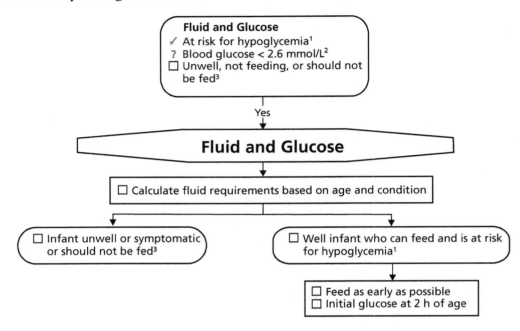

The baby has latched and is sucking well. She has breastfed twice, and mom believes that she has produced colostrum. The initial blood glucose screen, completed at 2 h of age, is 1.8 mmol/L.

7. What should the Response be?

- ☐ Initiate IV fluids and re-check blood glucose 30 min after starting IV.
- ☐ Encourage breastfeeding without supplementation. There is no need to recheck blood glucose.
- ☐ Give 0.5 mL/kg of 40% dextrose gel and check blood glucose after 60 minutes.
- ☐ Give a measured feed of 5 mL/kg expressed breast milk or formula, and recheck blood glucose 60 min after completing feed.
- ☐ Give 0.5 mL/kg of 40% dextrose gel, followed by breastfeeding, and recheck blood glucose 30 min after completing the feed.

With mom, you review the importance of normalizing blood glucose. Because the baby's blood sugar is low despite early breastfeeding, it is important to increase the baby's intake.

You recommend using dextrose gel, and explain that gel supports breastfeeding by keeping moms and babies together. You ask mom for permission to administer 0.5 mL of 40% dextrose gel to the baby's buccal mucosa before breastfeeding and make a plan to recheck the infant's blood glucose 30 min after the next breastfeed. You let her know that you will inform her doctor or midwife about using gel.

You draw up 2 mL (0.5 mL/kg) of 40% dextrose gel in a syringe and help mom to apply it to the inside of the baby's cheek, then encourage her to try breastfeeding again.

You document the use of dextrose gel and record feeding time.

The infant breastfeeds well and remains skin-to-skin.

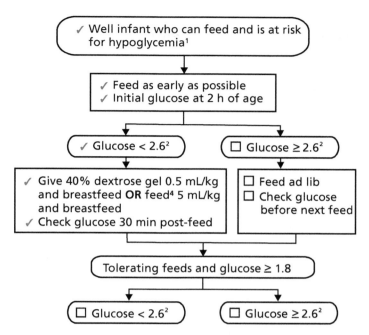

The baby remains asymptomatic 30 min after feeding is complete.

You obtain a repeat blood glucose. The result of the second screen is 2.3 mmol/L.

You inform mom that the baby's blood glucose is still low and explain that in an infant at risk for hypoglycemia, breast milk or dextrose gel alone may not be enough to support the elevated glucose utilization rate. You ask her:

- Has the infant spit up milk at any point?
- Could she express some milk to help you evaluate what volume she is currently producing?

The volume of colostrum that the mother expresses is 2 mL. You propose administering a second dose of dextrose gel, followed by a measured feed of 5 mL/kg (of expressed breast milk, donor milk, or formula), and continued breastfeeding.

Donor milk is not available at your centre, and mom is not happy about supplementing with formula. However, she understands the importance of maintaining blood glucose within the normal range.

You help her administer a second dose of gel, followed by the 2 mL of colostrum and a further 18 mLs of formula. You record this intake on the fluid balance sheet and document the blood glucose levels and use of dextrose gel.

The baby latches for further breastfeeding.

You update the infant's care provider and make a plan to check the infant's blood glucose level 30 min after the present feeding is completed. You also explain that IV fluids may be needed if blood sugar remains low.

The baby remains well. The glucose screen 30 min after feeding is 3.2 mmol/L. Mom is happy that the blood glucose has increased. She really wants to continue breastfeeding and asks whether additional doses of dextrose gel would make this possible.

You suggest that she try supplementing the next breastfeed with another 20 mL measured feed, with a plan to check blood glucose again. You do not recommend further dextrose gel applications.

The baby remains well. The glucose screen before the next feed is 2.8 mmol/L. Mom is delighted that her infant's blood glucose is now within target.

You suggest that she try breastfeeding within the next 2 h and explain that the blood glucose needs to be monitored until two consecutive samples are 2.6 mmol/L or greater 30 min after a feed is completed.

8. If this baby has a stable blood glucose equal to or greater than 2.6 mmol/L for two breastfeeds at 3-h intervals, what is the recommended monitoring period?

☐ 12 h

☐ 36 h

☐ 48 h

☐ 72 h

The baby's blood glucose levels, obtained every 3 to 6 h prior to feeding, remain ≥ 2.6 mmol/L with stable or increasing intake.

Mom and baby continue to do well and are discharged home the following day.

9. What Level of Risk is this baby at this time, and why?

☐ Green   ☐ Yellow   ☐ Red

_____

_____

Fluid and Glucose: Case 2—Persistent hypoglycemia

A baby boy is born by Caesarean section at 39 w GA to a mother with gestational diabetes and hypertension, who has been treated with labetalol. Caesarean section was necessary because of failure to progress and fetal distress. There was no need for resuscitation at birth.

The baby weighs 3500 g and appears well. He was placed skin-to-skin in the recovery room and latched and sucked at the breast within the first hour post-birth.

At 2 h of age, blood glucose was screened and was 1.6 mmol/L; 0.5 mL/kg (1.75 mL) of 40% dextrose gel was applied to the buccal mucosa, followed by breastfeeding.

The blood glucose 30 min after completion of feeding is 1.8 mmol/L.

0.5 mL/kg of 40% dextrose gel is again rubbed to the buccal mucosa, followed by 5 mL/kg (17.5 mL) of a measured feed and continued breastfeeding.

The blood glucose 30 min after completion of feeding is 2.0 mmol/L.

1. **Mark the pathway of care in the Fluid and Glucose Sequence segment below, including the next Response.**

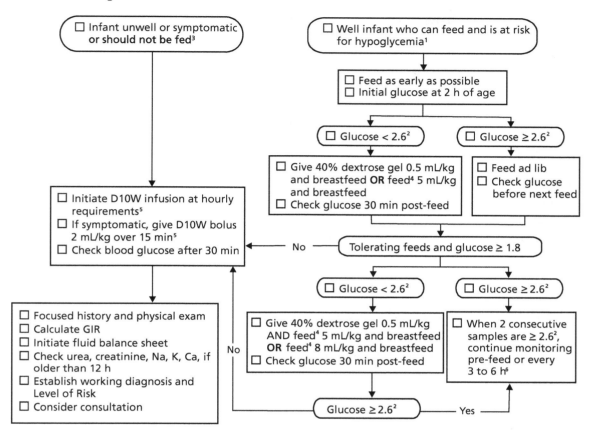

Because the response to dextrose gel, feeding, and supplementation has been insufficient, you discuss with mom the need for IV dextrose.

The baby looks well, with no jitteriness, tremors, or tachypnea. Therefore, you decide not to give a D10W bolus. You start a D10W infusion at 3 mL/kg/h and plan to check the blood glucose after 30 min.

2. **Calculate the GIR from the IV infusion.**

\
\

3. **Would the GIR calculated above meet the usual glucose needs of a newborn?**
   □ Yes   □ No

4. **Does the D10W infusion rate exceed the amount recommended in the Guidelines for Intake by Age Table to keep blood glucose within target range?**
   □ Yes   □ No

The baby's blood glucose 30 min after initiating the D10W infusion at 3 mL/kg/h is 2.3 mmol/L.

5. **What is the glucose target range for this baby, and why?**
   ☐ 2.6 to 5.0 mmol/L ☐ 3.3 to 5.0 mmol/L

   _____

   _____

6. **To increase the rate of glucose delivery to meet the glucose target range for this baby, you first:**
   ☐ Increase the infusion rate every 30 min by 1 mL/kg/h, checking glucose after 30 min, until within the target range.
   ☐ Increase the dextrose concentration to D12.5W.

The following table shows the glucose results after the increases in the D10W infusion rates in this infant:

Age in hours	D10W infusion rate	Blood glucose after 30 min
4:00	3 mL/kg/h	2.3 mmol/L
4:30	4 mL/kg/h	2.4 mmol/L
5:00	5 mL/kg/h	3.0 mmol/L

7. **What is the GIR at which the blood glucose was in the target range?**

   _____

   _____

8. **Based on the GIR above, what D%W concentration will be needed to maintain this baby within the target glucose and IV infusion rate range?**
   ☐ D12.5W at 4 mL/kg/h
   ☐ D15W at 3 mL/kg/h

9. **What Level of Risk is this baby, and why?**
   ☐ Green ☐ Yellow ☐ Red

   _____

   _____

10. **Does this baby need consultation and/or transfer to higher level care? Why or why not?**

   _____

   _____

Bibliography

Adamkin DH, AAP Committee on Fetus and Newborn. Postnatal glucose homeostasis in late-preterm and term infants. Pediatrics 2011;127(3):575–9.

Bagshaw SM, Bellomo R, Jacka MJ, Egi M, Hart GK, George C, ANZICS CORE Management Committee. The impact of early hypoglycemia and blood glucose variability on outcome in critical illness. Crit Care 2009;13(3):R91.

Ennis K, Dotterman H, Stein A, Rao R. Hyperglycemia accentuates and ketonemia attenuates hypoglycemia-induced neuronal injury in the developing rat brain. Pediatr Res 2015;77:84–90.

Harris DL, Weston PJ, Harding JE. Incidence of neonatal hypoglycemia in babies identified as at risk. J Pediatr 2012;161(5):787–91.

Harris DL, Weston PJ, Signal M, Chase JG, Harding JE. Dextrose gel for neonatal hypoglycaemia (the Sugar Babies Study): A randomised, double-blind, placebo-controlled trial. Lancet 2013;382(9910):2077–83.

Hay WW, Raju TN, Higgins RD, Kalhan SC, Devaskar SU. Knowledge gaps and research needs for understanding and treating neonatal hypoglycemia: Workshop report from Eunice Kennedy Shriver National Institute of Child Health and Human Development. J Pediatr 2009;155(5):612–7.

Kaiser JR, Bai S, Gibson N, et al. Association between transient newborn hypoglycemia and fourth-grade achievement test proficiency: A population-based study. JAMA Pediatr 2015;169(10):913–21.

McKinlay CJ, Alsweiler JM, Ansell JM, et al. Neonatal glycemia and neurodevelopmental outcomes at 2 years. N Engl J Med 2015;373(16):1507–18.

Narvey MR, Marks SD, Canadian Paediatric Society, Fetus and Newborn Committee. The screening and management of newborns at risk for low blood glucose. Paediatr Child Health 2019;24(8):536–54: www.cps.ca/en/documents/position/newborns-at-risk-for-low-blood-glucose.

Simmons R, Stanley C. Neonatal hypoglycemia studies—Is there a sweet story of success yet? N Engl J Med 2015;373(16):1567–9.

Solimano A, Kwan E, Osiovich H, Dyer R, Elango R. Dextrose gels for neonatal transitional hypoglycemia: What are we giving our babies? Paediatr Child Health 2019;24(2):115–8.

Solimano A, Osiovich H, Kwan E, Metzger DL, Everett R. Are there alternatives to over-the-counter diabetes care glucose gels for transitional neonatal hypoglycemia? Paediatr Child Helath 2020; online ahead of print DOI: doi.org/10.1093/pch/pxaa002.

Stanley CA, Rozance PJ, Thornton PS, et al. Re-evaluating 'transitional neonatal hypoglycemia': Mechanism and implications for management. J Pediatr 2015;166(6):1520–5.

Steinkrauss L, Lipman TH, Hendell CD, Gerdes M, Thornton PS, Stanley CA. Effects of hypoglycemia on developmental outcome in children with congenital hyperinsulinism. J Pediatr Nurs 2005;20(2):109–18.

Suh SW, Gum ET, Hamby AM, Chan PH, Swanson RA. Hypoglycemic neuronal death is triggered by glucose reperfusion and activation of neuronal NADPH oxidase. J Clin Invest 2007;117(4):910–8.

Thornton PS, Stanley CA, De Leon DD, et al. Recommendations from the Pediatric Endocrine Society for evaluation and management of persistent hypoglycemia in neonates, infants, and children. J Pediatr 2015;167(2):238–45.

van der Lugt NM, Smits-Wintjens VE, van Zwieten PH, Walther FJ. Short and long term outcome of neonatal hyperglycemia in very preterm infants: A retrospective follow-up study. BMC Pediatr 2010;10:52.

Vanhatalo T, Tammela O. Glucose infusions into peripheral veins in the management of neonatal hypoglycemia—20% instead of 15%? Acta Paediatr 2010;99(3):350–3.

Winnipeg Regional Health Authority. Neonatal clinical practice guideline: Parenteral fluid management for preterm and high risk neonates. June 2015. http://www.wrha.mb.ca/extranet/eipt/files/EIPT-035-018.pdf

Wintergerst KA, Buckingham B, Gandrud L, Wong BJ, Kache S, Wilson DM. Association of hypoglycemia, hyperglycemia, and glucose variability with morbidity and death in the pediatric intensive care unit. Pediatrics 2006;118(1):173–9.

Answer key: Fluid and Glucose Case 1—The infant of a diabetic mother

1. Complete the ACoRN Primary Survey and Consolidated Core Steps, and generate a Problem List.

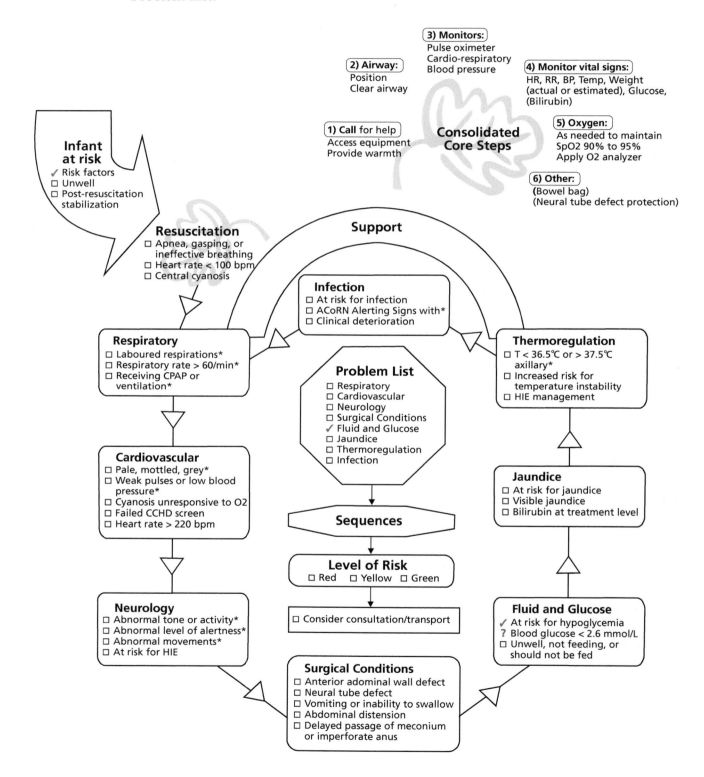

2. **This baby is at risk for hypoglycemia because her mother has diabetes. When should the first glucose screen occur?**
   - ☐ At birth, because glucose control during pregnancy was difficult.
   - ☐ At birth, as part of the Consolidated Core Steps in the first cycle through the Primary Survey.
   - ☐ At 1 h of age, because the baby has breastfed well.
   - ✓ At 2 h of age, because that is when blood glucose in infants at risk for hypoglycemia is best assessed.

The nadir or lowest level for blood glucose occurs at approximately 1 h post-birth. By 2 h, this infant should have been fed and, as a result, her glucose level should be on its way back up. Therefore, a test at 2 h is the better representation of expected glucose control.

3. **According to the Guidelines for Intake by Age Table, what are the recommended fluid requirements? (Enter a tick mark.)**

Age	Measured feeds (if not breastfeeding on cue)	IV fluids
✓ Day 1	Up to 6 mL/kg q 2 h or 9 mL/kg q 3 h	3 mL/kg/h
☐ Day 2	Up to 8 mL/kg q 2 h or 12 mL/kg q 3 h	4 mL/kg/h
☐ Day 3	Up to 10 mL/kg q 2 h or 15 mL/kg q 3 h	5 mL/kg/h
☐ ≥ Day 4	Up to 12 mL/kg q 2 h or 18 mL/kg q 3 h	6 mL/kg/h
Because free water excretion is limited during the normal pre-diuretic phase of neonatal transition, fluid volumes exceeding 4 mL/kg/h should not be administered before an infant is 24 to 48 h old.		

4. **Is there an indication to restrict breastfeeding at this time?**
   - ☐ Yes   ✓ No

5. **Is there an indication to restrict fluid intake at this time?**
   - ☐ Yes   ✓ No

6. **How do you Organize Care for this infant?**

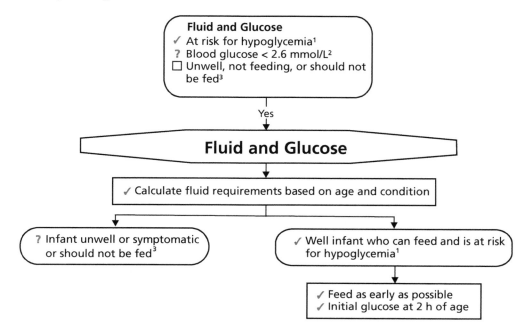

Organization of Care is based on the facts that this baby is well, can feed, and is at risk for hypoglycemia. You encourage early breastfeeding and put a blood glucose on your 'to-do' list for 2 h of age.

7. What should the Response be?

- ☐ Initiate IV fluids and recheck blood glucose 30 min after starting IV.
- ☐ Encourage breastfeeding without supplementation. There is no need to recheck blood glucose.
- ☐ Give 0.5 mL/kg of 40% dextrose gel and check blood glucose after 60 minutes.
- ☐ Give a measured feed of 5 mL/kg expressed breast milk or formula, and recheck blood glucose 60 min after completing feed.
- ✓ Give 0.5 mL/kg of 40% dextrose gel, followed by breastfeeding, and recheck blood glucose 30 min after completing the feed.

8. If this baby has a stable blood glucose equal to or greater than 2.6 mmol/L for two breastfeeds at 3-h intervals, what is the recommended monitoring period?

- ✓ 12 h
- ☐ 36 h
- ☐ 48 h
- ☐ 72 h

9. What Level of Risk is this baby at this time, and why?

    ✓ Green   ☐ Yellow   ☐ Red

The Level of Risk is Green because this baby is well and feeding, and her blood glucose entered target range with use of dextrose gel and/or measured feeds.

Answer key: Fluid and Glucose Case 2—Persistent hypoglycemia

1. Mark the pathway of care in the Fluid and Glucose Sequence segment below, including the next Response.

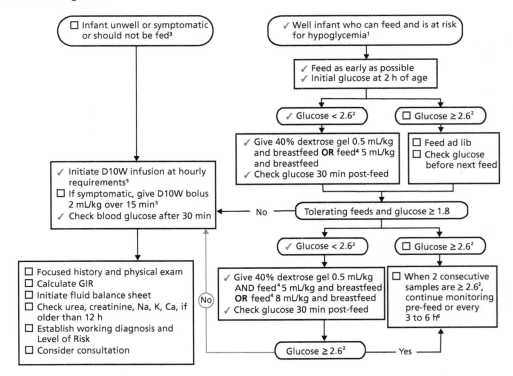

2. Calculate the GIR from the IV infusion.

The IV is D10W at 3 mL/kg/h. GIR = $(10 \times 3) / 6 = 5$ mg/kg/min

3. Would the GIR calculated above meet the usual glucose needs of a newborn?
 ✓ Yes   ☐ No

4. Does the D10W infusion rate exceed the amount recommended in the Guidelines for Intake by Age Table to keep blood glucose within target range?
 ☐ Yes   ✓ No

5. What is the glucose target range for this baby, and why?
 ✓ 2.6 to 5.0 mmol/L   ☐ 3.3 to 5.0 mmol/L

The baby is less than 72 h old.

6. To increase the rate of glucose delivery to meet the glucose target range for this baby, you first:
 ✓ Increase the infusion rate every 30 min by 1 mL/kg/h, checking glucose after 30 min, until glucose is within the target range.
 ☐ Increase the dextrose concentration to D12.5W.

7. What is the GIR at which the blood glucose was in the target range?

The blood glucose entered the target range at 5 h of age. The IV was D10W at 5 mL/kg/h. GIR = $(10 \times 5) / 6 = 8.3$ mg/kg/min

8. Based on the previous GIR, what D%W concentration will be needed to maintain this baby within the target glucose and IV infusion rate range?
 ✓ D12.5W at 4 mL/kg/h, GIR = 8.3 mg/kg/min
 ☐ D15W at 3 mL/kg/h, GIR = 7.5 mg/kg/min

D12.5W at 4 mL/kg/h yields a GIR of 8.3 mg/kg/min. D15W at 3 mL/kg/h yields a GIR of 7.5 mg/kg/min. Because the baby's blood glucose was *just below* the target range at 4.5 h of age (2.4 mmol/L; GIR 6.7 mg/kg/min), you opt to increase the concentration to D12.5W to allow the hourly rate to remain within recommended range for an infant in the first 24 to 48 h post-birth. The D12.5W infusion is running at the upper end of the volume you want to infuse on day 1 (4 mL/kg/h).

The D15W solution would require a central line for long-term infusion. A blood glucose will need to be drawn 30 min after the D12.5W is initiated.

9. What Level of Risk is the baby, and why?
 ☐ Green   ☐ Yellow   ✓ Red

The Level of Risk is Red. This baby requires IV D12.5W and a GIR greater than 8 mg/kg/min to maintain blood glucose in target range. No neurologic signs are present. This baby is at risk for persistent hyperglycemia and may require a higher concentration of dextrose and possibly a central line.

10. Does this baby need consultation and/or transfer to higher level care? Why or why not?

Yes. This baby is at risk for persistent hypoglycemia. To achieve blood glucose levels within target range, he currently requires D12.55W, a solution at the maximal recommended daily infusion rate. If D15W is needed, central access would be recommended. His hospital stay may exceed a week, and he may require additional workup, including critical hypoglycemia blood work to diagnose an underlying endocrine problem. He also requires close monitoring to avoid dilutional hyponatremia and other electrolyte abnormalities.

Jaundice

Educational objectives

Upon completion of this chapter, you will be able to:

- Recognize infants who are at increased risk for jaundice.
- Apply the Acute Care of at-Risk Newborns (ACoRN) Jaundice Sequence.
- Evaluate risk in term and late preterm infants with jaundice.
- Use the Predictive Nomogram for Hyperbilirubinemia and the Timed Bilirubin Decision-Making Table (Figure 8.3 and Table 8.2) to direct appropriate care for term and late preterm infants at risk for hyperbilirubinemia.
- Interpret and apply the Phototherapy Thresholds and Exchange Transfusion Thresholds nomograms (Figures 8.1 and 8.2) for jaundiced infants.
- Anticipate risk for severe hyperbilirubinemia and the need for consultation or care in a level 3 centre.
- Use the Bilirubin-induced Neurologic Dysfunction (BIND) Score (Table 8.1) to recognize and quantify severity of illness in acute bilirubin encephalopathy (ABE).
- Recognize when to exit the Jaundice Sequence to other ACoRN sequences.

Key concepts

1. The risk for developing severe hyperbilirubinemia is higher in late preterm infants who are discharged early and in infants who have difficulty feeding or excessive weight loss post-birth.
2. Severe hyperbilirubinemia should be anticipated in infants with red cell antigen incompatibilities (e.g., Rh or ABO incompatibility), glucose-6-phosphate dehydrogenase (G6PD) deficiency, hereditary spherocytosis, and other conditions that cause red cell breakdown or decreased bilirubin excretion.
3. The detection and management of hyperbilirubinemia in infants less than 35 weeks gestational age (GA) is different and should be directed in consultation with your regional centre.
4. The best method for predicting hyperbilirubinemia is a timed total serum bilirubin (TSB) measurement, analysed in the context of an infant's gestational age and direct antibody test (DAT).
5. Transcutaneous bilirubin (TcB) can be used as an initial screening tool.
6. TSB concentration is the standard that determines phototherapy and other treatments.
7. Neurologic symptoms occurring with hyperbilirubinemia may indicate the presence of BIND.
8. Symptomatic hyperbilirubinemia is a medical emergency.

Skills

- Plotting and interpreting nomograms
- TcB testing
- Phototherapy delivery

An estimated 60% of term infants develop jaundice, with approximately 2% developing severe hyperbilirubinemia, defined as a TSB concentration greater than 340 µmol/L. The prevention of long-term complications of hyperbilirubinemia in otherwise healthy infants remains a challenge. While jaundice is common, severe hyperbilirubinemia and its long-term complications are relatively rare.

Infants with jaundice can present in hospital or in the community. The prevention of severe hyperbilirubinemia involves a standardized assessment of risk at 24 to 48 h of age, or before discharge from the hospital if infants are less than 24 h old. Routine screening and the use of a validated predictive nomogram for assessment of risk, as well as optimal feeding support, predischarge education, and adequate postdischarge follow-up, are essential. Late preterm infants are at added risk for severe complications related to hyperbilirubinemia. Infants with known risk factors for hemolytic disease (maternal red blood cell [RBC] antibodies) are also at higher risk for early and severe hyperbilirubinemia.

The assessment of risk for hyperbilirubinemia should be conducted by trained individuals who can obtain a bilirubin measurement and arrange for timely treatment, when needed. The detection and management of hyperbilirubinemia in infants less than 35 weeks GA is different, and outside the scope of ACoRN. Management of hyperbilirubinemia in this population should be in consultation with your regional referral centre.

Sudden increases in TSB concentration occasionally occur beyond 2 to 3 days of age, and have been associated with feeding difficulties and dehydration, characterized by excessive postnatal weight loss (defined as greater than 10% of birth weight). Two-thirds of infants with jaundice, and most with severe or critical hyperbilirubinemia, present postdischarge, with readmissions peaking on days 3 to 8 post-birth.

Severe neonatal hyperbilirubinemia is defined as a TSB greater than 340 µmol/L, and critical neonatal hyperbilirubinemia as a TSB greater than 425 µmol/L and/or requiring an exchange transfusion.

ABE is the acute neurologic manifestation of bilirubin toxicity. Alerting Signs from the ACoRN Neurology Sequence occurring in the presence of hyperbilirubinemia may indicate ABE. ABE is rare in term infants whose peak TSB concentrations remain below 340 µmol/L, and uncommon unless concentrations exceed 425 µmol/L. However, ABE can occur at lower TSB levels in preterm infants, or in conditions which displace bilirubin from its carrying protein, albumin, or when the blood–brain barrier has been compromised, such as in acidosis or after hypoxic-ischemia.

The BIND score (Table 8.1) indicates mild, moderate, or severe abnormalities in an infant's mental status, muscle tone, or cry. Higher scores indicate worsening signs of neurotoxicity associated with hyperbilirubinemia. The BIND score provides a framework to estimate the severity of ABE. It is used whenever an infant presents with hyperbilirubinemia at or above the exchange transfusion threshold, or for infants with bilirubin levels above the phototherapy threshold and Alerting Signs from the Neurology Sequence.

Table 8.1.
Bilirubin-induced Neurologic Dysfunction (BIND) Score

Points	Cry pattern	Behaviour and mental status	Muscle tone
0	☐ Normal	☐ Normal	☐ Normal
1	☐ High-pitched	☐ Sleepy, poor feeding	☐ Variable hypotonia
2	☐ Piercing, shrill, frequency decreased or increased	☐ Lethargy, very poor feeding, irritable	☐ Moderate hyper- or hypotonia, posturing, 'bicycling', nuchal or truncal arching
3	☐ Inconsolable or cries only with stimulation	☐ Semi-coma, intermittent apnea, seizures	☐ Severe hyper- or hypotonia, opisthotonos, fever
Total points =			

BIND score	BIND stage	Interpretation
1 to 3	1A	Minimal signs; totally reversible with therapy
4 to 6	1B	Progressive signs but reversible with therapy
7 to 9	2	Irreversible signs but severity decreased with prompt and aggressive therapy

Adapted from Johnson L, Brown AK, Bhutani VK. BIND—A clinical score for bilirubin induced neurologic dysfunction in newborns. Pediatr 1999;104(Suppl):746–7.

Infants who are unwell with the following clinical conditions or symptoms are at increased risk for developing severe hyperbilirubinemia and BIND:

- Acidosis
- Dehydration
- Hydrops
- Hyperosmolarity
- Hypoalbuminemia
- Hypoxic-ischemic injury
- Prematurity
- Respiratory distress
- Seizures
- Sepsis

These conditions may indicate that an infant's blood–brain barrier permeability or bilirubin–albumin binding has been compromised.

Chronic bilirubin encephalopathy (CBE) is a sequela of ABE. CBE is characterized by athetoid cerebral palsy (with or without seizures), developmental delay, hearing deficit, oculomotor disturbances, dental dysplasia, and mental impairment. Early identification, monitoring, and treatment of infants at risk for severe hyperbilirubinemia can prevent the vast majority of cases from developing CBE. Severe hyperbilirubinemia in the absence of ABE may cause less severe long-term complications, such as hearing loss.

The ACoRN Jaundice Sequence promotes the early identification and management of infants who are at risk for developing clinically significant levels of hyperbilirubinemia, or who need treatment for hyperbilirubinemia.

ACoRN Jaundice Sequence

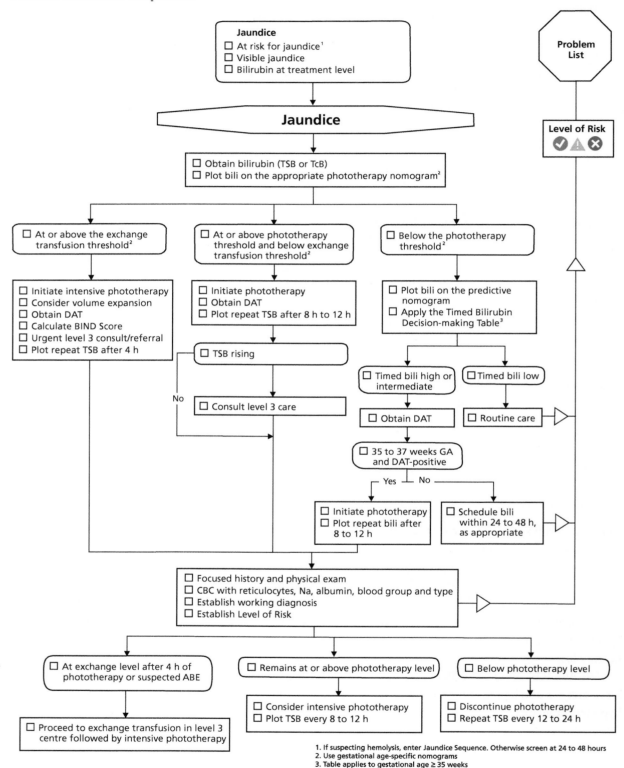

Jaundice
- ☐ At risk for jaundice[1]
- ☐ Visible jaundice
- ☐ Bilirubin at treatment level

Problem List

Level of Risk

Jaundice

- ☐ Obtain bilirubin (TSB or TcB)
- ☐ Plot bili on the appropriate phototherapy nomogram[2]

☐ At or above the exchange transfusion threshold[2]

☐ At or above phototherapy threshold and below exchange transfusion threshold[2]

☐ Below the phototherapy threshold[2]

- ☐ Initiate intensive phototherapy
- ☐ Consider volume expansion
- ☐ Obtain DAT
- ☐ Calculate BIND Score
- ☐ Urgent level 3 consult/referral
- ☐ Plot repeat TSB after 4 h

- ☐ Initiate phototherapy
- ☐ Obtain DAT
- ☐ Plot repeat TSB after 8 h to 12 h

- ☐ Plot bili on the predictive nomogram
- ☐ Apply the Timed Bilirubin Decision-making Table[3]

☐ TSB rising

No

☐ Consult level 3 care

☐ Timed bili high or intermediate

☐ Timed bili low

☐ Obtain DAT

☐ Routine care

☐ 35 to 37 weeks GA and DAT-positive

Yes — **No**

- ☐ Initiate phototherapy
- ☐ Plot repeat bili after 8 to 12 h

- ☐ Schedule bili within 24 to 48 h, as appropriate

- ☐ Focused history and physical exam
- ☐ CBC with reticulocytes, Na, albumin, blood group and type
- ☐ Establish working diagnosis
- ☐ Establish Level of Risk

☐ At exchange level after 4 h of phototherapy or suspected ABE

☐ Remains at or above phototherapy level

☐ Below phototherapy level

☐ Proceed to exchange transfusion in level 3 centre followed by intensive phototherapy

- ☐ Consider intensive phototherapy
- ☐ Plot TSB every 8 to 12 h

- ☐ Discontinue phototherapy
- ☐ Repeat TSB every 12 to 24 h

1. If suspecting hemolysis, enter Jaundice Sequence. Otherwise screen at 24 to 48 hours
2. Use gestational age-specific nomograms
3. Table applies to gestational age ≥ 35 weeks

Abbreviations: ABE - acute bilirubin encephalopathy, bili - bilirubin, BIND - bilirubin-induced neurologic dysfunction, CBC - complete blood count, DAT - direct antibody test, GA - gestational age, h - hours, Na - sodium, TcB - transcutaneous bilirubin, TSB - total serum bilirubin

Alerting Signs

An infant with one or more of the following Alerting Signs enters the ACoRN Jaundice Sequence.

> **Jaundice**
> ☐ At risk for jaundice[1]
> ☐ Visible jaundice
> ☐ Bilirubin at treatment level

At risk for jaundice

Universal screening using a timed bilirubin measurement plotted in the context of an infant's GA at birth and post-natal age in hours can reduce the risk for developing bilirubin levels known to place newborns at risk for bilirubin encephalopathy. Routine screening for bilirubin levels is recommended for all infants at 24 h to 48 h of age, or before discharge from hospital when they are less than 24 h old. For these at-risk infants, entry into the Jaundice Sequence occurs when the screening bilirubin value is known. Infants with risk factors for hemolysis or who present with visible jaundice before 24 h of age require a bilirubin measurement sooner. Infants at increased risk for severe hyperbilirubinemia include:

- Late-preterm infants aged 34 to 36 weeks GA who are discharged within 48 h of birth,
- Infants born to mothers with known RBC antibodies,
- Infants with significant bruising or cephalohematoma,
- Infants of Asian, Middle Eastern, and Mediterranean backgrounds, and
- Infants with a sibling who had severe hyperbilirubinemia.

Breastfed infants are at a higher risk for developing severe hyperbilirubinemia than formula-fed infants. Breastfeeding jaundice occurs early in the course of establishing feeds because enterohepatic circulation of bilirubin can increase in infants who have lower milk intake and dehydration. Breast milk jaundice is different from breastfeeding jaundice. It develops after 5 to 7 days of age and peaks at about 2 weeks of age. Breast milk jaundice is believed to be caused by an increased concentration of beta-glucuronidase in breast milk, causing an increase in the deconjugation and reabsorption of bilirubin. The slightly higher risk for hyperbilirubinemia in breastfed infants is insignificant when compared with the many health benefits of breastfeeding. Breast milk jaundice can be managed with appropriate post-discharge follow-up and breastfeeding support by knowledgeable individuals.

Routine formula supplementation of breastfed infants does not prevent hyperbilirubinemia.

Exclusively breastfed infants usually experience their maximum weight loss by day 3 of age and typically lose 6% to 8% of their birth weight. Infants who lose more than 8% to 10% of their birth weight are at increased risk of hyperbilirubinemia.

Risk factors associated with hemolytic jaundice include Rh isoimmunization, ABO incompatibility, other minor blood group antigen incompatibilities, RBC enzyme deficiencies (e.g., G6PD deficiency) and membranopathies (e.g., spherocytosis).

Visible jaundice

Many factors influence a care provider's ability to perceive jaundice. Therefore, relying on a visual estimation of jaundice in infants to determine risk for hyperbilirubinemia requiring treatment is inadequate.

- Jaundice may be noticeable with bilirubin at 85 μmol/L, but it can also remain undetected at levels as high as 204 μmol/L, even by experienced clinicians.

- False negative clinical assessments of jaundice have also been shown to be frequent in late preterm newborns (less than 37 weeks), in cases of early discharge (36 h or less), and in infants with darker skin tones.

Bilirubin levels should be measured by TcB or TSB in all infants with visible jaundice.

Bilirubin at treatment level

TSB concentration is the standard value that determines need for therapy. TSB is made up by two fractions: unconjugated or indirect bilirubin and conjugated or direct bilirubin. TSB fractionation is usually not required in neonatal jaundice, unless there is Rh hemolytic disease, jaundice persisting beyond days 7 to 10 post-birth, or repeatedly rebounding bilirubin levels. TSB fractions are required when there is suspicion of hepatobiliary or metabolic disease, hepatosplenomegaly, thrombocytopenia, or congenital infection.

In hyperbilirubinemia, the decision to treat is guided by graphs and nomograms (Figures 8.1 to 8.3) developed by the American Academy of Pediatrics and adapted for Canadian use:

- Figure 8.1, Phototherapy thresholds (term and late preterm infants)
- Figure 8.2, Exchange transfusion thresholds (term and late-preterm infants), and
- Figure 8.3, Predictive nomogram for hyperbilirubinemia (term and late preterm infants).

For infants born at less than 35 weeks gestation, GA-specific phototherapy graphs are required to direct management. Thresholds for starting phototherapy are different for these infants and treatment should be guided by your level 3 referral centre.

Core Steps

The essential Core Steps in the Jaundice Sequence are:

- Obtain a bilirubin measurement. Initial measurement can be either TcB or TSB.
- Plot bilirubin on the appropriate phototherapy graph (Figure 8.1 or 8.2).

Bilirubin levels are obtained and evaluated as either a universal timed bilirubin screen (TcB or TSB), or a diagnostic test (TSB) for infants with hemolytic risk factors or visible jaundice. Bilirubin can be measured using capillary or venous blood samples (TSB) or estimated by TcB testing.

TcB is noninvasive and can be used as an initial screen to identify need for more accurate blood sampling. It can also identify infants who need to be fast-tracked to receive rapid and aggressive therapy.

> For infants with mild jaundice, TcB testing may suffice to reassure providers that bilirubin levels are below the treatment threshold. For infants close to or above the threshold, a blood sample for TSB testing is needed.

TcB meters work by directing white light into a newborn's skin and measuring intensity of the specific wavelengths returned. TcB meters are increasingly used to screen newborns for jaundice, but devices vary widely in accuracy and are most accurate at lower bilirubin levels. TcB meters are less reliable in infants with darker skin pigmentation, with changes in skin colour and thickness, or after initiation of phototherapy.

All bilirubin values should be plotted on Figure 8.1 and interpreted according to the infant's GA at birth, age in hours, and risk factors.

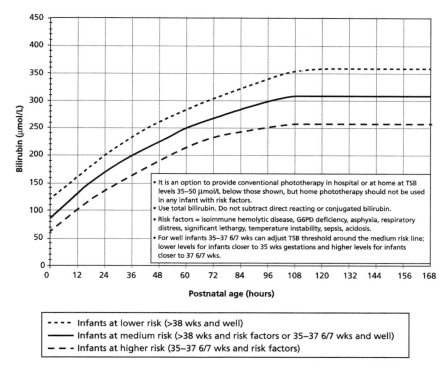

Figure 8.1. Phototherapy thresholds (term and late preterm infants)

Source: American Academy of Pediatrics Subcommittee on Hyperbilirubinemia. Management of hyperbilirubinemia in the newborn infant 35 or more weeks of gestation. Pediatrics 2004;114:297–316. Adapted and reproduced with permission.

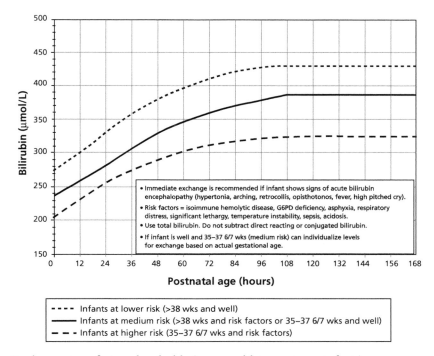

Figure 8.2. Exchange transfusion thresholds (term and late-preterm infants)

Source: American Academy of Pediatrics Subcommittee on Hyperbilirubinemia. Management of hyperbilirubinemia in the newborn infant 35 or more weeks of gestation. Pediatrics 2004;114:297–316. Adapted and reproduced with permission.

A TSB should be obtained if TcB is not available or whenever the value exceeds institutional or recommended TcB thresholds. A TSB is required whenever phototherapy is initiated, and for all subsequent samples, to monitor bilirubin levels in infants receiving treatment.

The TSB level at which phototherapy is recommended in well infants 35 to 37 weeks GA is lower than for infants older than 38 weeks GA. The lower an infant's GA, the higher the risk that TSB will rise at a rate that requires treatment, and the higher the potential permeability of the blood–brain barrier to free bilirubin.

If an infant's bilirubin level is above the threshold for starting phototherapy, it should also be plotted on Figure 8.2 to help determine the risk of progression to severe hyperbilirubinemia requiring exchange transfusion.

Organization of Care

Care in the Jaundice Sequence is organized based on plotting bilirubin levels on Figures 8.1 and 8.2.

- **Bilirubin is below the phototherapy threshold in Figure 8.1.** These infants are not presenting with hyperbilirubinemia but may be at risk for developing it in the future. Figure 8.3 and Table 8.2 are used to direct management.
- **Bilirubin is at or above the phototherapy threshold and below the exchange transfusion threshold in Figures 8.1 and 8.2.** These infants have hyperbilirubinemia. Bilirubin levels are plotted sequentially on Figure 8.1.
- **Bilirubin is at or above the exchange transfusion threshold in Figure 8.2.** These infants have severe hyperbilirubinemia and are at increased risk for BIND. Bilirubin levels are plotted sequentially on Figure 8.2.

When an infant's bilirubin level is within 50 μmol/L of phototherapy or exchange transfusion thresholds, close attention should be paid to risk factors for rapid progression. Early repeat bilirubin testing and/or initiation of the next level of intervention may be warranted.

Response

Bilirubin is below the phototherapy threshold

Response is first determined by plotting the infant's bilirubin level on Figure 8.3 to determine the infant's risk zone. Four **risk zones** (i.e., high, high intermediate, low intermediate, and low) in the **predictive nomogram for hyperbilirubinemia** estimate the potential for bilirubin levels to rise at rates that will require intervention.

- A TSB concentration between the 75th and 94th percentiles is associated with a fourfold risk of progression to bilirubin concentrations greater than 342 μmol/L in infants born 36 weeks GA (12%), versus 3% risk in infants born 40 weeks GA, and
- The lower an infant's gestational age, the higher the risk that TSB will rise at a rate that requires treatment.

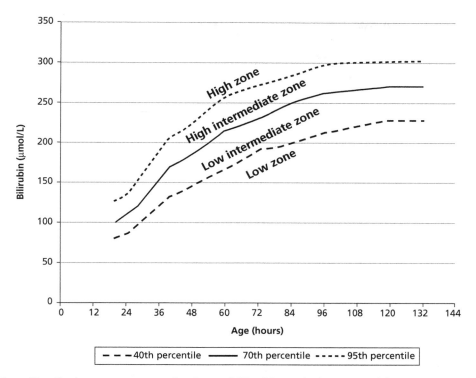

Figure 8.3. Predictive nomogram for hyperbilirubinemia (term and late preterm infants)

Source: American Academy of Pediatrics Subcommittee on Hyperbilirubinemia. Management of hyperbilirubinemia in the newborn infant 35 or more weeks of gestation. Pediatrics 2004;114:297–316. Adapted and reproduced with permission.

This risk zone identified from plotting the bilirubin value in Figure 8.3 is used in conjunction with Table 8.2 to determine appropriate follow-up, including routine care or repeat bilirubin levels, with recommended intervals for re-testing.

When maternal RBC antibodies are present, blood group and a direct antiglobulin test (DAT) are required. The DAT is positive when antibodies are attached to RBC surfaces and agglutinate when

Table 8.2.
Timed bilirubin decision-making (term and late preterm infants)

Risk zone	>37 weeks GA and DAT-negative	35 to 37 weeks GA *or* DAT-positive	35 to 37 weeks GA *and* DAT-positive
High	Test within 24 to 48 h if below phototherapy zone	Test within 24 h if below phototherapy zone	Needs phototherapy
High intermediate	Routine care	Test within 24 to 48 h	Test within 24 to 48 h
Low intermediate	Routine care	Routine care	Test within 24 to 48 h
Low	Routine care	Routine care	Routine care

DAT: direct antiglobulin test; GA: gestational age

incubated with antihuman globulin. The two most common conditions where DAT is positive are Rh incompatibility and severe ABO incompatibility. For jaundiced infants of mothers who are group O, or infants who fall within the high to intermediate risk zone, a DAT test helps determine level of risk and the threshold for therapy. A positive DAT does not necessarily predict hyperbilirubinemia, but the risk for needing phototherapy is greater in these infants.

Active hemolysis may be present with a negative DAT in mild ABO incompatibility and conditions where antibodies are not involved, such as in enzymopathies (e.g., G6PD deficiency) and red cell membrane defects (e.g., spherocytosis).

The recommended follow-up for infants who do not require phototherapy should be clearly communicated to parents. A written plan outlining next steps should be provided to parents and the infant's primary health care provider at discharge.

Bilirubin is at or above the phototherapy threshold and below the exchange transfusion threshold

The Response for these infants is to initiate phototherapy with maximal surface area coverage, obtain a DAT, repeat a TSB after 8 to 12 h, and plot it on Figure 8.1 to monitor the response to phototherapy.

When an infant's TSB is rising despite intensive phototherapy with maximal surface area coverage, a level 3 consult is recommended.

Phototherapy treatment

Phototherapy is a well-established and effective intervention for managing hyperbilirubinemia that has significantly reduced the need for exchange transfusions in infants with severe or even critical hyperbilirubinemia.

In phototherapy, light converts bilirubin into water-soluble isomers that can then be excreted in bile and urine. While light in the blue-green part of the spectrum is most active, the white light in current light-emitting diode (LED) phototherapy units is equally effective. The effectiveness of phototherapy relates to the area of skin exposed and the intensity of the light, measured in units of irradiance (μW/cm2/nm) at the relevant wavelengths, at skin level. There is a direct, linear relationship between irradiance (light intensity) and the 24-h decline in bilirubin levels to at least 55 μW/cm2/nm, with no evidence of a saturation point.

Most new phototherapy units use LED lighting. Advantages include high intensity, low power consumption, low heat production, and longer life span. LED-based phototherapy units are able to deliver an irradiance of 50 μW/cm2/nm or greater at skin level.

In jaundiced infants with lower risk of progressing to severe hyperbilirubinemia, phototherapy can be administered at an irradiance of less than 30 μW/cm2/nm. For these infants, a diaper can be left in place.

The type of phototherapy, and the resultant TSB measurements, should be routinely documented.

Intensive phototherapy, with a measured irradiance greater than 30 μW/cm2/nm, should be administered to infants at higher risk, including those who are DAT-positive or suspected to have hemolysis, or whose TSB is approaching or above the exchange transfusion threshold.

Maximal skin area should be exposed to light during phototherapy, and the covered diaper area minimized. Fibre optic phototherapy blankets, placed under or wrapped around the infant, help irradiate a large skin surface with high intensity light. They can also be used when breastfeeding infants during phototherapy, and during transport. Two phototherapy units may need to be placed around the infant to maximize surface area coverage. Eye shields protect the infant's developing retinas during phototherapy, including when breastfeeding or wrapped in a fibre optic blanket.

Breastfeeding should be continued as infants receive phototherapy.

The intensity of phototherapy can also be increased by moving the unit closer to the infant, but this may cause increased heat transfer and overheating. Manufacturer specifications for safe use should be followed.

Side effects of phototherapy include temperature instability, intestinal hypermotility, diarrhea, interference with maternal–infant interaction and, if conjugated bilirubin is elevated, bronze discolouration of the skin.

Supplemental fluids, including intravenous (IV) fluids, should only be administered to infants who are approaching the exchange transfusion threshold.

Bilirubin is at or above the exchange transfusion threshold

The goal of treatment is to maximize the rate of bilirubin clearance to prevent or minimize the neurotoxic effects of severe hyperbilirubinemia. Intensive phototherapy and supportive fluid management, including fluid expansion, should be initiated as soon as possible.

Volume expansion

Supplemental fluids can markedly reduce the frequency of exchange transfusions in infants whose bilirubin levels are near or at exchange levels, even when they are not obviously dehydrated. An IV bolus of 10 mL/kg 0.9% NaCl (normal saline) is administered initially, followed by a continuous dextrose infusion to supplement feeding. Fluids replace volume deficit, provide energy, and reduce the enterohepatic reuptake of bilirubin.

A **DAT** should be performed to better assess the risk of hemolytic anemia contributing to rapid and prolonged increase in bilirubin levels.

The **BIND score** should be calculated and documented as part of the neurologic assessment in infants with severe hyperbilirubinemia or in infants with hyperbilirubinemia and ACoRN Alerting Signs from the Neurology Sequence.

Urgent consultation

Exchange transfusion may be necessary. An exchange transfusion is a procedure that essentially replaces the infant's circulating blood volume. The goal is to remove not only the bilirubin but also the antibodies or defective RBCs causing hemolysis. The rapid reduction in serum bilirubin levels achieved with exchange transfusion, combined with the effects of intensive phototherapy, can reduce neurotoxicity risks significantly. The procedure is associated with substantial morbidity and should only be performed in centres with the appropriate expertise and monitoring ability. When a care provider anticipates that an infant's bilirubin could reach exchange transfusion levels, urgent consultation with a level 3 centre is essential to plan timely access to the procedure.

Symptomatic or severe hyperbilirubinemia (bilirubin greater than 340 µmol/L in the first 28 days post-birth) is a medical emergency. Infants with symptoms or signs of ABE should receive an exchange transfusion even if their bilirubin levels decline rapidly. The BIND score should be rechecked and documented regularly when bilirubin is at or near exchange transfusion levels, or if the infant shows any of the Alerting Signs from the Neurology Sequence in conjunction with hyperbilirubinemia.

Plot repeat bilirubin 4 h after starting phototherapy

Most infants with bilirubin above the exchange transfusion threshold respond to intensive phototherapy and supportive management for severe hyperbilirubinemia, thus avoiding an exchange transfusion. In cases of severe hyperbilirubinemia, the infant's TSB should be checked 4 h after initiating treatment to confirm response and determine whether the decrease in bilirubin levels is rapid enough to bring the TSB below exchange transfusion levels. The BIND score should be rechecked and documented regularly when bilirubin is at or near exchange transfusion levels.

Intravenous immunoglobulin

Intravenous immunoglobulin (IVIG) contains the pooled immunoglobulin G from the plasma of approximately a thousand or more blood donors. It is an immune-modulating agent that acts as a competitive inhibitor for antibodies that cause red cell destruction. IVIG has been shown to reduce bilirubin concentrations in newborns with rhesus hemolytic disease and other immune hemolytic jaundice, preventing the need for exchange transfusion. However, the evidence supporting the efficacy of IVIG for this use is limited.

Infants with a positive DAT who are at or progressing to exchange transfusion levels despite intensive phototherapy may benefit from IVIG at a dose of 1 g/kg. Level 3 consultation and direction before initiating this treatment is essential.

Next Steps

The Next Steps in the Jaundice Sequence include obtaining a focused history, conducting a physical examination, ordering necessary blood work, and establishing a working diagnosis and Level of Risk.

Focused history

Important information to gather for a focused jaundice history includes the following:

Antepartum

- Maternal blood group Rh negative or type O
- Blood group incompatibility or maternal RBC antibodies
- Evidence of hemolysis, fetal anemia studies, or intrauterine transfusions

- Intrauterine maternal infection (e.g., toxoplasmosis, cytomegalovirus, rubella, or herpes simplex virus)
- Previous infants with severe hyperbilirubinemia
- Family history of inherited disorders causing jaundice (e.g., G6P deficiency, spherocytosis, thalassemia)
- Splenectomy

Intrapartum

- High-dose oxytocin use
- Prolonged time before umbilical cord clamping

Neonatal

- Preterm or late preterm gestation
- Instrumented delivery, cephalohematoma, excessive bruising
- Poor feeding, decreased urine or stool output, or other signs of dehydration

Focused physical examination

In addition to the examination conducted during the ACoRN Primary Survey, a focused jaundice physical examination should include:

- Assessment of the infant's general appearance:
  - Unwell appearance or lethargy (possible sepsis or BIND)
  - Extent of jaundice
  - Plethora or ruddiness (polycythemia)
- Assessment of hydration status, intake and output, and fluid requirements:
  - Current weight compared with birth weight and percentage of weight loss
  - Feeding frequency, eagerness to feed, latch and suck, duration of feeds
  - Frequency of wet diapers, absence of (or excessive) stool output
- Presence of hepatosplenomegaly, ecchymosis, or petechiae (possible hemolysis)
- Presence of cephalohematoma, excessive bruising (increased bilirubin load)
- Neurologic signs consistent with ABE or BIND

Blood work

Complete blood count with reticulocytes

A complete blood count may document a high hemoglobin level in jaundice associated with high red cell mass (polycythemia) or low hemoglobin associated with either hemolysis or traumatic or concealed bleeding. The presence of reticulocytes may indicate ongoing hemolysis. An elevated white cell count or left shift may be seen in jaundice associated with infection.

Electrolytes

Elevated serum sodium may be present in jaundice associated with difficulty feeding, poor intake, and dehydration. Low serum sodium may be present in jaundice associated with excessive fluid losses and dehydration.

Albumin

Low serum albumin is rare in neonatal jaundice, but identifying hypoalbuminemia is important, because albumin binds unconjugated bilirubin in a 1:1 ratio. A low serum albumin may increase risk for neurotoxicity by increasing free unconjugated bilirubin. Consideration should be given to obtaining a serum albumin level when bilirubin levels are at or above exchange level, and in cases of hyperbilirubinemia in extremely premature infants.

Blood group-type

Maternal and neonatal blood group and type in conjunction with DAT testing is important to establish the presence or absence of alloimmune hemolytic disease.

Specific Diagnosis and Management

ACoRN deals with the identification and management of neonatal jaundice during the initial stabilization period. The specific diagnosis and underlying etiology for hyperbilirubinemia may involve additional testing and is outside the scope of ACoRN.

Infants whose TSB is at or exceeds the exchange transfusion threshold in Figure 8.2, or who are suspected of having ABE, should be managed in a level 3 centre. Intensive phototherapy with maximal body surface area coverage should be started as soon as possible and continued until transfer to a level 3 facility can be arranged. Early notification and consultation are important to ensure timely access to the services required.

Specifics related to the preparation for, or the performance of an exchange transfusion are outside the scope of ACoRN.

For infants whose bilirubin level remains at or above phototherapy level, continue intensive phototherapy. Plot serial TSBs, obtained every 8 to 12 h, until the level is below the phototherapy threshold.

Phototherapy can be discontinued once levels are below the appropriate phototherapy threshold identified in Figure 8.1. TSB levels should be assessed after discontinuing phototherapy to ensure that no rebound increase in bilirubin occurs.

Level of Risk: Jaundice

In the ACoRN Jaundice Sequence, level of risk is based on the assessed risk for hyperbilirubinemia, bilirubin level and trajectory, the level of treatment required, and the presence or absence of BIND.

Green:
- Risk for hyperbilirubinemia plotted in the low zone (per Table 8.2: Timed bilirubin decision-making)
- Bilirubin is stable, not needing phototherapy
- Rate of rise in bilirubin remains in the low zone (per Figure 8.3: Predictive nomogram for hyperbilirubinemia)

Yellow:
- Visible jaundice on day 1 or before bilirubin screening is completed
- Risk for hyperbilirubinemia plotted within the low-intermediate zone or higher (per Table 8.2: Timed bilirubin decision-making)
- Rate of rise in bilirubin with trajectory toward phototherapy zone (per Figure 8.1: Phototherapy thresholds)
- Jaundice in a preterm or late preterm infant
- Presence of bruising or cephalohematoma
- A DAT-positive infant responding to phototherapy
- Infant is receiving phototherapy but bilirubin level is under control (per Figure 8.1: Phototherapy thresholds)

Infants at a Yellow Level of Risk require increased levels of attention and may require consultation. Transfer is required if needs exceed site capabilities.

Red:
- Rate of rise in bilirubin with trajectory toward the exchange transfusion zone (per Figure 8.1: Phototherapy thresholds)
- Bilirubin at exchange transfusion level (per Figure 8.2: Exchange transfusion thresholds)
- Neurologic dysfunction with hyperbilirubinemia
- Infant is unwell
- Confirmed immune or non-immune hemolytic disease not responding to phototherapy

Infants at Red Level of Risk require level 3 care. Transfer is required if needs exceed site capabilities.

Jaundice: Case 1—The late preterm infant readmitted with severe jaundice

A late preterm baby boy is born at your hospital. The baby was born at 35 weeks GA, with a birth weight of 3000 g, to an 18-yo mother in her first pregnancy. The mother's blood group is O positive. There was no need for resuscitation at birth and overall, the baby has done well. The mother requested an early discharge from hospital because all her support systems are at or near home. The baby is latching and breastfeeding and behaving well. To facilitate this, a TSB is done at 24 h with the newborn screen. The TSB is 100 μmol/L.

1. Plot the infant's TSB level on the Phototherapy Thresholds nomogram (Figure 8.1).

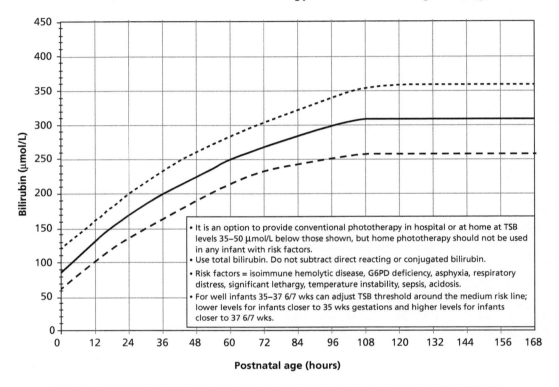

Source: American Academy of Pediatrics Subcommittee on Hyperbilirubinemia. Management of hyperbilirubinemia in the newborn infant 35 or more weeks of gestation. Pediatrics 2004;114:297–316. Adapted and reproduced with permission.

2. Which threshold line applies to this baby?
☐ Infant at lower risk (> 38 weeks and well).
☐ Infant at medium risk (> 37 weeks and risk factors, or 35 to 37 weeks and well).
☐ Infant at higher risk (35 to 37 6/7 weeks and risk factors).

3. **Because this baby is below the phototherapy threshold, you plot the bilirubin on the Predictive Nomogram for Hyperbilirubinemia (Figure 8.3).**

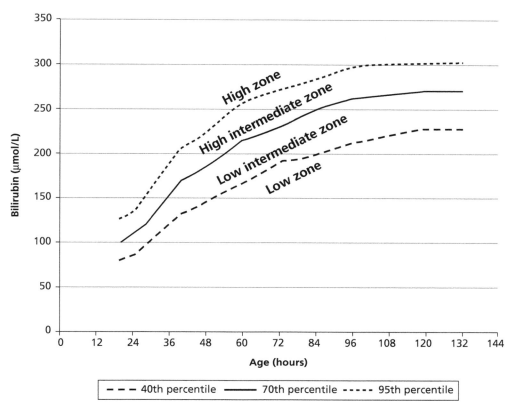

Source: American Academy of Pediatrics Subcommittee on Hyperbilirubinemia. Management of hyperbilirubinemia in the newborn infant 35 or more weeks of gestation. Pediatrics 2004;114:297–316. Adapted and reproduced with permission.

4. **You then use this information to complete your Timed Bilirubin Decision-making (Table 8.2).**

Table 8.2.
Timed bilirubin decision-making (term and late preterm infants)

Risk zone	>37 weeks GA and DAT-negative	35 to 37 weeks GA or DAT-positive	35 to 37 weeks GA and DAT-positive
High	Test within 24 to 48 h if below phototherapy zone	Test within 24 h if below phototherapy zone	Needs phototherapy
High intermediate	Routine care	Test within 24 to 48 h	Test within 24 to 48 h
Low intermediate	Routine care	Routine care	Test within 24 to 48 h
Low	Routine care	Routine care	Routine care

DAT: direct antiglobulin test; GA: gestational age

Baby is breastfeeding well and there is a 6% weight loss since birth. As the baby continues to look well, you provide routine care.

Based on the Timed Bilirubin Decision-making guidelines for term and late preterm infants, you arrange for follow-up with the community health nurse in the community in 48 h.

The clinic was closed on Sunday, so the baby was seen on Monday morning, about 48 h post-discharge. At 72 h of age, the baby arrives in the emergency room with jaundice, referred by the community health nurse. On arrival in the ER, the baby's weight is 2680 grams. He appears jaundiced but otherwise well.

5. **Complete the ACoRN Primary Survey, indicate the Consolidated Core Steps you would perform, and generate a Problem List.**

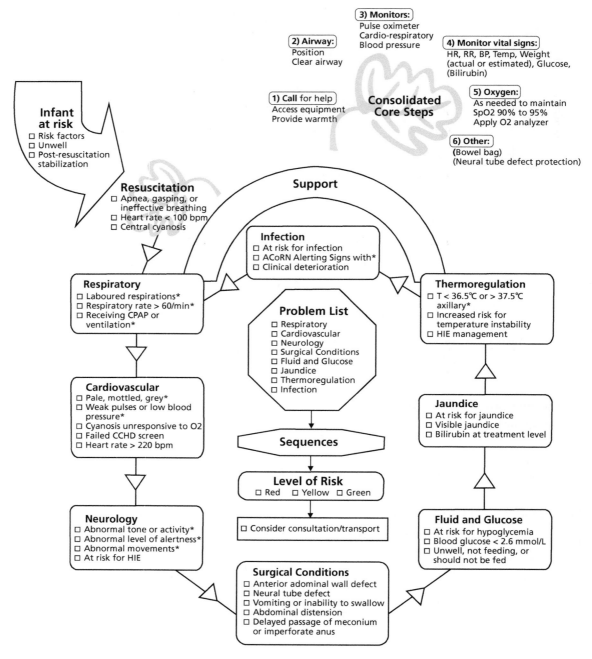

The Consolidated Core Steps add the following information: the baby's heart rate is 110 bpm, respiratory rate is 50 breaths/min, mean blood pressure is 45 mmHg, and axillary temperature 36.9°C. The glucose screen is 4.5 mmol/L and the TSB is 380 μmol/L. The estimated weight loss from birth is 11%.

The first Sequence identified in the Problem List is Jaundice.

6. Plot the re-admission TSB on Figure 8.1, the Phototherapy Thresholds nomogram, as indicated in Core Steps.

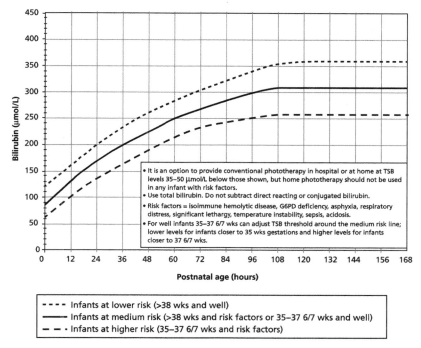

Source: American Academy of Pediatrics Subcommittee on Hyperbilirubinemia. Management of hyperbilirubinemia in the newborn infant 35 or more weeks of gestation. Pediatrics 2004;114:297–316. Adapted and reproduced with permission.

7. Because the value is above the phototherapy threshold, plot the TSB level on the Exchange Transfusion Thresholds nomogram (Figure 8.2).

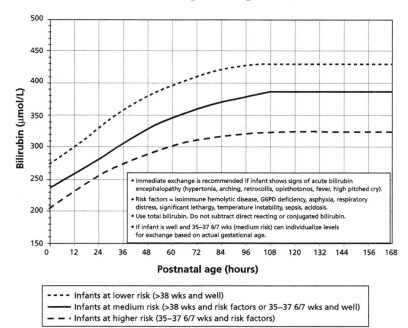

Source: American Academy of Pediatrics Subcommittee on Hyperbilirubinemia. Management of hyperbilirubinemia in the newborn infant 35 or more weeks of gestation. Pediatrics 2004;114:297–316. Adapted and reproduced with permission.

8. How do you Organize Care for this baby?

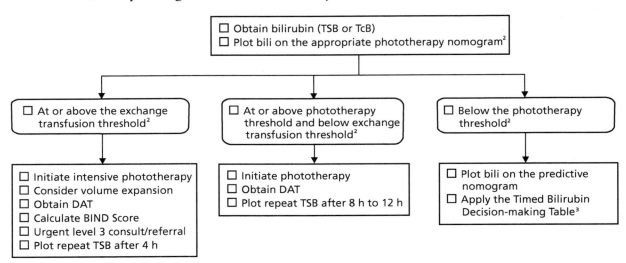

You initiate intensive phototherapy, obtain bloodwork, start an IV, and calculate a BIND score while the physician calls the regional referral centre for consult and transport: this baby's bilirubin is above the level for exchange.

9. What constitutes appropriate intensive phototherapy for this baby?
- ☐ One bank of phototherapy fluorescent or LED lights.
- ☐ Two banks of phototherapy fluorescent or LED lights.
- ☐ Three banks of phototherapy fluorescent or LED lights.
- ☐ Phototherapy with a light intensity at skin level of greater than 30 to 40 µW/cm2/nm.
- ☐ Phototherapy with a light intensity at skin level of greater than 30 to 40 µW/cm2/nm, plus a biliblanket under the infant.

10. While you are starting intensive phototherapy, you talk with mom about feeding. You recommend:
- ☐ Keeping the baby NPO to maximize time under the phototherapy light and avoid exchange transfusion.
- ☐ Keeping the baby NPO as he will likely need exchange transfusion because his TCB level is so high.
- ☐ Keeping the baby NPO to increase bilirubin excretion into the gut.
- ☐ Supported breastfeeding during phototherapy, and a biliblanket.

11. Why is the DAT assessed in severe hyperbilirubinemia? Tick all that apply.
- ☐ If positive, it indicates that antibodies are bound to the surface of RBC.
- ☐ If positive, it rules out the diagnosis of antibody–mediated hemolysis.
- ☐ The most common cause of severe hyperbilirubinemia due to hemolysis in newborns is alloimmunization involving the ABO, Rh, and minor group systems.

12. Why is it important to complete the BIND score for infants with severe hyperbilirubinemia? Tick all that apply.

☐ The BIND score focuses clinicians on the signs of ABE.

☐ The BIND score provides a structured means to document the presence or absence and severity of ABE.

☐ Infants with symptomatic severe hyperbilirubinemia should all receive an exchange transfusion.

☐ Infants with a BIND score of 0 to 3 are responsive to therapy and expected to develop mild chronic bilirubin encephalopathy.

You quickly assess the baby to determine the BIND score. He cried during his blood work and IV start but is now settled in the incubator and is sucking on his soother. He is positioned supine on the biliblanket, with arms and legs flexed.

13. Calculate and interpret the BIND Score:

Points	Cry pattern	Behaviour and mental status	Muscle tone
0	☐ Normal	☐ Normal	☐ Normal
1	☐ High-pitched	☐ Sleepy, poor feeding	☐ Variable hypotonia
2	☐ Piercing, shrill, frequency decreased or increased	☐ Lethargy, very poor feeding, irritable	☐ Moderate hyper- or hypotonia, posturing, bicycling, nuchal or truncal arching
3	☐ Inconsolable or cries only with stimulation	☐ Semi-coma, intermittent apnea, seizures	☐ Severe hyper- or hypotonia, opisthotonos, fever
Total points =			

BIND score	BIND stage	Interpretation
☐ 1 to 3	1A	Minimal signs; totally reversible with therapy
☐ 4 to 6	1B	Progressive signs but reversible with therapy
☐ 7 to 9	2	Irreversible signs but severity decreased with prompt and aggressive therapy

You initiate intensive phototherapy with two LED phototherapy lights and a fibre optic biliblanket.

You perform a focused history and physical examination.

The baby appears jaundiced and the whites of his eyes are yellowish (scleral icterus). His oral mucosa is dry, and his fontanelle is slightly sunken. You call your level 3 centre neonatologist for an urgent consult.

The consulting neonatologist requests a volume expansion of 10 mL/kg of 0.9% NaCl over 30 min. She advises to continue breastfeeding at regular intervals and to initiate a D10W infusion at 3 mL/kg/h.

Arrangements are made for transfer to the level 3 centre in case an exchange transfusion is needed. The transport coordinating physician advises that the transport time (before the baby arrives at the level 3 centre) will be at least 4 h.

Results from initial blood work show that the baby's hemoglobin is 170 g/L, serum sodium is 145 mEq/kg, and serum albumin is 35 g/L. The blood group and type are B positive, and the DAT is negative. The TSB after 4 h is 320 μmol/L, and the BIND score remains at 0. The baby has been to the breast twice and done well. The IV continues to infuse at 3 mL/kg/h. He has passed urine and stool.

14. How would you interpret the rate of TSB drop shown here?

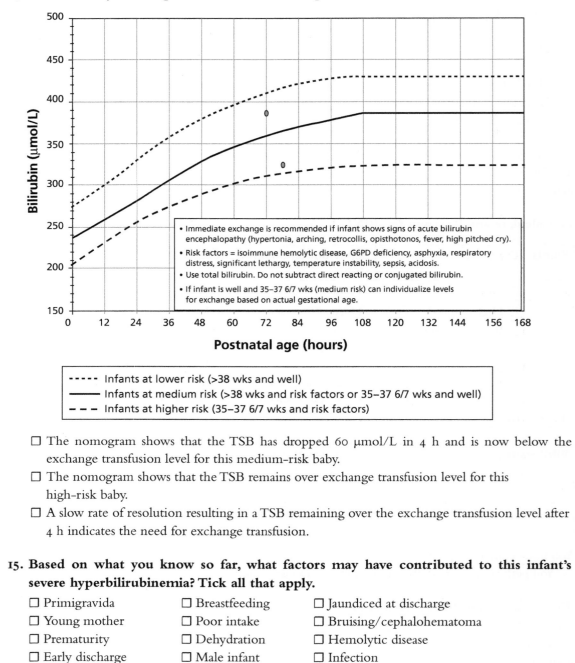

Postnatal age (hours)

----- Infants at lower risk (>38 wks and well)

——— Infants at medium risk (>38 wks and risk factors or 35–37 6/7 wks and well)

– – – Infants at higher risk (35–37 6/7 wks and risk factors)

☐ The nomogram shows that the TSB has dropped 60 µmol/L in 4 h and is now below the exchange transfusion level for this medium-risk baby.

☐ The nomogram shows that the TSB remains over exchange transfusion level for this high-risk baby.

☐ A slow rate of resolution resulting in a TSB remaining over the exchange transfusion level after 4 h indicates the need for exchange transfusion.

15. Based on what you know so far, what factors may have contributed to this infant's severe hyperbilirubinemia? Tick all that apply.

☐ Primigravida   ☐ Breastfeeding   ☐ Jaundiced at discharge

☐ Young mother   ☐ Poor intake   ☐ Bruising/cephalohematoma

☐ Prematurity   ☐ Dehydration   ☐ Hemolytic disease

☐ Early discharge   ☐ Male infant   ☐ Infection

16. What was this infant's Level of Risk before initial discharge?

☐ Green   ☐ Yellow   ☐ Red

17. What was this infant's Level of Risk when re-admitted?

☐ Green   ☐ Yellow   ☐ Red

The transport team arrives and mom and baby are transferred for higher level care. The infant is transported in a fibre optic biliblanket to allow phototherapy to continue in transit.

Bibliography

American Academy of Pediatrics Subcommittee on Hyperbilirubinemia. Management of hyperbilirubinemia in the newborn infant 35 or more weeks of gestation. Pediatrics 2004;114(1):297–316. Erratum in Pediatrics 2004;114(4):1138.

Barrington KJ, Sankaran K, Canadian Paediatric Society, Fetus and Newborn Committee. Guidelines for detection, management and prevention of hyperbilirubinemia in term and late preterm newborn infants. Paediatr Child Health 2007 (reaffirmed 2018);12(Suppl B):1B–12B: www.cps.ca/en/documents/position/hyperbilirubinemia-newborn

Bhutani VK, Johnson L, Sivieri EM. Predictive ability of a predischarge hour-specific serum bilirubin for subsequent significant hyperbilirubinemia in healthy term and near-term newborns. Pediatrics 1999;103(1):6–14.

Brodersen R, Friis-Hansen B, Stern L. Drug-induced displacement of bilirubin from albumin in the newborn. Dev Phamacol Ther 1983;6(4):217–29.

Dysart KC. Neonatal Hyperbilirubinemia (Jaundice in Neonates). Merck Manual: Professional Version: merckmanuals.com/professional/pediatrics/metabolic,-electrolyte,-and-toxic-disorders-in-neonates/neonatal-hyperbilirubinemia

Hansen TWR. Core concepts: Bilirubin metabolism. NeoReviews 2010;11(6):e316–22.

Johnson L, Brown AK, Bhutani VK. BIND—A clinical score for bilirubin induced neurologic dysfunction in newborns. Pediatr 1999;104(Suppl):746–7. (Abstract)

Kuzniewicz MW, Escobar GJ, Newman TB. Impact of universal bilirubin screening on severe hyperbilirubinemia and phototherapy use. Pediatrics 2009;124(4):1031–9.

Maisels MJ, McDonagh AF. Phototherapy for neonatal jaundice. N Engl J Med 2008;358(9):920–8.

Riskin A, Tamir A, Kugelman A, Hemo M, Bader D. Is visual assessment of jaundice reliable as a screening tool to detect significant neonatal hyperbilirubinemia? J Pediatr 2008;152(6):782–7.

Setia S, Villaveces A, Preet Dhillon P, Mueller BA. Neonatal jaundice in Asian, white, and mixed-race infants. Arch Pediatr Adolesc Med 2002;156(3):276–9.

Sgro M, Kandasamy S, Shah V, Ofner M, Campbell D. Severe neonatal hyperbilirubinemia decreased after the 2007 Canadian guidelines. J Pediatr 2016;171:43–7.

Sgro M, Campbell DM, Kandasamy S, Shah V. Incidence of chronic bilirubin encephalopathy in Canada, 2007–2008. Pediatrics 2012;130(4):e886–90.

Sgro M, Campbell D, Shah V. Incidence and causes of severe neonatal hyperbilirubinemia in Canada. CMAJ 2006;175(6):587–90.

Tan-Dy C, Moore A, Satodia P, Blaser S, Fallagh S. Predicting kernicterus in severe unconjugated hyperbilirubinemia. Paediatr Child Health 2004;9(Suppl A):17A. (Abstract)

Wennberg RP. The blood-brain barrier and bilirubin encephalopathy. Cell Mol Neurobiol 2000;20(1):97–109.

Answer key: Jaundice Case 1—The late preterm infant readmitted with severe jaundice

1. Plot the infant's TSB level on the Phototherapy Thresholds nomogram (Figure 8.1).

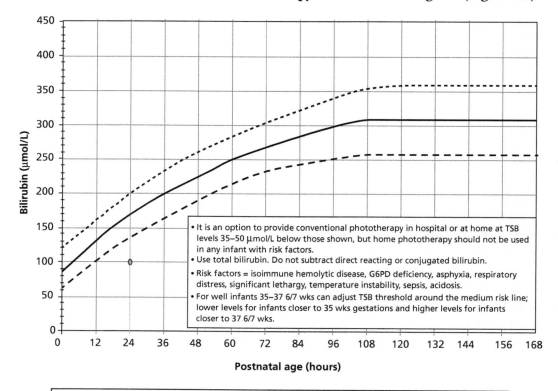

Y-axis: Bilirubin (µmol/L)

X-axis: Postnatal age (hours)

Text box within figure:
- It is an option to provide conventional phototherapy in hospital or at home at TSB levels 35–50 µmol/L below those shown, but home phototherapy should not be used in any infant with risk factors.
- Use total bilirubin. Do not subtract direct reacting or conjugated bilirubin.
- Risk factors = isoimmune hemolytic disease, G6PD deficiency, asphyxia, respiratory distress, significant lethargy, temperature instability, sepsis, acidosis.
- For well infants 35–37 6/7 wks can adjust TSB threshold around the medium risk line; lower levels for infants closer to 35 wks gestations and higher levels for infants closer to 37 6/7 wks.

Legend:
- - - - - Infants at lower risk (>38 wks and well)
- —— Infants at medium risk (>38 wks and risk factors or 35–37 6/7 wks and well)
- – – – Infants at higher risk (35–37 6/7 wks and risk factors)

2. Which threshold line applies to this baby?

☐ Infant at lower risk (> 38 weeks and well).

✓ Infant at medium risk (> 37 weeks and risk factors, or 35 to 37 weeks and well).

☐ Infant at higher risk (35 to 37 6/7 weeks and risk factors).

Because this baby was born at 35 weeks gestation and is well, with no known risk factors from the pregnancy history, we use the middle line on the predictive nomogram. Late preterm babies have a higher risk for hyperbilirubinemia because they package and clear bilirubin more slowly than term babies.

3. Because this baby is below the phototherapy threshold, you plot the bilirubin on the Predictive Nomogram for Hyperbilirubinemia (Figure 8.3).

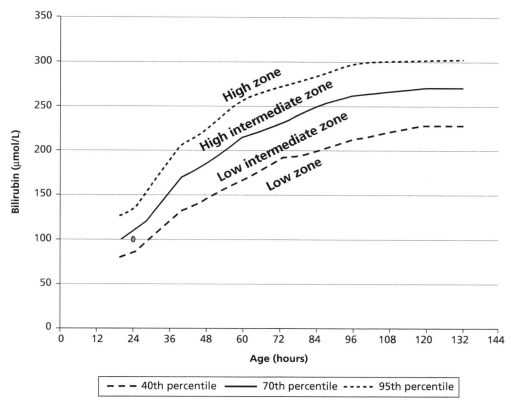

Low intermediate zone.

4. You then use this information to complete your Timed Bilirubin Decision-making (Table 8.2).

Risk zone	>37 weeks GA and DAT-negative	35 to 37 weeks GA or DAT-positive	35 to 37 weeks GA and DAT-positive
High	Test within 24 to 48 h if below phototherapy zone	Test within 24 h if below phototherapy zone	Needs phototherapy
High intermediate	Routine care	Test within 24 to 48 h	Test within 24 to 48 h
Low intermediate	Routine care	Routine care	Test within 24 to 48 h
Low	Routine care	Routine care	Routine care

DAT: direct antiglobin test; GA: gestational age

5. **Complete the ACoRN Primary Survey, indicate the Consolidated Core Steps you would perform, and generate a Problem List.**

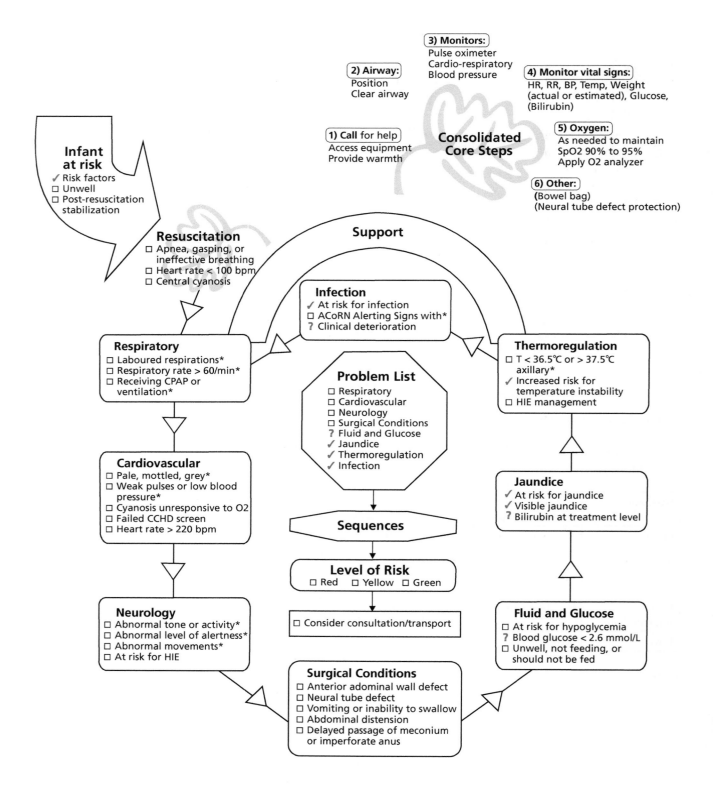

Consolidated Core Steps

1) Call for help:
Access equipment
Provide warmth

2) Airway:
Position
Clear airway

3) Monitors:
Pulse oximeter
Cardio-respiratory
Blood pressure

4) Monitor vital signs:
HR, RR, BP, Temp, Weight
(actual or estimated), Glucose,
(Bilirubin)

5) Oxygen:
As needed to maintain
SpO2 90% to 95%
Apply O2 analyzer

6) Other:
(Bowel bag)
(Neural tube defect protection)

Infant at risk
✓ Risk factors
☐ Unwell
☐ Post-resuscitation stabilization

Resuscitation
☐ Apnea, gasping, or ineffective breathing
☐ Heart rate < 100 bpm
☐ Central cyanosis

Support

Infection
✓ At risk for infection
☐ ACoRN Alerting Signs with*
? Clinical deterioration

Respiratory
☐ Laboured respirations*
☐ Respiratory rate > 60/min*
☐ Receiving CPAP or ventilation*

Problem List
☐ Respiratory
☐ Cardiovascular
☐ Neurology
☐ Surgical Conditions
? Fluid and Glucose
✓ Jaundice
✓ Thermoregulation
✓ Infection

Thermoregulation
☐ T < 36.5℃ or > 37.5℃ axillary*
✓ Increased risk for temperature instability
☐ HIE management

Cardiovascular
☐ Pale, mottled, grey*
☐ Weak pulses or low blood pressure*
☐ Cyanosis unresponsive to O2
☐ Failed CCHD screen
☐ Heart rate > 220 bpm

Jaundice
✓ At risk for jaundice
✓ Visible jaundice
? Bilirubin at treatment level

Sequences

Level of Risk
☐ Red   ☐ Yellow   ☐ Green

Neurology
☐ Abnormal tone or activity*
☐ Abnormal level of alertness*
☐ Abnormal movements*
☐ At risk for HIE

☐ Consider consultation/transport

Fluid and Glucose
☐ At risk for hypoglycemia
? Blood glucose < 2.6 mmol/L
☐ Unwell, not feeding, or should not be fed

Surgical Conditions
☐ Anterior adominal wall defect
☐ Neural tube defect
☐ Vomiting or inability to swallow
☐ Abdominal distension
☐ Delayed passage of meconium or imperforate anus

This baby appears well in the ER, with no abnormalities noted other than visible jaundice. His weight is 2680 g, down from 3000 g, an 11% weight loss, suggestive of mild dehyration and poor feeding. Jaundice is common in the neonatal period and when it occurs after 2 to 3 days of age, is often associated with feeding difficulties and dehydration.

An important cause of jaundice that must be ruled out is an infectious etiology. Although the Primary Survey did not identify any Alerting Signs with an asterisk (*), it is important to consider this baby at risk for infection until further information is obtained or infection is ruled out.

Infection can be a cause in infants with prolonged or later onset jaundice. At this early stage, it is uncertain whether there are additional risk factors for infection or if this presentation represents a clinical deterioration. You put a tick mark in risk factors for infection and a **?** beside clinical deterioration to remind you to explore these items

If the baby is undressed in the ER or on an overbed warmer and not skin-to-skin in parents' arms, he is also considered at increased risk for temperature instability.

6. Plot the re-admission TSB on Figure 8.1, the Phototherapy Thresholds nomogram, as indicated in Core Steps.

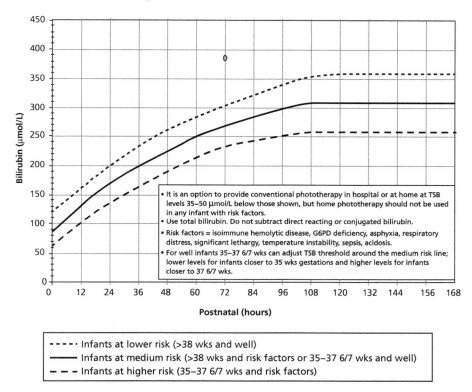

Re-admission bilirubin was 380 μmol/L at 72 h of age. This reading is above the phototherapy nomogram line for treatment, and requires plotting on the Exchange Transfusion Thresholds nomogram to determine whether an exchange transfusion may be needed.

7. **Because the value is above the phototherapy threshold, plot the TSB level on the Exchange Transfusion Threshold nomogram (Figure 8.2).**

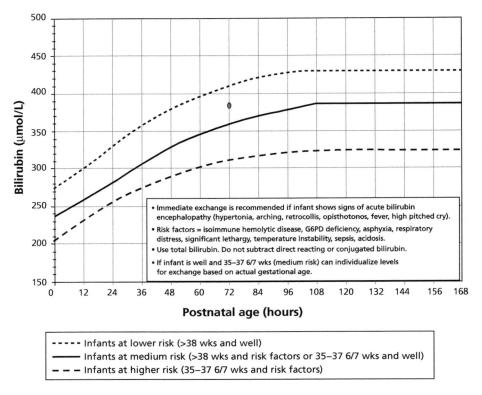

Infants at lower risk (>38 wks and well)
Infants at medium risk (>38 wks and risk factors or 35–37 6/7 wks and well)
Infants at higher risk (35–37 6/7 wks and risk factors)

This infant was assessed to at medium risk (35 weeks and well). His re–admission bilirubin (380 μmol/L) is above the threshold for exchange transfusion.

8. How do you Organize Care for this baby?

Care in the Jaundice Sequence is organized based on plotting bilirubin levels on the Phototherapy Thresholds and Exhange Transfusion Thresholds nomograms (Figures 8.1 and 8.2).

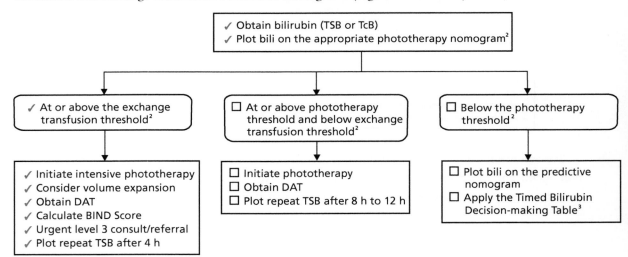

The bilirubin is above exchange transfusion threshold and this baby is at risk for progression of hyperbilirubinemia and ABE. The appropriate response is to initiate intensive phototherapy with maximal surface area coverage. Anticipate the need for more intensive management, including a double volume exchange transfusion.

9. **What constitutes appropriate intensive phototherapy for this baby?**
   ☐ One bank of phototherapy fluorescent or LED lights.
   ☐ Two banks of phototherapy fluorescent or LED lights.
   ☐ Three banks of phototherapy fluorescent or LED lights.
   ☐ Phototherapy with a light intensity at skin level greater than 30 to 40 µW/cm2/nm.
   ✓ Phototherapy with a light intensity at skin level greater than 30 to 40 µW/cm2/nm, plus a biliblanket under the infant.

The last two options constitute intensive phototherapy as defined by light intensity greater than 30 µW/cm2/nm. The final option maximizes surface area coverage and has a greater chance of decreasing the baby's TSB level over the next 4 h, and is the better choice.

10. **While you are starting intensive phototherapy, you talk with mom about feeding. You recommend:**
    ☐ Keeping the baby NPO to maximize time under the phototherapy light and avoid exchange transfusion.
    ☐ Keeping the baby NPO as he will likely need exchange transfusion because his TCB level is so high.
    ☐ Keeping the baby NPO to increase bilirubin excretion into the gut.
    ✓ Supported breastfeeding during phototherapy, and a biliblanket.

Whenever possible, breastfeeding should be maintained during phototherapy to support maternal–infant bonding and help establish milk supply. It is important to maintain, as much as possible, the level of phototherapy that the infant requires during feeding.

11. **Why is the DAT assessed in severe hyperbilirubinemia?**
    ✓ If positive, it indicates that antibodies are bound to the surface of RBC.
    ☐ If positive, it rules out the diagnosis of antibody-mediated hemolysis.
    ✓ The most common cause of severe hyperbilirubinemia due to hemolysis in newborns is alloimmunization involving the ABO, Rh, and minor group systems.

Babies that are DAT-positive with TSB at or approaching phototherapy levels are more likely to progress to severe hyperbilirubinemia and require close monitoring and early intervention.

12. **Why is it important to complete the BIND score for infants with severe hyperbilirubinemia?**
    ✓ The BIND score focuses clinicians on the signs of ABE.
    ✓ The BIND score provides a structured means to document the presence or absence and severity of ABE.
    ✓ Infants with symptomatic severe hyperbilirubinemia should all receive an exchange transfusion.
    ☐ Infants with a BIND score of 0 to 3 are responsive to therapy and expected to develop mild chronic bilirubin encephalopathy.

13. Calculate and interpret the BIND Score.

Points	Cry pattern	Behaviour and mental status	Muscle tone
0	✓ Normal	✓ Normal	✓ Normal
1	☐ High-pitched	☐ Sleepy, poor feeding	☐ Variable hypotonia
2	☐ Piercing, shrill, frequency decreased or increased	☐ Lethargy, very poor feeding, irritable	☐ Moderate hyper- or hypotonia, posturing, bicycling, nuchal or truncal arching
3	☐ Inconsolable or cries only with stimulation	☐ Semi-coma, intermittent apnea, seizures	☐ Severe hyper- or hypotonia, opisthotonos, fever
Total points = 0			

BIND score	BIND stage	Interpretation
☐ 1 to 3	1A	Minimal signs; totally reversible with therapy
☐ 4 to 6	1B	Progressive signs but reversible with therapy
☐ 7 to 9	2	Irreversible signs but severity decreased with prompt and aggressive therapy

He does not have any signs of ABE at this time.

14. How would you interpret the rate of TSB drop shown here?

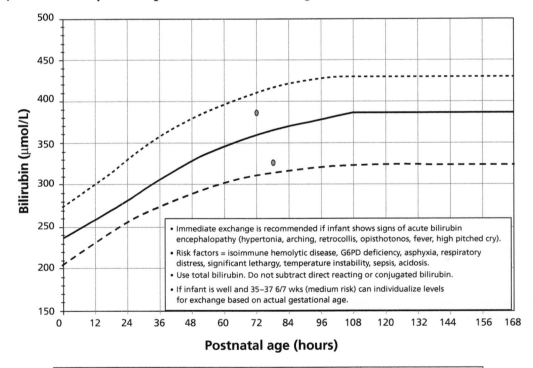

- Immediate exchange is recommended if infant shows signs of acute bilirubin encephalopathy (hypertonia, arching, retrocollis, opisthotonos, fever, high pitched cry).
- Risk factors = isoimmune hemolytic disease, G6PD deficiency, asphyxia, respiratory distress, significant lethargy, temperature instability, sepsis, acidosis.
- Use total bilirubin. Do not subtract direct reacting or conjugated bilirubin.
- If infant is well and 35–37 6/7 wks (medium risk) can individualize levels for exchange based on actual gestational age.

----- Infants at lower risk (>38 wks and well)
—— Infants at medium risk (>38 wks and risk factors or 35–37 6/7 wks and well)
- - - Infants at higher risk (35–37 6/7 wks and risk factors)

✓ The nomogram shows that the TSB has dropped 60 µmol/L in 4 h and is now below the exchange transfusion level for this medium-risk baby.

☐ The nomogram shows that the TSB remains over exchange transfusion level for this high-risk baby.

☐ A slow rate of resolution resulting in a TSB remaining over the exchange transfusion level after 4 h indicates the need for exchange transfusion.

15. Based on what you know so far, what factors may have contributed to this infant's severe hyperbilirubinemia?

✓ Primigravida	✓ Breastfeeding	☐ Jaundiced at discharge
✓ Young mother	✓ Poor intake	☐ Bruising/cephalohematoma
✓ Prematurity	✓ Dehydration	☐ Hemolytic disease
✓ Early discharge	✓ Male infant	☐ Infection

16. What was this infant's Level of Risk for jaundice before initial discharge?
☐ Green ✓ Yellow ☐ Red

The infant's Level of Risk was Yellow before initial discharge because he was preterm and his predischarge bilirubin plotted in the low-intermediate zone.

17. What was this infant's Level of Risk for jaundice when re-admitted?
☐ Green ☐ Yellow ✓ Red

The infant's Level of Risk is now Red because his bilirubin levels are above exchange transfusion levels. He requires intensive phototherapy, IV fluids, and close monitoring while awaiting transport.

Thermoregulation

Educational objectives

Upon completion of this chapter, you will be able to:

- Explain the importance of a thermally controlled environment.
- Define neutral thermal environment (NTE).
- Identify risk factors for and causes of temperature instability.
- Recognize and manage infants with or at risk for hypothermia or hyperthermia.
- Recognize the critical importance of thermal management in infants with or at risk of hypoxic ischemic encephalopathy (HIE).
- Consider principles of management for therapeutic hypothermia and strict normothermia in the infant with or at risk for HIE.
- Apply the ACoRN Thermoregulation Sequence.
- Recognize when to exit the Thermoregulation Sequence to other ACoRN Sequences.

Key concepts

1. All newborns are at risk for temperature instability.
2. Infants at increased risk for hypothermia include those born:
   - Preterm (less than 37 weeks gestational age [GA]),
   - Small for GA (SGA) (less than the 10th percentile),
   - With low birth weight (LBW; less than 2500 g),
   - With exposed lesions, such as abdominal wall or neural tube defects,
   - Unwell, and
   - In a suboptimal or uncontrolled thermal environment, such as a prehospital birth.
3. In an NTE, infants maintain normal body temperature efficiently, using the least energy, oxygen, and calories possible.
4. Cold stress can interfere with resuscitation and stabilization.
5. Hypothermia and hyperthermia can cause morbidity and mortality.
6. Temperature controls to prevent hypothermia and hyperthermia should be provided in all settings where newborns are cared for.
7. Temperature instability can be a sign of infection.
8. Maintaining a steady temperature in infants with HIE helps control metabolic rate and reduces risk for long-term neurodevelopmental injury.
9. Therapeutic hypothermia is a tertiary care treatment. It should be initiated with level 3 supervision, close monitoring, and a rehearsed clinical protocol.

Skills

- Accurate temperature measurement
- Use of an incubator
- Use of a radiant warmer

From the moment of birth, newborns use developmentally regulated mechanisms to control body temperature. These mechanisms become more effective as gestation approaches term. Temperature control is a delicate balance between heat production, conservation, and losses, and all infants are at risk for temperature instability. Infant body temperature needs to be supported for environmental and, sometimes, for illness-related reasons. Maintaining body temperature is an essential aspect of newborn care that requires minimizing heat loss and providing warmth, while avoiding overheating. Temperature support becomes especially important when stabilizing preterm or unwell infants.

Infants need to be nursed in an NTE, defined as the environmental air temperature range in which an infant can produce heat and maintain normal body temperature with minimal metabolic expenditure and oxygen consumption. Maintaining the infant's NTE is key to temperature control and management. Supporting infant and environmental temperatures appropriately can:

- Prevent hypothermia and hyperthermia,
- Maintain valuable energy stores, and
- Help prevent hypoglycemia, metabolic acidosis, and pulmonary hypertension.

Ongoing temperature monitoring is essential to avoid both hypothermia and hyperthermia.

> Infection should be considered when an infant's temperature remains elevated after controlling for environmental factors, or when the temperature of a previously normothermic infant increases, becomes unstable, or decreases.

Cold stress

Cold stress is the infant's physiological response to excessive heat loss. Cold-stressed infants can become hypermetabolic as they attempt to control body temperature. Cold stress increases caloric expenditure and oxygen consumption, depleting the infant's energy stores of brown fat and glycogen. Even when the cold stress response succeeds in preventing hypothermia, the physiological effects of increased caloric expenditure and oxygen consumption remain. Preventing hypothermia is important for infant survival and outcomes (Table 9.1).

Cold-stressed infants can show one or more of the following clinical signs:

- Bradycardia
- Irritability
- Tachycardia
- Tachypnea
- Vasoconstriction

Table 9.1.
Mechanism-specific strategies to prevent heat loss

Heat loss mechanism	Strategy
Conduction	Prewarm the radiant warmer or incubator Cover weigh scales or X-ray plate with a warm blanket Change wet for dry bedding and diapers as soon as possible Use a thermal mattress covered with a blanket for infants < 32 weeks GA
Evaporation	Dry well, if infants are ≥ 32 weeks GA Use wet-in-bag resuscitation if infant is < 32 weeks GA Cover exposed abdominal wall defect (e.g., gastroschisis) or other lesion Warm and humidify oxygen/air supplied to the incubator or ventilator circuit Delay bathing until temperature is normal and stable
Convection	Maintain room temperature at 23°C to 25°C (very LBW infants may require a higher room temperature) Prevent drafts created by air vents, windows, doors or fans 'Nest' by placing blankets or rolls around the infant Place the infant in an incubator and close portholes Raise the sides on the radiant warmer
Radiation	Keep the infant in a flexed position Place warm blankets under the infant, especially if the radiant warmer is not preheated Once dried, place a pre-warmed hat on the infant's head Avoid blocking the heat source in a radiant warmer Use the servo control setting on a radiant warmer Use a double-walled incubator, if possible, or put a transparent shield over the infant in a single-walled incubator Place a cover over a transport incubator and use servo control

Extended periods of cold stress can cause harmful side effects, including apnea, hypoglycemia, respiratory distress, hypoxia, metabolic acidosis, necrotizing enterocolitis, and failure to gain weight. Infants with sepsis, respiratory distress, shock, or hypoxia often experience the effects of hypothermia quickly and severely, as do infants who are experiencing heat loss from more than one mechanism (e.g., a wet infant in a drafty environment).

Taking a single temperature may not indicate whether an infant is cold-stressed, hypermetabolic, or consuming oxygen at an accelerated rate. A newborn who is not cared for within an NTE will experience cold stress and become hypermetabolic, even while managing to maintain a normal body temperature. An infant who is thermally supported while undergoing therapeutic hypothermia or being rewarmed will not be hypermetabolic.

Heat stress

Heat stress occurs when environmental or other demands exceed an infant's thermoregulatory mechanisms for staying cool, raising body temperature beyond the normothermic range. An elevated temperature immediately following birth is usually caused by maternal hyperthermia. Early hyperthermia can also have an iatrogenic cause, such as overheating by a radiant warmer. Other causes of hyperthermia to consider include chorioamnionitis, dehydration, infection, administration of prostaglandin E1, and central nervous system disorders.

The ACoRN Thermoregulation Sequence

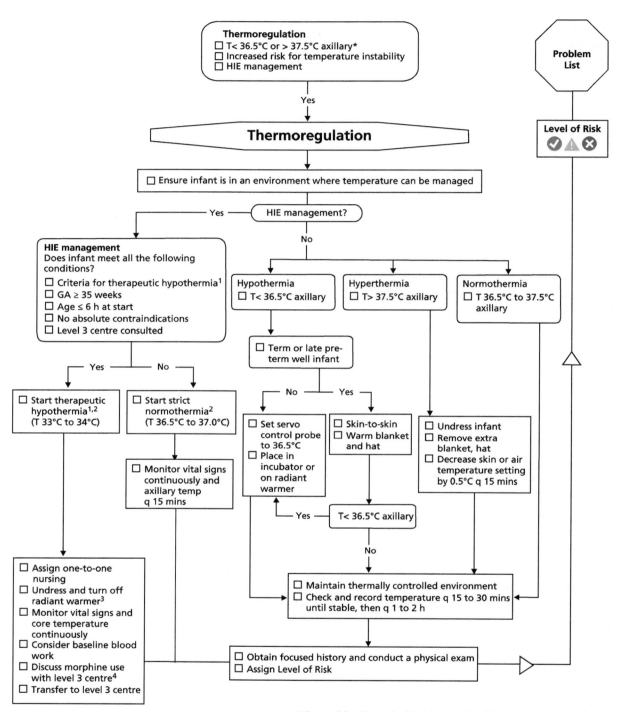

Thermoregulation
- ☐ T< 36.5°C or > 37.5°C axillary*
- ☐ Increased risk for temperature instability
- ☐ HIE management

Yes

Problem List

Level of Risk
✓ ⚠ ✗

Thermoregulation

☐ Ensure infant is in an environment where temperature can be managed

Yes — **HIE management?**

No

HIE management
Does infant meet all the following conditions?
- ☐ Criteria for therapeutic hypothermia[1]
- ☐ GA ≥ 35 weeks
- ☐ Age ≤ 6 h at start
- ☐ No absolute contraindications
- ☐ Level 3 centre consulted

Yes — No

Hypothermia
- ☐ T< 36.5°C axillary

Hyperthermia
- ☐ T> 37.5°C axillary

Normothermia
- ☐ T 36.5°C to 37.5°C axillary

☐ Term or late pre-term well infant

No — Yes

☐ Start therapeutic hypothermia[1,2] (T 33°C to 34°C)

☐ Start strict normothermia[2] (T 36.5°C to 37.0°C)

☐ Monitor vital signs continuously and axillary temp q 15 mins

☐ Set servo control probe to 36.5°C
☐ Place in incubator or on radiant warmer

☐ Skin-to-skin
☐ Warm blanket and hat

☐ Undress infant
☐ Remove extra blanket, hat
☐ Decrease skin or air temperature setting by 0.5°C q 15 mins

Yes — T< 36.5°C axillary

No

☐ Maintain thermally controlled environment
☐ Check and record temperature q 15 to 30 mins until stable, then q 1 to 2 h

☐ Assign one-to-one nursing
☐ Undress and turn off radiant warmer[3]
☐ Monitor vital signs and core temperature continuously
☐ Consider baseline blood work
☐ Discuss morphine use with level 3 centre[4]
☐ Transfer to level 3 centre

☐ Obtain focused history and conduct a physical exam
☐ Assign Level of Risk

1. Therapeutic hypothermia should only be attempted with trained personnel and under a rehearsed clinical protocol–the "low tech" method in this Sequence is adapted from the ICE Trial Protocol. See also the Neurology Chapter and Appendix A
2. Poorly administered hypothermia may be worse than maintaining normothermia
3. Passive hypothermia is not meant to replace servo controlled therapeutic hypothermia
4. Hypothermia is stressful; stress may worsen outcomes

Abbreviations: GA - gestational age, h - hours, HIE - hypoxic ischemic encephalopathy, mins - minutes, q - every, T - temperature

Clinical features may help to distinguish whether an infant's elevated temperature is caused by overheating or an increase in heat production. The overheated infant uses heat-reducing mechanisms, such as vasodilation (having a flushed appearance and warm hands and feet), an extended posture, tachypnea and, in the term infant, sweating. The febrile infant produces heat with rising body temperature and is vasoconstricted (having pale or mottled skin and cool hands and feet). Irritability, tachycardia, and a bounding pulse may be present in either situation of hyperthermia.

If heat stress is severe, the infant may also experience apnea or seizures. When hyperthermia is untreated, increased metabolic rate and evaporative water loss will ultimately lead to dehydration and shock.

Alerting Signs

An infant who shows any of the following Alerting Signs enters the ACoRN Thermoregulation Sequence.

> **Thermoregulation**
> ☐ T< 36.5℃ or > 37.5℃ axillary*
> ☐ Increased risk for temperature instability
> ☐ HIE management

Temperature less than 36.5℃ or greater than 37.5℃ axillary*

Axillary temperature should be maintained in the normothermic range between 36.5℃ and 37.5℃, inclusive.

Obtaining an infant's temperature

Axillary:

- Ensure the infant's armpit is dry.
- Place the tip of an electronic thermometer mid-armpit and adduct the arm.
- Hold this position until the electronic thermometer beeps and the temperature is displayed.

When proper technique is used, axillary temperature measurement is safe, convenient, and comparable to rectal temperature measurement.

Rectal:

- Not recommended for routine readings due to risk for rectal or sigmoid trauma.

Core temperature monitoring for therapeutic hypothermia:

- A rectal probe is inserted to 5 cm and marked with tape at that length. Each time a temperature is recorded, check the probe position to ensure it has not moved.
- Though ideal for continuous monitoring in infants receiving therapeutic hypothermia, this method may not be practical or available in many community hospital settings.

Glass mercury and tympanic thermometers are not recommended for use in newborns.

A newborn with an infection is more likely to be hypothermic than hyperthermic.

Increased risk for temperature instability

Infants have a surface area-to-body mass ratio that is four times that of an adult, yet their ability to increase heat production is only one-third as efficient.

All infants are at increased risk of temperature instability. Consider infant body temperature in the context of GA, birth weight, birth history, physical exam findings, and the environment.

Some medications (e.g., prostaglandin E1) and interventions (e.g., phototherapy) can impact infant temperature and need to be considered when assessing and managing thermoregulation.

Temperature is especially labile during transition from the intrauterine to extrauterine environment. Although minor variances from normal are common, a fluctuating temperature can trigger a hypermetabolic response.

Whenever possible, thermal management using skin-to-skin ('kangaroo') care is strongly encouraged.

Infants at increased risk for hypothermia include those born:

- Preterm—Hypothermia risk increases with decreasing GA and birth weight. These infants have not yet developed adequate stores of heat-generating brown fat or insulating white fat. Preterm infants are less able to increase their metabolic rate than weight-matched SGA infants.
- SGA—They have used up their stores of heat-generating brown fat and have less white fat.
- LBW (less than 2500 g) and SGA—These infants have larger surface area in relation to their body weight and experience greater heat loss than term, appropriate for GA infants.
- Unwell—They are unable to break down their stores of brown fat, and have lower heat production rates, especially if they are infected or hypoxic.
- With congenital anomalies—They will experience excessive evaporative heat loss, if they have an open lesion or exposed organ.
- With central nervous system injury.
- With decreased activity or hypotonia related to medication exposure, such as paralytics, anaesthesia, or sedatives.
- In a suboptimal thermal environment, such as prehospital birth. These infants may have heat loss from multiple mechanisms (e.g., a cold environment, wet linens, insufficient drying, or drafts).

Although infants less than 35 weeks GA can produce heat and respond to changes in their thermal environment, they have difficulty regulating and overcoming heat loss.

Infants born less than 32 weeks GA may benefit from a combination of temperature management strategies immediately after birth, such as:

- Using a thermal mattress covered with a blanket.
- Placing a prewarmed hat after drying the infant's head.

- Placing the infant in a transparent polyethylene plastic bag or wrap:
  - When umbilical catheters are being inserted, make an X-shaped cut in the polyethylene bag over the cord. This allows the infant to remain in the bag and benefit from temperature management strategies.
  - Heart rate and breath sounds can be auscultated over the plastic.
  - The bag or wrap remains in place until the infant is admitted to an incubator and the axillary temperature is within target.
  - Dry the infant when the bag or wrap is removed.

HIE management

HIE is often unanticipated, and many infants are cared for initially in community hospitals. Hyperthermia increases risk for adverse neurodevelopmental outcomes in infants with HIE. Following resuscitation and reperfusion, there is a latent period of 1 to 6 h when impairment of an infant's cerebral oxidative metabolism can recover, at least partially, before irreversible mitochondrial dysfunction occurs. This latent phase is the therapeutic window for neuroprotective interventions.

> Preventing hyperthermia is critical in infants with HIE. Strict normothermia should be routinely provided in all newborn care settings. Hyperthermia or swings in temperature increase an infant's metabolic rate and risk for long-term injury.

Therapeutic hypothermia to prevent or decrease brain injury is a standard of care for infants 35 weeks GA or greater with moderate to severe HIE. In community hospitals, passive hypothermia with close monitoring of the infant's temperature should only be initiated in consultation with a tertiary care centre. When passive cooling cannot be safely performed, strict normothermia should be maintained.

Core Steps

There is only one Core Step in the ACoRN Thermoregulation Sequence, and that is to ensure the infant is in an environment where temperature can be managed.

Use an incubator or a radiant warmer when an infant is unwell. (For procedures related to radiant warmer or incubator use, see Appendix A.) An infant who is at risk or requires observation may be cared for skin-to-skin.

Organization of Care

Newborns at risk for HIE have specific management recommendations described in Chapter 5, Neurology, and outlined in the ACoRN Thermoregulation Sequence. The first step in the Organization of Care is to determine whether the infant requires HIE management.

When the infant requires HIE management (as identified in Chapter 5, Neurology), the next action is to determine whether criteria are met for initiating therapeutic hypothermia). Eligible infants meet Criteria A or B (page 168) and have:

- Moderate to severe HIE as identified in the Encephalopathy Assessment Table (pages 161, 168, Criteria C)
- A GA of 35 weeks or greater
- A postnatal age of 6 h or less
- No absolute contraindications, and
- Agreement from consultation with the level 3 centre that therapeutic hypothermia can be initiated.

When infants require HIE management but do not meet all treatment criteria for therapeutic hypothermia, they receive strict normothermia. The aim of strict normothermia is to minimize risk for overheating.

When the infant does not require HIE management, the next action is to determine whether the axillary temperature is within normal or abnormal range.

- In hypothermia, axillary temperature is less than 36.5°C.
- In hyperthermia, axillary temperature is greater than 37.5°C.
- In normothermia, axillary temperature is 36.5°C to 37.5°C.

Response

HIE management

Infants being managed for HIE require monitoring for cardiorespiratory instability, abnormal movements or seizures, and hypoglycemia. These infants require level 3 NICU care. Their body temperature should be maintained within target range and kept as stable as possible. Temperature swings increase the metabolic rate and risk for brain injury. As much as possible, these infants need one-to-one nursing.

In therapeutic hypothermia, the infant's core temperature is kept as stable as possible, within the range of 33°C to 34°C for 72 h (see Appendix A).

- Passive hypothermia can be initiated in community hospitals by undressing the infant and turning off the radiant heater. Passive hypothermia does not replace servo controlled therapeutic hypothermia, and transfer to a level 3 centre remains mandatory.
- Vital signs must be monitored continuously.
- The infant's core temperature needs continuous monitoring. When this is not possible, the axillary temperature should be rechecked every 15 min.
- Hypothermia is stressful, and stress can worsen outcomes. Administering morphine should be discussed with your level 3 centre.

Rewarming post-therapeutic hypothermia is accomplished in level 3 centres and is outside the scope of ACoRN.

> Therapeutic hypothermia must be administered with close monitoring and supervision. Specific staff training and a rehearsed clinical protocol are recommended. Infants with severe HIE may drop their temperature very quickly. Care must be taken to avoid overcooling.

The goal of strict normothermia is to keep the infant's core temperature within the target range of 36.5°C to 37°C and as stable as possible, to avoid temperature swings and hyperthermia. Frequent temperature monitoring (every 15 to 30 min) is essential when attempting to maintain normothermia in infants.

Hypothermia

Well term, late preterm, and LBW infants can be warmed using kangaroo care—skin-to-skin contact with their mothers or fathers. A few simple interventions may be sufficient to warm mildly hypothermic (35.0°C to 36.4°C) well infants:

Table 9.2.
Degrees of hypothermia

Degree of hypothermia	Body temperature
Mild	35.0°C to 36.4°C
Moderate	32.0°C to 34.9°C
Severe	< 32.0°C

Adapted from: WHO, Thermal protection of the newborn: A practical guide. Geneva: Author; 1997.

- Place the infant—naked except for a dry diaper and a warm hat—in an upright position between the mother's breasts (or on the father's chest). Skin-to-skin contact maximizes heat transfer from parent to infant. Cover both with a warm blanket.
- Recheck the infant's temperature every 15 to 30 min to ensure it is rising.
- Raise the room temperature to the 23°C to 25°C range.

If the infant's temperature does not respond within 30 min (Table 9.2), place the infant in an incubator or under a radiant warmer.

If kangaroo care cannot be provided because the infant is unstable or too premature (less than 34 weeks gestation), warming should occur in a servo-controlled incubator or radiant warmer.

There is little evidence to guide rewarming after unintentional, moderate hypothermia.

- A rewarming rate of 1°C to 2°C every hour is generally recommended.
- Temperature should be monitored every 15 to 30 min.
- Vital signs, level of consciousness, and acid–base balance should also be monitored.

In cases of extreme hypothermia (less than 32.0°C), consultation with a tertiary centre is advised to guide rate and method of rewarming.

Interventions to restore normothermia in a warm or cool newborn depend on whether the infant is sick or well, the degree of variance from normal temperature range, and GA.

When adjusting the ambient temperature to achieve normothermia, the infant's temperature should be checked and recorded every 15 to 30 min until it is stable.

Hyperthermia

Hyperthermia increases an infant's metabolic rate. In infants with HIE, hyperthermia greater than 38.5°C can have negative, irreversible neurodevelopmental effects. In the newly born, hyperthermia is usually caused by environmental factors, but in a term or older infant, it can also be infection-related.

The cause of infant hyperthermia (extrinsic or intrinsic) and its timing relative to birth determine approach to management. It is important to:

- Identify and remove potential causes of overheating before making a judgment about whether the elevated temperature is a sign of sepsis, and

- Consider sepsis when risk factors for infection are present, or an infant's condition is changing in the absence of environmental factors.

Controlling the environment to cool an infant with hyperthermia is the essential first step:

- Establish an NTE (e.g., place the infant away from direct sources of heat, such as sunlit windows) to minimize heat gain.
- Undress the infant, partially or fully, and remove extra blankets and hat to facilitate heat loss.
- For a radiant warmer or incubator, select the servo control setting and place the skin probe flat on the infant's upper abdomen. On a radiant warmer, the skin probe is shielded with a reflective cover.
- Set the servo control temperature 0.5°C to 1.0°C below the infant's temperature, with alarms set 0.5°C above and below the set temperature. Decrease the pre-set skin temperature by 0.5°C to 1.0°C every 15 min, until the infant's temperature is in normothermia range.
- Do not turn off an incubator to reduce temperature below its lowest setting, because this also turns off the airflow.

> Managing an infant's temperature with servo control can mask a fever by lowering heat output or incubator temperature in response to the infant's increasing skin temperature.
>
> When heat output from a radiant warmer or incubator decreases in response to a previously stable newborn's skin temperature, it suggests that a fever is being masked.

Next Steps

ACoRN Next Steps for the Thermoregulation Sequence include maintaining a thermally controlled environment, monitoring infant temperature, obtaining a focused history, conducting a physical exam, and assessing Level of Risk.

The frequency with which an infant's temperature should be rechecked depends on:

- Whether the infant is receiving therapeutic hypothermia or strict normothermia,
- How widely the infant's temperature has diverged from normal,
- The stability of the infant's condition, and
- The mechanism(s) being used to warm or cool the infant.

Focused history

Important information to gather in the Thermoregulation Sequence includes the following.

Intrapartum

- Maternal fever
- Fetal surveillance during labour (e.g., for tachycardia)
- Epidural use (which may cause maternal and/or neonatal hyperthermia)
- Risk factors for infection

Neonatal

- Care under a radiant warmer or incubator
- Environmental temperature requirement
- Temperature instability
- Being managed with therapeutic hypothermia or strict normothermia for HIE
- Prematurity, including late preterm, intrauterine growth restriction, SGA
- Postnatal age
- Requirement for neonatal resuscitation

Focused physical examination

A focused physical examination in the Thermoregulation Sequence includes assessment of:

- Axillary or core temperature in relation to environmental temperature,
- Vasoconstriction: appearing pale, mottled, cold extremities,
- Vasodilation: appearing plethoric (flushed), and
- Signs of dehydration.

There are no diagnostic tests specific to the ACoRN Thermoregulation Sequence because care is principally concerned with maintaining the infant's body temperature within normal range. While many underlying medical conditions can affect body temperature, their presentation, diagnosis, and laboratory evaluation are addressed in other ACoRN Sequences.

Level of Risk: Thermoregulation
In the ACoRN Thermoregulation Sequence, level of risk is based on whether the infant is receiving HIE management, the degree of hypothermia or hyperthermia, environmental temperature control (ambient, incubator, or radiant warmer), and risk factors for temperature instability.

Green:
- Infant's temperature is within the normal range (36.5°C to 37.5°C) with only skin-to-skin care for support

Yellow:
- Incubator or radiant warmer care is needed
- Infant is preterm, SGA, or IUGR
- Hypothermia or hyperthermia that responds to thermal management

Infants at Yellow Level of Risk require increased levels of attention and consultation. Transfer is required if needs exceed site capabilities.

Red:
- HIE management with therapeutic hypothermia or strict normothermia

Infants at Red Level of Risk infants require level 3 care. Transfer is required if needs exceed site capabilities.

Thermoregulation: Case 1—The cold, outborn baby

A baby boy is born in a car on a winter night and arrives at the rural nursing station at about 15 min of age. You are working alone. As the father passes you the baby, wrapped in a damp sweater, he tells you the birth was 3 weeks early. The baby is breathing spontaneously and is peripherally cyanosed. He appears sleepy, although his tone is normal. The baby appears small for 37 weeks GA. He is breathing easily in room air, with no signs of respiratory distress. As you easily palpate the brachial and femoral pulses, you notice that his limbs are cool to touch and that he has acrocyanosis. There are no obvious congenital defects and the baby has not been fed.

I. Does this baby present with any Alerting Signs for Resuscitation?

☐ Yes   ☐ No

The baby's heart rate is 130 bpm and his respiratory rate 40 bpm. Pulse oximetry shows SpO2 is greater than 95%. His axillary temperature is 35.5°C, and his weight is 2400 grams. The point-of-care blood glucose is 3.4 mmol/L.

2. Complete the ACoRN Primary Survey and Consolidated Core Steps, and generate a Problem List.

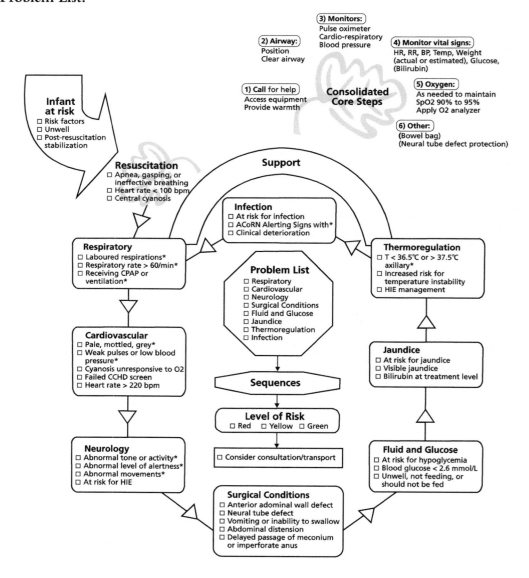

Ideally, you would perform the Primary Survey and Consolidated Core Steps with a colleague, but in this case, you are working alone.

3. **When you enter the Thermoregulation Sequence, which of the following actions should you consider? Tick all that apply.**
   ☐ Ensure the sweater is wrapped around the infant to keep him warm.
   ☐ Place the infant skin-to-skin on his mother's or father's chest.
   ☐ Place the infant in an extended position to allow maximum heat absorption.
   ☐ Start a heating lamp to warm up mother and infant.
   ☐ After gentle drying, put a warm hat on the infant's head.
   ☐ Cover infant and mother with a warm blanket.
   ☐ Turn up the thermostat to 25°C.
   ☐ Plug in an incubator to warm it up.
   ☐ Maintain therapeutic hypothermia to prevent this baby from developing HIE.

Over the next 20 min, you have the opportunity to talk with the parents while continuing to monitor their baby. There are no maternal risk factors for sepsis, and you decide there are no contraindications to breastfeeding this baby.

The physical examination reveals a term newborn that appears growth restricted, but otherwise healthy.

4. **In caring for this baby, which of the following are important to keep in mind? Tick all that apply.**
   ☐ Axillary temperature is difficult to measure because mercury thermometers are no longer used.
   ☐ To measure axillary temperature accurately, a baby's armpit should be dry, the thermometer positioned mid-armpit, and the arm adducted.
   ☐ Normal axillary temperature is between 36.5°C and 37.5°C.
   ☐ All infants are at risk for temperature instability.
   ☐ Risk for hypothermia increases in proportion to an infant's weight and GA.

You check the axillary temperature every 15 min and observe at 30 min that it has risen to 36.3°C.

5. Outline your pathway of care in the Thermoregulation Sequence.

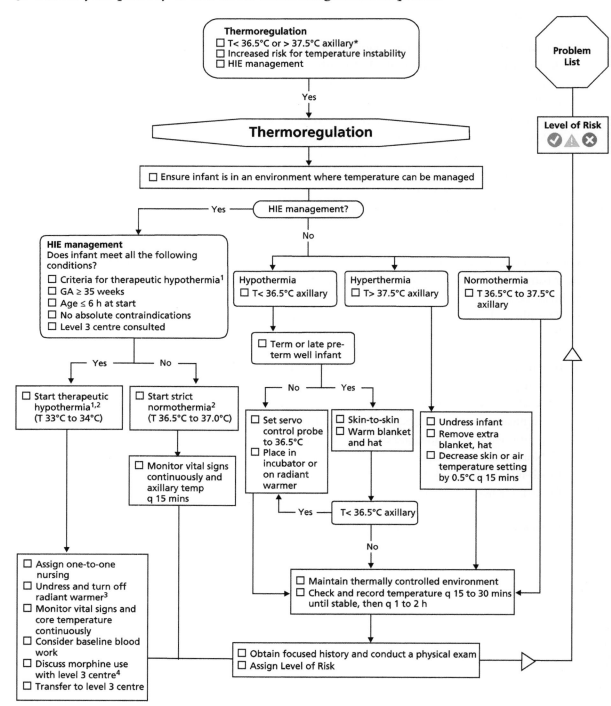

1. Therapeutic hypothermia should only be attempted with trained personnel and under a rehearsed clinical protocol—the "low tech" method in this Sequence is adapted from the ICE Trial Protocol. See also the Neurology Chapter and AppendixA
2. Poorly administered hypothermia may be worse than maintaining normothermia
3. Passive hypothermia is not meant to replace servo controlled therapeutic hypothermia
4. Hypothermia is stressful; stress may worsen outcomes

Abbreviations: GA - gestational age, h - hours, HIE - hypoxic ischemic encephalopathy, mins - minutes, q - every, T - temperature

6. In reviewing the Thermoregulation and Infection Sequences, you decide to:
   (Tick all that apply.)
   ☐ Perform a lumbar puncture and initiate antibiotics.
   ☐ Keep the infant skin-to-skin, if the mother wants to and if his temperature is increasing.
   ☐ Place the infant in a thermal-neutral environment in an incubator if temperature is not increasing or if skin-to-skin care is not feasible (e.g., the mother requires care or is fatigued).
   ☐ Stop feeds because the infant arrived hypothermic.
   ☐ Discharge the infant now that his temperature has normalized.

At 2 h, the baby is active, alert, and wanting to feed. His axillary temperature is 36.8°C.

You repeat a Primary Survey and find no Alerting Signs. You reassure his mother that he is progressing well and discuss when the baby will be ready for discharge.

Bibliography

Allen K. Neonatal thermal care: A discussion of two incubator modes for optimizing thermoregulation. A care study. J Neonatal Nurs 2011;17(2):43–8.

American Academy of Pediatrics, Committee on Fetus and Newborn, Papile LA, et al. Hypothermia and neonatal encephalopathy. Pediatrics 2014;33(6):1146–50.

American Heart Association, American Academy of Pediatrics. Neonatal Resuscitation Textbook, 7th ed. Elk Grove Village, IL: American Academy of Pediatrics; 2016.

Association of Women's Health, Obstetric and Neonatal Nurses. Neonatal Skin Care: Evidence Based Clinical Practice Guidelines, 3rd ed. Washington, DC: Johnson & Johnson; 2013.

Baley J, Committee on Fetus and Newborn. Skin-to-skin care for term and preterm infants in the neonatal ICU. Pediatrics 2015;136(3):596–9.

Battin M, Bennet L, Gunn AJ. Rebound seizures during rewarming. Pediatrics 2004;114(5):1369.

Bhat SR, Meng NF, Kumar K, Nagesh KN, Kawale A, Bhutani, VK. Keeping babies warm: A non-inferiority trial of a conductive thermal mattress. Arch Dis Child Fetal and Neonatal Ed 2015;100(4):F309–12.

Bissinger RL, Annibale DJ. Thermoregulation in very low-birth-weight infants during the golden hour: Results and implications. Adv Neonatal Care 2010;10(5):230–8.

Champlain Maternal Newborn Regional Program. Newborn thermoregulation: Self-learning module, June 2013. www.cmnrp.ca/uploads/documents//Newborn_Thermoregulation_SLM_2013_06.pdf

Conde-Agudelo A, Díaz-Rossello JL. Kangaroo mother care to reduce morbidity and mortality in low birthweight infants. Cochrane Database Syst Rev 2016;8:CD002771.

DiMenna L. Considerations for implementation of a neonatal kangaroo care protocol. Neonatal Netw 2006;25(6):405–12.

Fawcett K. Preventing admission hypothermia in very low birth weight neonates. Neonatal Netw 2014;33(3):143–9.

Gardner SL, Hernandez JA. Heat balance. In: Gardner SL, Carter BS, Enzman-Hines M, Hernandez JA, eds. Merenstein & Gardner's Handbook of Neonatal Intensive Care, 8th ed. St. Louis, MO: Mosby; 2015.

Jaimovich DG, Vidyasagar D. Handbook of Pediatric and Neonatal Transport Medicine, 2nd ed. Philadelphia, PA: Hanley & Belfus; 2005.

Janes M, Pinelli J, Landry S, Downey S, Paes B. Comparison of capillary blood sampling using an automated incision device with and without warming the heel. J Perinatology 2002;22(2):154–8.

Jefferies AL, Canadian Paediatric Society, Fetus and Newborn Committee. Kangaroo care for the preterm infant and family. Paediatr Child Health 2012;17(3):141–3. www.cps.ca/documents/position/kangaroo-care-for-preterm-infant

Knobel RB. Fetal and neonatal thermal physiology. Newborn Infant Nurs Rev 2014;14(2):45–9.

Knobel RB. Thermal stability of the premature infant in neonatal intensive care. Newborn Infant Nurs Rev 2014;14(2):72–6.

Knobel-Dail RB. Role of effective thermoregulation in premature neonates. Res Rep Neonatol 2014;4:147–56.

Koh KH, Yu CW. Comparing the accuracy of skin sensor temperature at two placement sites to axillary temperature in term infants under radiant warmers. J Neonatal Nurs 2016;22(4):196–203.

Leduc D, Woods S, Canadian Paediatric Society, Community Paediatrics Committee, 2000 (updated 2015). Temperature measurement in paediatrics. www.cps.ca/documents/position/temperature-measurement

Lemyre B, Chau V, Canadian Paediatric Society, Fetus and Newborn Committee. Hypothermia for newborns with hypoxic-ischemic encephalopathy. Paediatr Child Health 2018;23(4):285–91.

Loring C, Gregory K, Gargan B, et al. Tub bathing improves thermoregulation of the later preterm infant. J Obstet Gynecol Neonatal Nurs 2012;41(2):171–9.

Manani M, Jegatheesan P, DeSandre G, Song D, Showalter L, Govindaswami B. Elimination of admission hypothermia in preterm very low-birth-weight infants by standardization of delivery room management. Perm J 2013;17(3):8–13.

McCall EM, Alderdice F, Halliday HL, Jenkins JG, Vohra S. Interventions to prevent hypothermia at birth in preterm and/or low birthweight infants. Cochrane Database Syst Rev 2010;3:CD004210.

Molgat-Seon Y, Daboval T, Chou S, Jay O. Assessing neonatal heat balance and physiological strain in newborn infants nursed under radiant warmers in intensive care with fentanyl sedation. Eur J Appl Physiol 2014;114(12):2539–49.

Morris I, Adappa R. Early care of the preterm infant—Current evidence. Paediatr Child Health 2015;26(4):157–61.

Mosalli R. Whole body cooling for infants with hypoxic-ischemic encephalopathy. J Clin Neonatol 2012;1(2):101–6.

Nimbalkar SM, Patel VK, Patel DV, Nimbalkar AS, Sethi A, Phatak A. Effect of early skin-to-skin contact following normal delivery on incidence of hypothermia in neonates more than 1800 g: Randomized control trial. J Perinatol 2014;34(5):364–8.

Petty J. Fact sheet: Normal post natal adaptation to extrauterine life –b) Thermoregulation and glucose homeostasis. J Neonatal Nurs 2010;16(5):198–99.

Schafer D, Boogaart S, Johnson L, Keezel C, Ruperts L, Vander Laan KJ. Comparison of neonatal skin sensor temperatures with axillary temperature: Does skin sensor placement really matter? Adv Neonatal Care 2014;14(1):52–60.

Sethi A, Patel D, Nimbalkar A, Phatak A, Nimbalkar S. Comparison of forehead infrared thermometry with axillary digital thermometry in neonates. Indian Pediatr 2013;50(12):1153–4.

Shankaran S. Therapeutic hypothermia for neonatal encephalopathy. Curr Treat Options Neurol 2012;14(6):608–19.

Shankaran S, Laptook AR, Ehrenkranz RA, et al. Whole-body hypothermia for neonates with hypoxic-ischemic encephalopathy. New Engl J Med 2005;353(15):1574–84.

Smith J, Alcock G, Usher K. Temperature measurement in the preterm and term neonate: A review of the literature. Neonatal Netw 2013;32(1):16–25.

Stokowski LA. Fundamentals of phototherapy for neonatal jaundice. Adv Neonatal Care 2011;11(5 Suppl):S10–21.

Thoresen M, Whitelaw A. Cardiovascular changes during mild therapeutic hypothermia and rewarming in infants with hypoxic-ischemic encephalopathy. Pediatrics 2000;106(1 Pt 1):92–9.

Trays G, Banerjee S. Fetal and neonatal hyperthermia. Paediatr Child Health 2014;24(9):419–23.

World Health Organization. Thermal protection of the newborn: A practical guide. Geneva: World Health Organization; 1997.

Waldren S, MacKinnon R. Neonatal thermoregulation. Infant 2007;3(3):101–4.

Answer key: Thermoregulation Case 1—The cold, outborn baby

1. Does this baby present with any Alerting Signs for Resuscitation?

☐ Yes ✓ No

This baby has acrocyanosis but is not centrally cyanosed. His heart rate and breathing are normal. He does not demonstrate any of the Alerting Signs requiring resuscitation.

2. Complete the ACoRN Primary Survey and Consolidated Core Steps, and generate a Problem List.

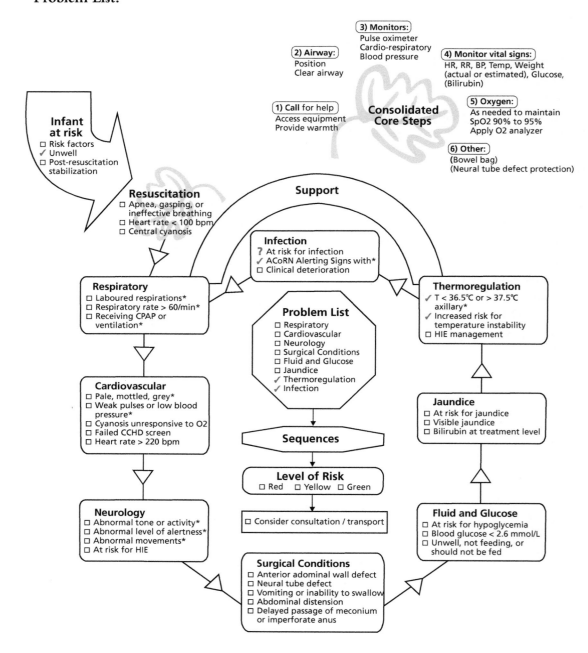

You mark the Alerting Signs, resulting in a Problem List that prioritizes Thermoregulation and Infection. You may also have marked 'Unwell, not feeding or should not be fed' in the Fluid and Glucose Sequence with a **?** reminding you to gather more information and assess readiness for feeding.

3. When you enter the Thermoregulation Sequence, which of the following actions should you consider?

☐ Ensure the sweater is wrapped around the infant to keep him warm.

✓ Place the infant skin-to-skin on his mother's or father's chest.

☐ Place the infant in an extended position to allow maximum heat absorption.

☐ Start a heating lamp to warm up mother and infant.

✓ After gentle drying, put a warm hat on the infant's head.

✓ Cover infant and mother with a warm blanket.

✓ Turn up the thermostat to 25°C.

✓ Plug in an incubator to warm it up.

☐ Maintain therapeutic hypothermia to prevent this baby from developing HIE.

Removing sources of potential heat loss is an important thermoregulation step, and keeping parents and infant is together is a key component of supportive care. Skin-to-skin contact with a parent, covering both with a warm blanket, applying a warm hat, and removing any wet blankets or clothing from the infant are simple but essential steps for infant thermoregulation.

Using a heating lamp is not recommended because it provides an unpredictable source of heat and can lead to hyperthermia. Turning the room temperature to 25°C can be helpful. Plugging the incubator in to warm up may be useful in the event that the infant needs additional warming, should skin-to-skin prove to be ineffective or not feasible.

4. In caring for this baby, which of the following are important to keep in mind?

☐ Axillary temperature is difficult to measure because mercury thermometers are no longer used.

✓ To measure axillary temperature accurately, a baby's armpit should be dry, the thermometer positioned mid-armpit, and the arm adducted.

✓ Normal axillary temperature is between 36.5°C and 37.5°C.

✓ All infants are at risk for temperature instability.

☐ Risk for hypothermia increases in proportion to an infant's weight and GA.

Axillary temperature-taking is a safe, convenient method for assessing an infant's temperature, and is comparable to rectal temperature for accuracy. Rectal temperature-taking is not recommended due to risk for trauma.

Infants who are preterm, SGA, or growth restricted are at greater risk for hypothermia due to their greater surface skin area in relation to body weight. Risk for hypothermia decreases as birth weight and GA increase.

5. Outline your pathway of care in the Thermoregulation Sequence.

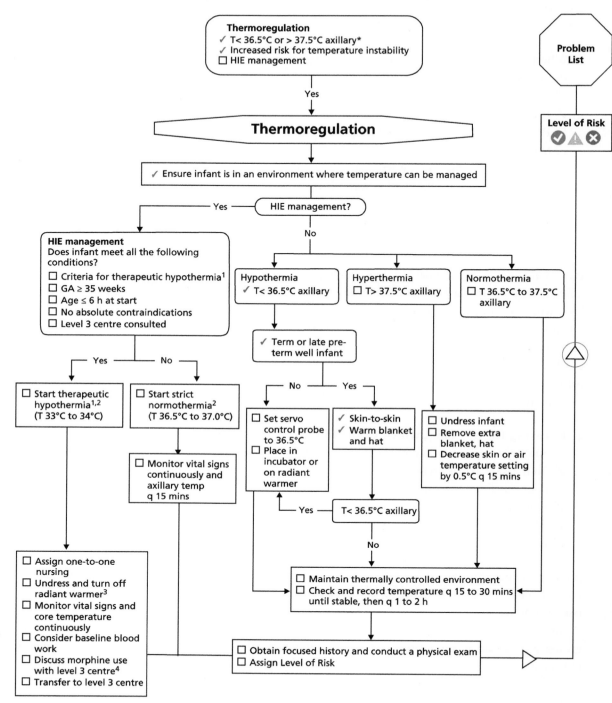

Thermoregulation
- ✓ T< 36.5°C or > 37.5°C axillary*
- ✓ Increased risk for temperature instability
- ☐ HIE management

Yes

Thermoregulation

Problem List

Level of Risk
✓ ⚠ ✗

✓ Ensure infant is in an environment where temperature can be managed

Yes — HIE management? — No

HIE management
Does infant meet all the following conditions?
- ☐ Criteria for therapeutic hypothermia[1]
- ☐ GA ≥ 35 weeks
- ☐ Age ≤ 6 h at start
- ☐ No absolute contraindications
- ☐ Level 3 centre consulted

Yes — No

☐ Start therapeutic hypothermia[1,2] (T 33°C to 34°C)

☐ Start strict normothermia[2] (T 36.5°C to 37.0°C)

☐ Monitor vital signs continuously and axillary temp q 15 mins

Hypothermia
- ✓ T< 36.5°C axillary

✓ Term or late pre-term well infant

No — Yes

☐ Set servo control probe to 36.5°C
☐ Place in incubator or on radiant warmer

✓ Skin-to-skin
✓ Warm blanket and hat

Yes — T< 36.5°C axillary — No

Hyperthermia
- ☐ T> 37.5°C axillary

Normothermia
- ☐ T 36.5°C to 37.5°C axillary

☐ Undress infant
☐ Remove extra blanket, hat
☐ Decrease skin or air temperature setting by 0.5°C q 15 mins

☐ Assign one-to-one nursing
☐ Undress and turn off radiant warmer[3]
☐ Monitor vital signs and core temperature continuously
☐ Consider baseline blood work
☐ Discuss morphine use with level 3 centre[4]
☐ Transfer to level 3 centre

☐ Maintain thermally controlled environment
☐ Check and record temperature q 15 to 30 mins until stable, then q 1 to 2 h

☐ Obtain focused history and conduct a physical exam
☐ Assign Level of Risk

1. Therapeutic hypothermia should only be attempted with trained personnel and under a rehearsed clinical protocol–the "low tech" method in this Sequence is adapted from the ICE Trial Protocol. See also the Neurology Chapter and AppendixA
2. Poorly administered hypothermia may be worse than maintaining normothermia
3. Passive hypothermia is not meant to replace servo controlled therapeutic hypothermia
4. Hypothermia is stressful; stress may worsen outcomes

Abbreviations: GA - gestational age, h - hours, HIE - hypoxic ischemic encephalopathy, mins - minutes, q - every, T - temperature

6. In reviewing the Thermoregulation and Infection Sequences, you decide to:

☐ Perform a lumbar puncture and initiate antibiotics.

✓ Keep the infant skin-to-skin, if the mother wants to and if his temperature is increasing.

✓ Place the infant in a thermal-neutral environment in an incubator if his temperature is not increasing or if skin-to-skin care is not feasible (e.g., the mother requires care or is fatigued).

☐ Stop feeds because the infant arrived hypothermic.

☐ Discharge the infant now that his temperature has normalized.

This baby's hypothermia was identified as environmental. He has no other Alerting Signs with a* and no risk factors were identified for infection. His Level of Risk is Green. Procedures such as a lumbar puncture, initiating antibiotics, or stopping feeds are not indicated. He will continue to need monitoring, which can be done during skin-to-skin care with the mother or father. Discharge of this infant should be delayed to ensure that his temperature remains within normal limits and breastfeeding is established.

Infection

Educational objectives

Upon completion of this chapter, you will be able to:

- Identify infants at increased risk for infection.
- Apply the Acute Care of at-Risk Newborns (ACoRN) Infection Sequence.
- Recognize that ACoRN Alerting Signs identified with an asterisk (*) may be clinical signs of neonatal infection.
- Use the ACoRN Infection Assessment Table to guide management of neonatal infection.
- Perform and interpret appropriate diagnostic evaluations for neonatal sepsis.
- Initiate appropriate antibiotic treatment and supportive care.
- Recognize when to exit the Infection Sequence to other ACoRN sequences.

Key concepts

1. Signs and symptoms of sepsis in the neonate are often subtle and non-specific.
2. Infection should be suspected in infants who:
   - Have recognized risk factors for infection
   - Have Alerting Signs identified with * in the ACoRN Primary Survey, or
   - Show clinical deterioration.
3. Early-onset sepsis (EOS) and late-onset sepsis (LOS) have different risk factors and microbial etiologies.
4. Risk for EOS with Group B *Streptococcus* (GBS) is low, but not zero, in infants whose mothers have received appropriate intrapartum antibiotics.
5. EOS with GBS can occur in infants whose mothers had negative GBS swabs.
6. Chorioamnionitis increases risk for EOS and is strongly associated with spontaneous onset of labour in decreasing gestational age (GA). However, risk for sepsis is low in the late preterm or term infant with a normal physical examination.
7. Premature infants, infants admitted to intensive care settings, and infants with in-dwelling catheters and tubes are at higher risk for LOS.
8. Screening investigations, such as total white blood cell count (WBC), immature-to-total neutrophil count (I:T) ratio, immature granulocyte (IG) count, C-reactive protein (CRP), and procalcitonin, have limited predictive value.
9. When sepsis is suspected clinically, obtain appropriate cultures and initiate antibiotics without delay.

Skills

- Interpretation of complete blood count (CBC), differential WBC (I:T ratio and IG count), and biochemical markers of neonatal sepsis

All infants are born in environments that contain microorganisms. In most cases, these organisms are harmless. The infant is protected from infection by antibodies that are passively transferred from mother to baby, by their own developing immune system, and by nonspecific defence mechanisms such as mucosal and skin barriers. The newborn's defences against infection improve as the immune system matures and the skin and gut are colonized with appropriate microbial flora. Immune function is enhanced by early skin-to-skin contact with parents and protective factors found in colostrum and breast milk.

Approximately 1 in 1000 liveborn infants present with infection in the perinatal period. The incidence is higher in preterm infants compared with those born at term. EOS is defined as invasive infection in the first 72 h of life. EOS usually results from vertical transmission of pathogens from mother to infant. Bacterial flora from the maternal gastrointestinal or genitourinary tract can ascend to the amniotic fluid, or the infant may become colonized during passage through the vagina. The risk of EOS increases when a mother is colonized with organisms that are potentially pathogenic to the newborn, such as GBS, and when infection of the amniotic fluid is suspected, as evidenced by maternal fever or prolonged rupture of membranes. However, many infants exposed to risk factors for infection remain well and do not develop EOS. The challenge for clinicians is to identify and treat infants who are likely to be infected and require antibiotic therapy, while protecting others from unnecessary investigations and treatment.

Intrapartum maternal antibiotics have been shown to decrease the incidence of EOS from GBS, without a concomitant decrease in other pathogens. Intrapartum antibiotic prophylaxis (IAP) should be administered at least 4 h before delivery to mothers who:

- Have a positive GBS screen or have had GBS bacteriuria at any time during pregnancy,
- Have had a previous infant with invasive GBS infection,
- Have unknown GBS status and have risk factors such as preterm labour or premature rupture of membranes (PROM) greater than or equal to 18 h,
- Develop a fever of greater than 38°C during labour, *or*
- Have suspected or definitive chorioamnionitis.

Adequate IAP for GBS consists of at least one dose of either intravenous (IV) penicillin or cefazolin, administered at least 4 h before birth. IAP is inadequate if antibiotics are administered less than 4 h before birth. Women who are allergic to penicillin and at high risk for anaphylaxis usually are treated with IV clindamycin, erythromycin, or vancomycin. Although these alternate regimes are likely to be effective and therefore should be used, their efficacy compared with penicillin has not been proven in clinical trials. Consequently, their use in mothers is still considered inadequate for newborn prophylaxis.

Appropriate IAP reduces risk for early-onset GBS sepsis significantly but does not reduce the incidence of late-onset GBS disease.

Negative maternal GBS cultures or the use of intrapartum antibiotics should not change management of symptomatic infants. GBS disease occurs in the presence of negative maternal GBS cultures and, occasionally, following adequate IAP. IAP does not affect the frequency of sepsis caused by organisms other than GBS.

LOS is defined as infection occurring after the first 72 h post-birth. In LOS, the source of infection is typically nosocomial (hospital-acquired) or community-acquired. The incidence of LOS increases in the presence of factors that impair host defences, such as prematurity and admission to hospital, or that disrupt the host's natural barriers, such as indwelling lines or tubes. LOS may affect up to 20% in preterm infants admitted to a NICU.

The term 'sepsis' can denote bacteremia, pneumonia, meningitis, and urinary tract or bone and joint infections. The early signs of sepsis may be subtle or nonspecific, making it difficult to diagnosis. The presenting features do not reliably identify source or site of infection. Infants needing resuscitation at birth may already have an underlying infection, but sepsis may also present later in initially well-appearing newborns with or without risk factors. Approximately 95% of newly born infants who have sepsis show clinical signs within 24 h of infection onset. Closely monitoring newborns that have risk factors is crucial for detecting early, developing signs of sepsis.

Regular assessment of the infant's condition using the ACoRN Primary Survey (every 30 to 60 min until stable) is essential to ensure an organized approach to, and timely recognition of, sepsis.

Neonatal sepsis is most commonly bacterial, though viral or fungal infections can present in the neonatal period. The content of this chapter is directed primarily toward the early detection and management of serious bacterial infections.

Key management steps include starting empiric antibiotic therapy while waiting for cultures, and providing supportive treatment for infants with suspected sepsis.

Noninfectious conditions can present with sepsis-like signs. These conditions include:

- Ductus-dependent congenital heart disease,
- Congenital adrenal hyperplasia,
- Inborn errors of metabolism, and
- Abdominal catastrophe (e.g., bowel malrotation with volvulus).

ACoRN Infection Sequence

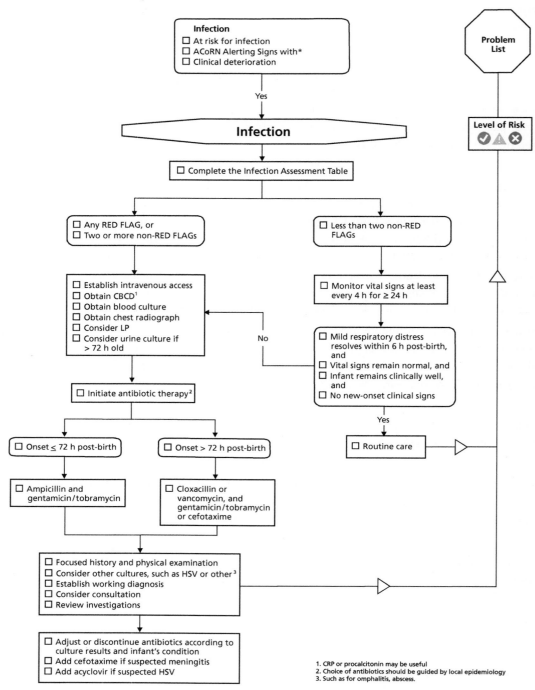

Abbreviations: CBCD - complete blood count and differential, CRP - C-reactive protein, h - hours, HSV - herpes simplex virus, LP - lumbar puncture

Alerting Signs

An infant with one or more of the following Alerting Signs enters the ACoRN Infection Sequence.

> **Infection**
> ☐ At risk for infection
> ☐ ACoRN Alerting Signs with*
> ☐ Clinical deterioration

At risk for infection

Specific risk factors for sepsis may be identified in the antenatal period, during labour, or after birth. Maternal risk factors associated with bacterial EOS in newborns are:

- GBS colonization during the current pregnancy,
- GBS bacteriuria during the current pregnancy,
- A previous infant with invasive GBS disease,
- PROM greater than or equal to 18 h before delivery,
- Prelabour rupture of membranes,
- Preterm birth (before 37 weeks GA) following spontaneous onset of labour,
- Intrapartum maternal fever (temperature greater than or equal to 38°C),
- Chorioamnionitis, and
- Suspected or confirmed invasive bacterial infection in the mother, treated during labour or in the 24-h-period before or after delivery.

Chorioamnionitis has been defined historically as inflammation and/or infection of the maternal–fetal membranes. Recently, more refined clinical definitions have been proposed:

- Suspected chorioamnionitis:
  - Maternal fever (two oral temperature readings of 38°C to 39°C at least 30 min apart *or* one oral temperature greater than 39°C) *plus*
  - Any one of the following:
    - Baseline fetal heart rate greater than 160 bpm for 10 min or longer
    - Maternal WBC greater than 15×10^9/L
    - Purulent fluid from the cervical os.
- Definite chorioamnionitis:
  - ALL of the previously listed signs *plus*
  - At least one of the following laboratory findings of infection:
    - Positive Gram stain of amniotic fluid
    - Low amniotic fluid glucose
    - High amniotic fluid white count
    - Positive amniotic fluid bacterial culture
    - Placental and/or fetal membrane histopathology with diagnostic features of inflammation and/or infection.

Chorioamnionitis risk factors are additive: the presence of more than one risk factor further increases the likelihood of EOS in the newborn. Also, the higher the maternal temperature, the longer the duration of ruptured membranes, or the younger the infant's GA, the greater the risk for EOS.

PROM, fever, or chorioamnionitis are risk factors for sepsis with GBS and non-GBS organisms.

Risk factors associated with LOS in the neonate include:

- Low birth weight,
- Prematurity,
- Admission to an intensive care unit or special care nursery,
- Mechanical ventilation,
- Invasive procedures, and
- Invasive therapies (particularly indwelling IV catheters and endotracheal or chest tubes).

ACoRN Alerting Signs identified with*

Alerting Signs with an asterisk (*) are recognized clinical signs that may indicate sepsis. They include:
- Respiratory Sequence:
  - Laboured respirations
  - Respiratory rate > 60/min
  - Receiving continuous positive airway pressure (CPAP) or ventilation
- Cardiovascular Sequence:
  - Pale, mottled, grey
  - Weak pulses or low blood pressure
- Neurology Sequence:
  - Abnormal tone or activity
  - Abnormal level of alertness
  - Abnormal movements
- Thermoregulation Sequence:
  - T < 36.5°C or > 37.5°C axillary

Sepsis should be suspected in any newborn who shows an ACoRN Alerting Sign with * in the ACoRN Primary Survey.

Clinical deterioration

Clinical deterioration in a previously well infant or worsening condition in an unwell infant is an indicator of possible sepsis and requires entry into the Infection Sequence.
Possible indicators of clinical deterioration include:

- Temperature instability. Sepsis can present with hypothermia, hyperthermia, or labile temperature control. Persistent high temperatures (greater than 38.5°C in infants, especially in the first week of life, may indicate a viral infection (e.g., herpes simplex virus [HSV]).
- Onset of apnea.
- Feeding problems (poor feeding, vomiting, excessive gastric aspirates, or abdominal distension).
- Metabolic abnormalities (hyper- or hypoglycemia, or metabolic acidosis with base deficit greater than 10).

Any local signs of infection, such as skin, wound, or eye drainage, must also be considered as indicators of possible infection requiring further investigation and possible treatment.

Core Steps

The essential Core Step in the ACoRN Infection Sequence is to complete the Infection Assessment (Table 10.1, below). Accurate assessment depends on knowledge of the infant's risk factors for infection and clinical presentation, as identified by the ACoRN Primary Survey and preceding sequences.

Items in the Infection Assessment Table are risk factors or clinical indicators of infection. They are defined either as 'red flags'—which indicate high risk for infection, or as 'non-red flags'—which

Table 10.1.
Infection Assessment

Risk factors		Clinical indicators	
Red flag	**Non-red flag**	**Red flag**	**Non-red flag**
☐ Invasive maternal infection requiring IV antibiotic therapy 24 h before or after birth ☐ Infection in co-twin (multiple pregnancy)	☐ Invasive GBS in previous infant and inadequate IAP ☐ Maternal GBS colonization or UTI in current pregnancy and inadequate IAP ☐ Rupture of membranes > 18 h ☐ Intrapartum maternal fever (> 38°C) or confirmed or suspected chorioamnionitis ☐ Preterm (< 37 weeks) birth following spontaneous labour	☐ New-onset respiratory distress[1] ☐ Term infant receiving ventilation ☐ Shock ☐ Seizures	☐ Laboured respirations, respiratory rate > 60/min ☐ Preterm infant receiving ventilation ☐ New-onset apnea in a preterm infant[1] ☐ Abnormal tone or activity and/or abnormal level of alertness ☐ New-onset[1] feeding problems: feeding poorly, vomiting, excessive gastric aspirates, abdominal distension ☐ New-onset[1] metabolic abnormalities, such as hyper-/hypoglycemia or metabolic acidosis (BD ≥ 10 mmol/L) ☐ Bilirubin at treatment level before 24 h of age ☐ Axillary temperature < 36.5°C or > 37.5°C, unexplained by environmental factors ☐ Local signs of infection (eye, skin, umbilicus)

BD: base deficit; CPAP: continuous positive airway pressure; GBS: Group B *Streptococcus*; IAP: intrapartum antibiotic prophylaxis; IV: intravenous; UTI: urinary tract infection

[1]'New onset' is defined as any clinically significant change after a previous period of stability.

Source: Adapted from NICE Guideline CG149. Neonatal infection (early-onset): Antibiotics for prevention and treatment, 2012 (updated 2017).

indicate lower risk for infection when present in isolation. The presence of 2 or more non-red flags indicates higher risk for infection in the newborn.

> Respiratory distress is a common initial presentation of many term newborns, especially after Caesarean section, and often resolves within several hours. Infants who appear stable and lack perinatal risk factors for sepsis can be observed closely for up to 6 h to determine whether respiratory distress resolves before investigating for sepsis and starting antibiotics.

Organization of Care

In the ACoRN Infection Sequence, Organization of Care is determined by the presence and number of **red flags** and **non-red flags** in the Infection Assessment Table.

- Infants with **any red flag or 2 or more non-red flags** are considered at higher risk of sepsis, and require additional investigations and immediate management.
- Infants with **less than 2 non-red flags** and no red flags are at a lower risk for sepsis. They require close observation and clinical judgement to determine appropriate management.

Response

Infants with any red flag or 2 or more non-red flags

Infants in this category require immediate IV access, diagnostic testing, and antibiotic therapy as per the Infection Sequence.

There are no screening laboratory tests, including WBC indices and serum biomarkers, sensitive enough to preclude treatment of the unwell infant. Similarly, unwell infants must be investigated and treated regardless of maternal GBS status and IAP.

> Clinicians should not wait for results from any laboratory test before starting treatment for symptomatic infants who meet criteria as per the Infection Assessment Table.

Laboratory and diagnostic tests

Microbial cultures are critical for determining the site and causative organism in infants with suspected sepsis. Other laboratory tests may aid in determining likelihood of infection.

Complete blood count with differential

Septic infants frequently have abnormalities in the number or distribution of WBCs or in their platelet count. Various WBC indices (total WBC count, absolute neutrophil count, IG counts, and I:T ratio) are used to aid diagnosis of neonatal sepsis. However, while the predictive value of these tests improves with the hours post-birth, it remains low overall. A low WBC count (less than 5×10^9/L) or a low absolute neutrophil count (less than 1.5×10^9/L) are more likely to be associated with sepsis than an elevated I:T ratio (greater than 20% to 30%) or a high WBC count (greater than 30×10^9/L). For more information on interpreting CBC results, see Appendix B.

Blood cultures

A minimum sample volume of 1 mL should be placed into an aerobic culture bottle to optimize growth in low-colony-count sepsis. Multiple cultures drawn from different sites have not been shown to improve detection rates. Blood can be taken from a newly inserted catheter or by venipuncture or arterial puncture. Most infections in the neonatal/perinatal period are bacterial in origin. The causative agents and the antibiotic treatment of choice can change depending on the timing of presentation.

Radiographs (X-rays)

A CXR should be obtained whenever respiratory signs or symptoms are present. When gastrointestinal signs are present, an abdominal radiograph (AXR) is suggested.

Lumbar puncture (LP)

Although meningitis is uncommon in newly born infants, a small number may have meningitis when the blood culture is negative. The LP can be deferred when the infant is experiencing cardiovascular or respiratory instability, presenting with early respiratory signs only, or when a trained, experienced clinician is not available to perform the procedure. The LP must be performed if the infant has signs of encephalopathy or seizures, or if the blood culture is positive.

Urine culture

A urine culture by catheter or suprapubic aspiration should be obtained in infants more than 72 h old. Urine culture is not necessary for younger infants because urinary tract infection is rare in newly born infants.

Cultures from other sites

Consider cultures from other sites (e.g., vesicle, wound, fluid, stool) or viral/fungal cultures when clinically indicated.

Serum biomarkers

Testing other serum biomarkers, including CRP and procalcitonin, may be useful when evaluating a neonate for sepsis. A single CRP is not helpful in diagnosing EOS in the newly born infant. Serial negative CRPs have a high negative predictive value for sepsis. Emerging evidence suggests that procalcitonin may be a better marker than CRP for EOS in the neonate.

Antibiotics

Antibiotics should be administered intravenously and targeted to cover the most likely organisms associated with the timing of the sepsis (Table 10.2).

EOS

In EOS, the most likely organisms are those acquired from the maternal gastrointestinal or genitourinary tracts. These include GBS, other streptococci (e.g., *S. viridans*), *Listeria monocytogenes*, and enteric gram-negative organisms like *E. coli, Klebsiella*, and *Enterobacter* species. First-line antibiotics for these organisms are ampicillin and an aminoglycoside (gentamicin or tobramycin). Initial antibiotic choice may be modified if maternal cultures and sensitivities are known.

Table 10.2.
Common bacterial organisms in neonatal infection

Early-onset sepsis	Late-onset sepsis
Gram-positive bacteria • *Streptococcus agalactiae* (GBS) • *Listeria monocytogenes*	Gram-positive bacteria • *Streptococcus agalactiae* (GBS) • *Streptococcus pneumoniae* • *Staphylococcus aureus** • Coagulase-negative *Staphylococcus* species* • *Enterococcus species**
Gram-negative bacteria • *Escherichia coli (E. coli)* • *Klebsiella pneumoniae* • *Enterobacter species* • *Proteus* species • *Salmonella* species	Gram-negative bacteria • *Escherichia coli (E. coli)* • *Klebsiella pneumoniae* • *Enterobacter* species • *Proteus* species • Other (*Citrobacter, Serratia, Pseudomonas, Haemophilus, Neisseria*)

*Indicates organisms more commonly associated with nosocomial infections

LOS

Organisms likely to cause LOS can differ depending on whether a neonate is being cared for in a NICU or special care nursery (hospital-acquired) or at home (community-acquired). In LOS, gram-positive organisms predominate, with coagulase-negative *Staphylococcus* infections accounting for one-half of all cases. Other organisms implicated in late-onset bacterial sepsis include GBS, *Staphylococcus aureus*, enterococci, other streptococci (e.g., *S. pneumonae*), *E. coli, Klebsiella* species, and *Pseudomonas* species.

First-line antibiotics for LOS are cloxacillin or vancomycin with an aminoglycoside (gentamicin or tobramycin) or cefotaxime. The initial choice of antibiotics may be modified depending on local microbiograms and sensitivity patterns.

Infants with less than 2 non-red flags

Infants in this category present with either a single risk factor for neonatal infection or one nonspecific symptom and no known risk factors. These infants require close monitoring because 95% of infants with EOS demonstrate symptoms within 24 h regardless of maternal IAP coverage. Vital signs should be monitored at least every 4 h over the next 24 h to ensure early recognition and management of infection.

Persistence of mild respiratory distress beyond 6 h of age in a newly born infant, abnormality in vital signs, clinical deterioration, or new-onset clinical signs during the monitoring period require a shift in the Organization of Care to the treatment arm, as per the Infection Sequence.

Infants who remain well, with normal vital signs and no new-onset clinical signs after 24 h of observation, may exit the ACoRN Infection Sequence.

Next Steps

Next Steps in the ACoRN Infection Sequence are to obtain a focused history and conduct a detailed physical examination.

Focused infection history

The focused infection history should:

- Clarify any necessary details relating to the antepartum, intrapartum, and neonatal risk factors.
- Document any mitigating strategies for EOS, such as adequacy of IAP.

- Explore additional risks for infection, such as HSV history, new illness contacts and exposures, and the use of indwelling catheters or invasive procedures.

Focused physical examination

In addition to the examination conducted during the ACoRN Primary Survey and applicable sequences, a focused physical examination for infection should include ongoing measurement of vital signs: respiratory rate, heart rate, blood pressure, temperature, and pulse oximetry. Attention to signs that suggest a site or source of infection (e.g., pneumonia, meningitis, abscess, or skin lesions) may help to direct specific diagnostic interventions and management.

In general, EOS is usually characterized by respiratory distress, apnea, signs of distributive shock, pneumonia, and meningitis. LOS commonly presents with temperature instability, decreased activity levels, apnea, poor feeding, jaundice, and signs of distributive shock. Additional signs and symptoms may point to infections or complications in a particular organ system:

- Pneumonia: Respiratory distress, cyanosis responsive to oxygen, abnormal CXR
- Hematological: Petechiae from low platelet count or disseminated intravascular coagulation
- Meningitis: Seizures, high-pitched cry, bulging fontanels
- Gastrointestinal: Abdominal distension or discolouration, bilious vomiting, blood in stools

Consider other cultures

Local site cultures (e.g., swabs or aspiration) may be warranted.

Establish a working diagnosis

A working diagnosis is based on the timing of onset and suspected location of infection.

Consider consultation and review investigations

To help direct specimen collection and additional management, consult with your referral centre. Review investigations as they become available, to help identify the source of infection and optimize antibiotic therapy.

> Infants with sepsis can become unstable or develop complications rapidly. Close observation, and frequent assessment using the ACoRN Primary Survey and Sequences, are recommended. Supportive therapy is provided in accordance with other ACoRN sequences, while managing other complications (e.g., disseminated intravascular coagulation). Early consultation is advised.

Specific Diagnosis and Management

When establishing a diagnosis, the clinician must consider whether an infection is localized to a specific organ or tissue (e.g., pneumonia, meningitis, urinary tract infection) or involves the bloodstream. Risk factors for unusual organisms or non-bacterial sepsis must also be considered. Although bacterial infection is the most common cause of neonatal sepsis, viral and fungal infections must be considered.

Bacterial sepsis

Suspected bacterial sepsis is treated with broad-spectrum antibiotics until results from Gram stain and cultures are known. Antibiotic therapy should be modified to optimize treatment, depending on the organism identified, its sensitivity profile, and the site of infection. For example, when meningitis is suspected or confirmed, antibiotics that penetrate into the cerebrospinal fluid are required. Cefotaxime is started, and gentamicin discontinued, pending culture reports. Specific management includes:

- Reviewing culture results and antibiotic sensitivities,
- Adjusting the antibiotic agents and dosage, and monitoring response, as required, and
- Determining duration of antibiotic therapy.

Viral sepsis

Viral infections, particularly those caused by HSV or enteroviruses, should be considered if there is a history of recent maternal infection, active vaginal lesions, or diarrhea at the time of birth. Vesicular lesions on mother or infant should be investigated for HSV, but diagnosis does not depend on the presence of vesicles, which are absent in about 50% of cases.

HSV infection should be suspected in infants younger than 4 weeks of age with signs of CNS infection, persistent fevers, or clinical sepsis that does not respond to antibiotics, even when maternal history or symptoms are absent.

Treatment with acyclovir should be initiated urgently when HSV infection is suspected, especially in the presence of high fevers or neurologic signs.

Some 80% of neonatal HSV cases present without maternal symptoms or history. Special cultures and investigations (e.g., PCR testing of cerebrospinal fluid and skin lesions) are necessary for diagnosis. Urgent consultation, treatment, and isolation of the infant are necessary for infection control.

Fungal sepsis

Fungal (most commonly *Candida*) infections may be vertically acquired from a maternal vaginal infection, but they are more often late-onset, nosocomial infections. Risk factors for invasive fungal infection include recent or prolonged broad-spectrum antibiotic use, known colonization of the skin or mucous membranes, and endotracheal tube use. Treatment of invasive fungal infections is beyond the scope of ACoRN.

Level of Risk: Infection
In the ACoRN Infection Sequence, level of risk is based on presumed infection, clinical stability, and access to necessary investigations and treatment.
Green: • Infant has no signs of infection and the ongoing monitoring requirements do not exceed site capability
Yellow: • Infant has risk factors for infection but is clinically stable and within the site's capability to provide necessary monitoring and investigations • Infant has a presumed or confirmed infection but is clinically stable and within the site's capability to provide necessary monitoring, investigations, and ongoing management **Infants at a Yellow Level of Risk require increased levels of attention and consultation. Transfer is required if needs exceed site capabilities.**
Red: • Infant has a presumed or confirmed infection and is clinically unstable • Infant has a presumed or confirmed infection and requires specialty investigations or consultation **Infants at a Red level of Risk require level 3 care. Transfer is required if needs exceed site capabilities.**

Infection: Case 1—A term infant with mild respiratory distress

A baby girl is born in the operative birthing room. She is 30 min old. She was born by Caesarean section at 38 weeks for breech presentation approximately 60 min after the onset of contractions. Her mother has been healthy with no fevers. The GBS swab was negative, and membranes were intact at the time of delivery.

She is lying flexed skin-to-skin on dad's chest. She is grunting occasionally with mild subcostal retractions and a respiratory rate of 65 breaths/min. She is pink in room air.

You complete the ACoRN Primary Survey and the Consolidated Core Steps. You identify Alerting Signs with * in the Respiratory Sequence (laboured respirations* and respiratory rate > 60/min*). There are no other ACoRN Alerting Signs for this baby, and no additional risk factors for infection are noted in the mother's history or chart.

The Consolidated Core Steps provide the following information: airway is clear, heart rate is 140 beats/min, SpO2 in room air is 95%, BP is 68/35 mean of 46. The baby's temperature is 37°C. In the absence of significant risk factors, and given a clinically stable infant with minimal respiratory findings after a Caesarean birth, the health care team has decided to allow dad to continue skin–to–skin care and will reassess the infant's status in 15 min. If respiratory symptomatology worsens and a decision is made not to feed this baby, blood glucose will be drawn. In the Respiratory Sequence, you assign her a Respiratory Score of 3.

Based on her history (Caesarean section at 38 weeks in the absence of established labour) and your evaluation of mild respiratory distress, you assign a working diagnosis of mild respiratory distress. This baby requires close observation and monitoring to see whether her respiratory symptoms worsen and persist beyond 6 h of age, but no additional respiratory supports are needed at this point.

1. Do you need to enter the Infection Sequence? Why or why not?

☐ Yes ☐ No

2. How do you Organize Care for this infant? Tick all that apply.

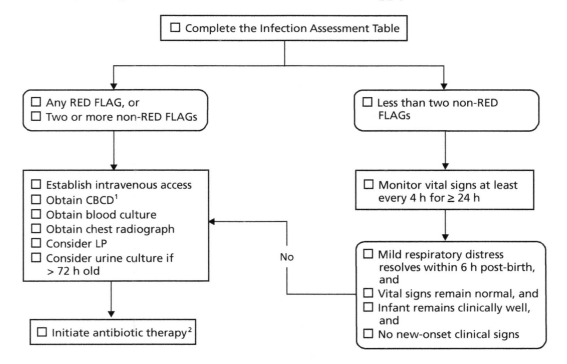

Thirty min later, you reassess the baby.

Her HR is 140 bpm and her respiratory rate is now 58 breaths/min, with a decrease in grunting and an oxygen saturation of 98% in room air. She has gone to breast to attempt a latch. Her temperature is 37.2°C skin-to-skin with mom.

You confirm that there are no additional risk factors for infection.

3. **What are your Next Steps? Tick all that apply.**
   ☐ Monitor vital signs at least q 4 h.
   ☐ Reassess if clinical deterioration OR respiratory distress persists > 6 h.
   ☐ Continue assessment using the Respiratory Score as long as respiratory distress persists and the infant is spontaneously breathing.
   ☐ Discharge home.
   ☐ Perform a complete blood count with differential and start antibiotics.

Infection: Case 2—A late preterm baby with respiratory distress and risk for infection

A baby boy presents with respiratory distress at 30 min of age. He was born by spontaneous vaginal delivery at 36 weeks GA to a 25-yo primiparous woman who is GBS-negative. Membranes were ruptured for 19 h, and the mother developed a fever in labour (temperature 38.5°C) with a WBC of 15.8 × 10⁹/L. Mild tachypnea was present at birth (RR = 70 breaths/min), and the infant has been admitted to the observation area for ongoing care and monitoring. Over the next 30 min, his respirations have become increasingly laboured. He is pink in room air and well-perfused, with HR at 170 beats/min and normal blood pressure for age. He has a normal neurologic exam. His weight is 3 kg. The point-of-care glucose is 3.0 mmol/L. His axillary temperature is 36.5°C.

1. **Complete the ACoRN Primary Survey (facing page) and Consolidated Core Steps, and generate a Problem List.**

On assessment, the baby continues to be tachypneic, with a respiratory rate of 65 to 70 breaths/min, mild subcostal retractions, and grunting with stimulation. You feel that the breath sounds are decreased to the bases, but he is not requiring oxygen.

You have calculated a Respiratory Score of 4, placing him in the mild respiratory distress category. You establish a working diagnosis of 'mild respiratory distress' and exit to your next priority sequence.

In Fluid and Glucose, you are not certain whether this baby should be fed. You are concerned about the degree of tachypnea and the risk of hypoglycemia associated with late preterm infants.

Blood glucose, at this point, is normal, and the baby is just over an hour of age.

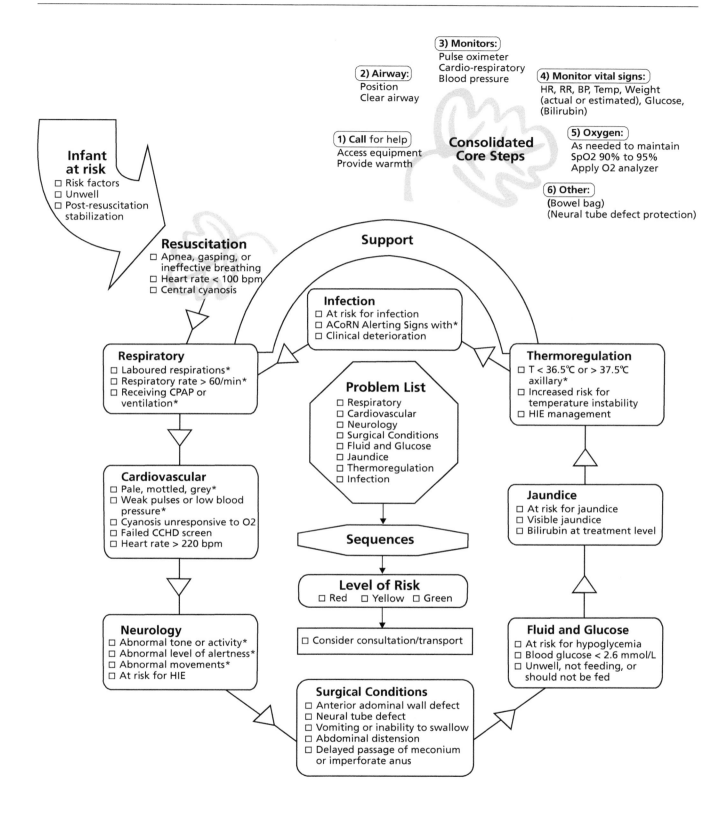

Infant at risk
- ☐ Risk factors
- ☐ Unwell
- ☐ Post-resuscitation stabilization

Consolidated Core Steps

1) Call for help
Access equipment
Provide warmth

2) Airway:
Position
Clear airway

3) Monitors:
Pulse oximeter
Cardio-respiratory
Blood pressure

4) Monitor vital signs:
HR, RR, BP, Temp, Weight
(actual or estimated), Glucose,
(Bilirubin)

5) Oxygen:
As needed to maintain
SpO2 90% to 95%
Apply O2 analyzer

6) Other:
(Bowel bag)
(Neural tube defect protection)

Resuscitation
- ☐ Apnea, gasping, or ineffective breathing
- ☐ Heart rate < 100 bpm
- ☐ Central cyanosis

Support

Infection
- ☐ At risk for infection
- ☐ ACoRN Alerting Signs with*
- ☐ Clinical deterioration

Respiratory
- ☐ Laboured respirations*
- ☐ Respiratory rate > 60/min*
- ☐ Receiving CPAP or ventilation*

Thermoregulation
- ☐ T < 36.5°C or > 37.5°C axillary*
- ☐ Increased risk for temperature instability
- ☐ HIE management

Problem List
- ☐ Respiratory
- ☐ Cardiovascular
- ☐ Neurology
- ☐ Surgical Conditions
- ☐ Fluid and Glucose
- ☐ Jaundice
- ☐ Thermoregulation
- ☐ Infection

Cardiovascular
- ☐ Pale, mottled, grey*
- ☐ Weak pulses or low blood pressure*
- ☐ Cyanosis unresponsive to O2
- ☐ Failed CCHD screen
- ☐ Heart rate > 220 bpm

Jaundice
- ☐ At risk for jaundice
- ☐ Visible jaundice
- ☐ Bilirubin at treatment level

Sequences

Level of Risk
- ☐ Red ☐ Yellow ☐ Green

☐ Consider consultation/transport

Fluid and Glucose
- ☐ At risk for hypoglycemia
- ☐ Blood glucose < 2.6 mmol/L
- ☐ Unwell, not feeding, or should not be fed

Neurology
- ☐ Abnormal tone or activity*
- ☐ Abnormal level of alertness*
- ☐ Abnormal movements*
- ☐ At risk for HIE

Surgical Conditions
- ☐ Anterior adominal wall defect
- ☐ Neural tube defect
- ☐ Vomiting or inability to swallow
- ☐ Abdominal distension
- ☐ Delayed passage of meconium or imperforate anus

2. Should this infant be fed?

☐ Yes ☐ No

3. In the Jaundice Sequence, this baby is at risk for hyperbilirubinemia because of prematurity. Do you need to do a bilirubin level at this time?

☐ Yes ☐ No

For Thermoregulation, you recognize that although this baby's temperature is normal, he is at risk for temperature instability.

4. What do you need to do? Tick all that apply.

☐ Apply skin probe and ensure servo control mode is selected on the over-bed warmer.

☐ Record temperature every 4 h.

☐ Monitor temperature regularly and observe for temperature instability.

The final sequence on your Problem List is Infection. You recognize that you have 2 Alerting Signs for Infection.

5. What Alerting Signs are present for Infection? Tick all that apply.

☐ Risk factor for infection.

☐ ACoRN Alerting Sign with*

    ☐ Laboured respirations*   ☐ Respiratory rate > 60/min*

    ☐ Receiving CPAP or ventilation*   ☐ Pale, mottled, grey*

    ☐ Weak pulses or low blood pressure*   ☐ Abnormal tone or activity*

    ☐ Abnormal level of alertness*   ☐ Abnormal movements

    ☐ Temperature <36.5 or >37.5 axillary*

☐ Clinical deterioration

6. You enter the Infection Sequence and perform the Core Step, completing the Infection Assessment Table. Tick all that apply.

Risk factors		Clinical indicators	
Red flag	**Non-red flag**	**Red flag**	**Non-red flag**
☐ Invasive maternal infection requiring IV antibiotic therapy 24 h before or after birth ☐ Infection in co-twin (multiple pregnancy)	☐ Invasive GBS in previous infant and inadequate IAP ☐ Maternal GBS colonization or UTI in current pregnancy and inadequate IAP ☐ Rupture of membranes > 18 h ☐ Intrapartum maternal fever (> 38°C) or confirmed or suspected chorioamnionitis ☐ Preterm (< 37 weeks) birth following spontaneous labour	☐ New-onset respiratory distress[1] ☐ Term infant receiving ventilation ☐ Shock ☐ Seizures	☐ Laboured respirations, respiratory rate > 60/min ☐ Preterm infant receiving ventilation ☐ New-onset apnea in a preterm infant[1] ☐ Abnormal tone or activity and/or Abnormal level of alertness ☐ New-onset[1] feeding problems: feeding poorly, vomiting, excessive gastric aspirates, abdominal distention ☐ New-onset[1] metabolic abnormalities, such as hyper-/hypoglycemia or metabolic acidosis (BD ≥ 10 mmol/L) ☐ Bilirubin at treatment level before 24 h of age ☐ Axillary temperature < 36.5°C or > 37.5°C, unexplained by environmental factors ☐ Local signs of infection (eye, skin, umbilicus)

BD: base deficit; CPAP: continuous positive airway pressure; GBS: Group B *Streptococcus*; IAP: intrapartum antibiotic prophylaxis; IV: intravenous; UTI: urinary tract infection

[1]'New onset' is defined as any clinically significant change after a previous period of stability.

Based on the Infection Assessment Table, your Organization of Care is based on the presence of 2 or more non-red flag items.

7. How do you Organize Care for this infant?

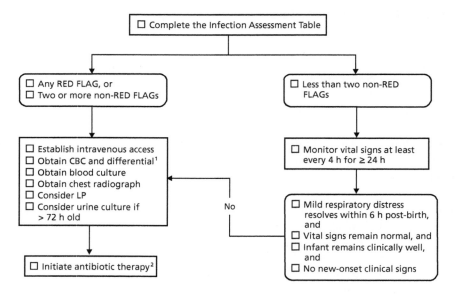

8. What organisms are you considering as the cause for this presumed EOS? Tick all that apply.

☐ *E. coli* ☐ GBS ☐ Coagulase-negative *Staphylococcus* species

☐ *Enterobacter* ☐ *Staphylococcus aureus* ☐ *Klebsiella*

9. What antibiotic orders will you write?

☐ Vancomycin 45 mg IV q 12 h *and* gentamycin OR tobramycin 10.5 mg IV q 24 h

☐ Ampicillin 150 mg IV q 12 h *and* gentamycin OR tobramycin 12 mg IV q 24 h

☐ Ampicillin 150 mg IV q 8 h *and* cefotaxime 150 mg IV q 8 h

10. What is the working diagnosis?

☐ EOS ☐ LOS ☐ Congenital pneumonia

11. What is this baby's Level of Risk?

☐ Green ☐ Yellow ☐ Red

Bibliography

Benitz WE, Wynn JL, Polin RA. Reappraisal of guidelines for management of neonates with suspected early-onset sepsis. J Pediatr 2015;166(4):1070–4.

Brady MT, Polin RA. Prevention and management of infants with suspected or proven neonatal sepsis. Pediatrics 2013;132(1):166–8.

Døllner H, Vatten L, Austgulen R. Early diagnostic markers for neonatal sepsis: Comparing C-reactive protein, interlukin-6, soluable tumour necrosis factor receptors and soluable adhesion molecules. J Clinic Epidemiol 2001;54(12):251–7.

Escobar GJ, Puopolo KM, Wi S, et al. Stratification of risk of early-onset sepsis in newborns ≥34 weeks' gestation. Pediatrics 2014;133(1):30–6.

Higgins RD, Saade G, Polin RA, et al. Evaluation and management of women and newborns with a maternal diagnosis of chorioamnionitis: Summary of a workshop. Obstet Gynecol 2016;127(3):426–36.

Jan IA, Ramanathan R, Cayabyab RG. Chorioamnionitis and management of asymptomatic infants ≥35 weeks without empiric antibiotics. Pediatrics 2017;140(1):pii:e20162744. Erratum in Pediatrics 2017;140(4):pii:e20172212.

Jefferies AL, Canadian Paediatric Society, Fetus and Newborn Committee. Management of term infants at increased risk for early-onset bacterial sepsis. Paediatr Child Health 2017;22(4):223–8: www.cps.ca/en/documents/position/management-infant-sepsis

Radcliffe A. NICE Guideline CG149. Neonatal infection (early-onset): Antibiotics for prevention and treatment. August 2012. Updated January 2017: www.nice.org.uk/guidance/cg149 (Accessed November 12, 2018).

Randis TM, Polin RA, Saade G. Chorioamnionitis: Time for a new approach. Curr Opin Pediatr 2017;29(2):159–64.

Sarkar S, Bhagat I, DeCristofaro JD, Wiswell TE, Spitzer AR. A study of the role of multiple site blood cultures in the evaluation of neonatal sepsis. J Perinatol 2006;26(1):18–22.

Schelonka RL, Chai MK, Yoder BA, Hensley D, Brockett RM, Ascher DP. Volume of blood required to detect common neonatal pathogens. J Pediatr 1996;129(2):275–8.

Stocker M, van Herk W, El Helou S, et al. Procalcitonin-guided decision making for duration of antibiotic therapy in neonates with suspected early-onset sepsis: A multicentre, randomised controlled trial (NeoPIns). Lancet 2017;390(10097):871–81.

Answer key: Infection Case 1—A term infant with mild respiratory distress

1. Do you need to enter the Infection Sequence? Why or why not?

    ✓ Yes   ☐ No

This baby has 2 Alerting Signs with a * and does need to enter the Infection Sequence. Additional surveillance will ensure other risk factors for infection are identified and assist practitioners to further organize her care.

2. How do you Organize Care for this infant?

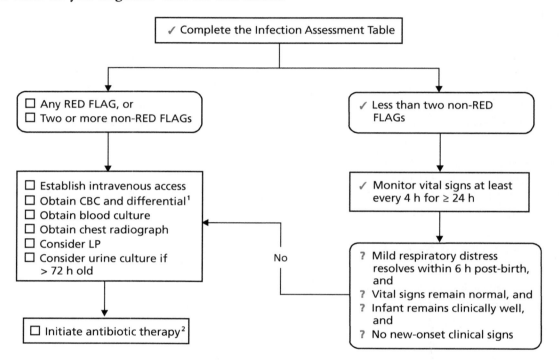

This baby has only one non-Red flag clinical indicator for infection. Care is organized based on this finding and the absence of other risk factors. You check in frequently with the parents as they remain in the recovery room post–Caesarean section, and take this opportunity to review the maternal history and risk factors that may not have been known.

3. What are your Next Steps?

    ✓ Monitor vital signs at least q 4 h.

    ✓ Reassess if clinical deterioration OR respiratory distress persists > 6 h.

    ✓ Continue assessment using the Respiratory Score as long as respiratory distress persists and the infant is spontaneously breathing.

    ☐ Discharge home.

    ☐ Perform a complete blood count with differential and start antibiotics.

The team is comfortable that this baby's mild respiratory distress is stable and presumes that she has transient tachypnea of the newborn. Without a CXR to confirm findings, your working diagnosis is mild respiratory distress. You have orders to monitor vital signs regularly and plan to inform the paediatrician if there is evidence of clinical deterioration or persistence of respiratory distress beyond 6 h of life. This child is not a candidate for early discharge based on the respiratory signs.

Answer key: Infection Case 2—A late preterm baby with respiratory distress and risk for infection

1. **Complete the ACoRN Primary Survey and Consolidated Core Steps, and generate a Problem List.**

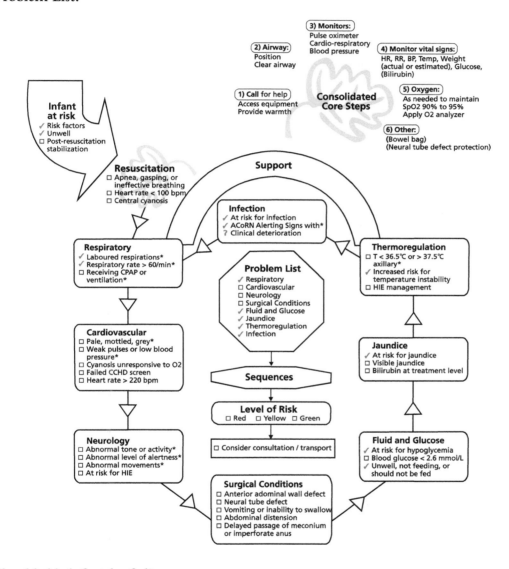

2. **Should this infant be fed?**

☐ Yes   ✓ No

This infant has mild respiratory distress evidenced by a Respiratory Score of 4. He has laboured respirations* and a respiratory rate >60 breaths/min*, which will make it difficult for this late-preterm infant to feed successfully. Both of these parameters also indicate risk for infection.

You decide to work through the Problem List, to see what additional interventions are required. You make a note on your 'to-do' list to determine whether the baby can be fed orally. You will continue to monitor his respiratory status to see if enteral feeds could be initiated.

You are not sure, at this time, if the baby's clinical presentation represents a clinical deterioration, so mark this Alerting Sign with a **?** to remind you to assess. As there are already Alerting Signs for Infection, it will not alter your Problem List or the need to enter the Infection Sequence.

3. In the Jaundice Sequence, this baby is at risk for hyperbilirubinemia because of prematurity. Do you need to do a bilirubin level at this time?

☐ Yes   ✓ No

Although the baby is at risk for hyperbilirubinemia based on GA, he is only 30 min of age and has no visible jaundice, so a sample is not warranted at this time. You do, however, add a 24-h bilirubin to your 'to-do' list and exit the sequence.

For Thermoregulation, you recognize that although this baby's temperature is normal, he is at risk for temperature instability.

4. What do you need to do?

✓ Apply skin probe and ensure servo control mode is selected on the over-bed warmer.
☐ Record temperature every 4 h.
☐ Monitor temperature regularly and observe for temperature instability.

Until the baby's temperature has stabilized, it is recommended to measure it more frequently (every 15 to 30 min until stable) and then every 1 to 2 h. You add temperature checks to the 'to-do' list.

5. What Alerting Signs are present for Infection?

✓ Risk factor for infection
✓ ACoRN Alerting Sign with*

     ✓ Laboured respirations*   ✓ Respiratory rate > 60/min*
     ☐ Receiving CPAP or ventilation*   ☐ Pale, mottled, grey*
     ☐ Weak pulses or low blood pressure*   ☐ Abnormal tone or activity*
     ☐ Abnormal level of alertness*   ☐ Abnormal movements
     ☐ Temperature < 36.5 or >37.5 axillary*
   ? Clinical deterioration

PROM (rupture of membranes for 19 h), maternal fever (temperature 38.5°C), maternal WBC of 15.8×10^9/L, and preterm birth (36 weeks GA) following spontaneous onset of labour, are all risk factors for neonatal infection.

The baby exhibited 2 Respiratory Alerting Signs, both with a *.

The baby has mild respiratory distress (ACoRN Respiratory Score of 4) and remains pink in room air. You decide to place a **?** beside Clinical deterioration, because the baby's respirations were reported to be more laboured in the last 30 min. You are reassured by the classification of mild respiratory distress. You make a note to reassess vital signs within the next 30 min, including a Respiratory Score, and continue to monitor the baby closely for signs that his condition is improving or deteriorating.

6. You enter the Infection Sequence and perform the Core Step, completing the Infection Assessment Table.

Risk factors		Clinical indicators	
Red flag	**Non-red flag**	**Red flag**	**Non-red flag**
☐ Invasive maternal infection requiring IV antibiotic therapy 24 h before or after birth ☐ Infection in co-twin (multiple pregnancy)	☐ Invasive GBS in previous infant and inadequate IAP ☐ Maternal GBS colonization or UTI in current pregnancy and inadequate IAP ✓ Rupture of membranes > 18 h ✓ Intrapartum maternal fever (> 38°C) or confirmed or suspected chorioamnionitis ✓ Preterm (< 37 weeks) birth following spontaneous labour	☐ New-onset respiratory distress[1] ☐ Term infant receiving ventilation ☐ Shock ☐ Seizures	✓ Laboured respirations, respiratory rate > 60/min ☐ Preterm infant receiving ventilation ☐ New-onset apnea in a pre-term infant[1] ☐ Abnormal tone or activity and/or Abnormal level of alertness ☐ New-onset[1] feeding problems: feeding poorly, vomiting, excessive gastric aspirates, abdominal distention ☐ New-onset[1] metabolic abnormalities, such as hyper-/hypoglycemia or metabolic acidosis (BD ≥ 10 mmol/L) ☐ Bilirubin at treatment level before 24 h of age ☐ Axillary temperature < 36.5°C or > 37.5°C, unexplained by environmental factors ☐ Local signs of infection (eye, skin, umbilicus)

BD: base deficit; CPAP: continuous positive airway pressure; GBS: Group B *Streptococcus*; IAP: intrapartum antibiotic prophylaxis; IV: intravenous; UTI: urinary tract infection.

[1]'New onset' is defined as any clinically significant change after a previous period of stability.

7. How do you Organize Care for this infant?

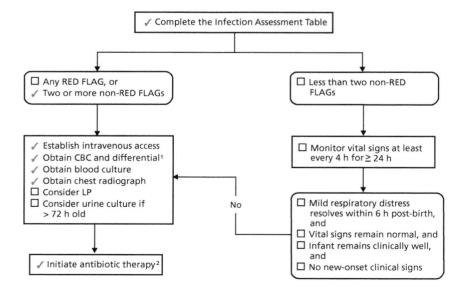

Your Organization of Care is based on the presence of 2 or more non-red flags. An infant with two or more non-red flags is considered at higher risk for sepsis, and this baby will require additional investigations (CBC and differential; blood culture; CXR) and immediate management. This infant will need IV access for administration of antibiotics.

You decide not to enterally feed the baby until you reassess his respiratory status, knowing that an IV has been started and you will be able to provide the baby with maintenance fluid intake. You refer to the Fluid and Glucose Sequence to determine the IV solution and rate needed to meet the infant's glucose needs (GIR).

Initiation of treatment (i.e., antibiotics) should not be delayed while waiting for laboratory results.

Completion of an LP as part of an initial sepsis work-up for EOS is controversial. This baby did not present with any Alerting Signs in the Neurology Sequence. Because his Alerting Signs were exclusively in the Respiratory Sequence, it would be reasonable not to perform an LP at this time. If the blood culture is positive or the baby presents with new-onset neurologic signs, an LP may be warranted.

A urine culture is not usually diagnostic in infants less than 72 h of age.

8. What organisms are you considering as the cause for this presumed EOS?

✓ *E. coli*   ✓ GBS   ☐ Coagulase-negative *Staphylococcus* species

✓ *Enterobacter*   ☐ *Staphylococcus aureus*   ✓ *Klebsiella*

The most likely organisms for this case are *E. coli, Klebsiella*, and *Enterobacter*. GBS is still possible despite negative swabs.

9. What antibiotic orders will you write?

☐ Vancomycin 45 mg IV q 12 h *and* gentamycin OR tobramycin 10.5 mg IV q 24 h

✓ Ampicillin 150 mg IV q 12 h *and* gentamycin OR tobramycin 12 mg IV q 24 h

☐ Ampicillin 150 mg IV q 8 h *and* cefotaxime 150 mg IV q 8 h

10. What is the working diagnosis?

✓ EOS   ☐ LOS   ✓ Congenital pneumonia

Based on the history and the infant's presentation of clinical signs in the first hour post-birth, the working diagnosis could be EOS or congenital neonatal pneumonia. The latter will be confirmed or ruled out based upon the CXR findings and ongoing respiratory symptoms.

11. What is this baby's Level of Risk?

☐ Green   ✓ Yellow   ☐ Red

You feel this baby is currently stable and your facility has a special care nursery with space, staff, and the capacity to support IV antibiotics, nasogastric feeds, and mild to moderate respiratory distress with CPAP, in case of deterioration.

Transport

Educational objectives

Upon completion of this chapter, you will be able to:

- Recognize factors that determine the decision to transport a sick infant.
- Describe the information needed by the receiving hospital.
- Use a standardized communication tool for information handover.
- Describe the roles of the sending hospital, the receiving physician, the transport coordinating physician, and the transport team.

Key concepts

1. In utero transport is recommended, whenever possible.
2. Early consultation facilitates timely advice and early initiation of transport, if necessary, to optimize care.
3. Consultation with a referral centre does not always imply a need for transport.
4. Effective stabilization before transport minimizes morbidity and mortality.
5. Communication and support of the family is an integral part of the transfer process.

Skills

- Determining Level of Risk
- Use of the SBARR communication tool

Neonatal transport is a process that requires special training, equipment, and coordination. The use of a specialized transport team is associated with improved infant outcomes and survival. Policies and procedures must be in place to guide team performance. A single access point, with provincial/territorial or regional coordination and integrated modes of transport, must ensure the immediate availability of medical advice, the rapid dispatch of a transport team, and the identification of the receiving hospital.

The Acute Care of at-Risk Newborns (ACoRN) program helps to standardize the identification and assessment of at-risk or unwell newborns by generating a prioritized Problem List and guiding initial stabilization. It also prompts ACoRN providers to consider early consultation and transport for these infants.

Determining factors for transport

Requesting a consult does not necessarily mean you want or need to transport an infant to another facility. However, if an infant's current or anticipated problems cannot be managed locally, the earlier the need for more specialized care is identified, the sooner the transport process can be initiated.

The decision to consult on, or transport, an at-risk or unwell infant to another facility is based on discussions between the sending hospital or facility and the transport coordinating physician. A number of factors are considered, including:

- The infant's current condition and anticipated course,
- Sending hospital resources (i.e., on-site personnel, expertise, equipment, and specialized services),
- Regional referral patterns,
- Transport team availability,
- Mode and availability of transport, and
- Current or impending weather conditions.

Each of the ACoRN Sequences indicates when to consider obtaining consultation for management and possible transport.

Level of Risk

Establishing an infant's Level of Risk can help the ACoRN provider to decide whether transfer to a higher level of care is warranted. It considers the ongoing care needs for the infant, the stability achieved and the need for early consultation and/or transport. Each sequence assigns a Level of Risk for the infant. The highest level of risk assigned in any ACoRN sequence determines the final Level of Risk for this infant and is indicated on the ACoRN Primary Survey.

Establishing an infant's Level of Risk

Level of Risk: Transport
In the ACoRN Primary Survey, level of risk is based on the highest level of risk assigned in any of the ACoRN sequences.

Green:
- Infant is 35 weeks gestation or greater, clinically stable, and needs a low level of intervention and ongoing monitoring, **AND**
- Ongoing requirements do not exceed site capability

Yellow:
- Infant is clinically stable but needs a higher level of observation or intervention, **OR**
- Infant is clinically stable but a worsening clinical course is anticipated, **AND**
- Site can provide appropriate management, investigations, and monitoring for the infant's condition

Infants at a Yellow Level of Risk require increased levels of attention and may require consultation. Transfer is required if needs exceed site capabilities.

Red:
- Infant is unstable or unwell, needs a high level of observation or intervention, **OR**
- Infant is anticipated to become unstable or unwell, **OR**
- Infant requires care that is beyond the site's capacity to manage or monitor safely

Infants at a Red Level of Risk are considered unstable, and require level 3 care. Transfer is required if infant or care team needs exceed site capabilities.

The objective is to anticipate early which infants require or are likely to require an increased level of attention, early consultation, and timely transfer to a higher level of care.

The timeline for transports is critical. When safe to do so, an in utero transport, using the regional transfer network, is prioritized to enable delivery at a centre that can provide an appropriate level of care to mother and infant. However, not all mothers and fetuses with high-risk conditions are identified or deemed transportable in the prenatal period. Additionally, an infant may become unwell at or just after birth. These infants need initial stabilization and assessment for transport to a facility able to provide higher level care.

The primary reason to initiate early consultation is to improve infant outcomes. For infants requiring transport, the length of time it takes to get to the patient (the response time) and the time it takes to arrive at the receiving hospital (the transport time) should be minimized.

> The essential role of a perinatal transport system is to safely transfer newborns and/or their mothers to the hospital closest to home that is able to provide the care they require.

Initiating a consultation or transport request

A centralized process, with a single telephone number for accessing medical advice, triaging requests, and activating a specialized transport team, is the most efficient practice. These duties are often handled by a transport coordinating or logistics centre.

> Staff working in every health care facility should know how to access the regional maternal/neonatal transport system at any hour of the day or night.

A physician, midwife, or delegate caring for an infant at the sending hospital is responsible for initiating the consultation process. When a transport request is made, a triage process is initiated that prioritizes level of need with available resources. All communications should use a structured tool, such as SBARR, to achieve maximal clarity.

1. **Communicate the essentials:** Start with identifying yourself, your location and phone number, then give the patient's name and basic demographics.
2. **Make a clear statement of need:** Use the SBARR Communication Tool (Table 11.1) to focus the encounter, initiate consultation or triage, and direct specific attention to the needs of the patient and care providers.
3. **Provide specifics:** Collating the information required to assess, triage, and advise on ongoing care or transport can be difficult. Information that the transport coordinator will need includes:
   ☐ Essential demographics.
   ☐ The ACoRN Primary Survey and Problem List, which reflect the most recent assessments and examinations.
   ☐ A brief, relevant background history of the mother, along with perinatal events, the infant's initial condition, and early interventions.
   ☐ A description of current management, interventions (e.g., ventilation, boluses, infusions), and additional findings not captured elsewhere.

☐ Conditions that may determine need for isolation, including a history of infections or colonization by antibiotic-resistant organisms (i.e., MRSA).

☐ Level of risk, transport needs, and urgency.

Table 11.1.
How to use SBARR in transport scenarios

Item	Verbalize	Description and example
S—situation	'This is my chief concern'	A one-line descriptor of the situation and whether the infant is stable or unstable 'I am calling about a 1-h-old, 31-w-GA infant with respiratory distress. The baby is stable.'
B—background	'I want you to know'	Date and time of birth, gestational age and birth weight, condition. State the ACoRN Problem List and describe positive findings in the Primary Survey, Sequences, Focused History and Physical Exam. '1-h-old, 31-w gestation, 1500-g, female, with ACoRN Alerting Signs in Respiratory, Fluid and Glucose, Thermoregulation and Infection Sequences. She is in moderate respiratory distress, CPAP 5 with T-piece, 35% O2, SpO2 94%. D10W at 3 mL/kg/h via peripheral IV. Last glucose 3.6 mmol/L. On ampicillin and gentamicin. Mother had no antenatal steroids, MgSO4 or antibiotics; GBS negative, ROM 8 h.'
A—assessment	'This is the infant's condition'	Working diagnosis. Stable/unstable. Risk level assessment. 'Baby is stable now, but we cannot sustain level of care and her condition may worsen. Risk level is Red, as we are a level 1 unit.'
R—recommendation	'I need'	Consult only? Or transfer need? Identify how long care needs can be sustained in the sending hospital. 'Please send transport team ASAP.'
R—readback/response	'Are there any questions?'	Caller responds to questions, referring to the NICU Telephone Consultation form (page 343). Transport coordinating physician asks specific questions based on the information provided.

Use of the NICU Telephone Consultation form (page 343) can aid health care providers in organizing and transmitting the necessary information.

Transport coordination

Coordinating the transport of a sick newborn involves interactions and communication among multiple individuals with varying roles and responsibilities (Figure 11.1). A clear understanding of the process is essential.

A successful transport involves early identification by the sending hospital, relaying accurate assessments, advice, and support between the sending and receiving hospitals, and ensuring that transport logistics match the standards of care and timelines required by the infant's condition. The process requires knowledge of both the clinical situation and regional/provincial/territorial processes for transport (i.e., the mechanics of transport).

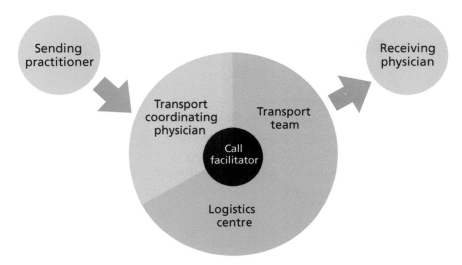

Figure 11.1. Components of a neonatal transport.

All communication among the sending practitioner, transport coordinating physician, logistics centre, transport team, and receiving physician constitute medical acts that require documentation.

Responsibilities of the sending hospital

The health care team at the sending hospital plays an integral role in neonatal transfer. They:

- Provide resuscitation and ongoing stabilization.
- Identify the need for early consultation and transport.
- Initiate contact with the transport coordination centre.
- Communicate up-to-date information on the infant's condition and the stabilization process to both the health care team and the family.
- Inform the transport coordinating physician of significant changes in the infant's condition (i.e., worsening respiratory distress, need for intubation), so that the transport team can be updated before they arrive.
- Remain with the infant to provide ongoing care and help the transport team with stabilization until departure.
- Identify infection control risk factors.
- Provide copies of maternal and infant charts.
- Prepare breast milk, if available, to transport with the infant.

Use a regional or provincial/territorial Neonatal Transfer Record (page 344) to ensure the information needed by the receiving hospital is complete. It is also useful to copy any nursing or physician notes and completed ACoRN tools in preparation for transfer.

Responsibilities of the transport coordinating physician

The transport coordinating physician is the medical supervisor and primary communicator with the transport team. This physician:

- Determines the level of hospital care needed.
- Identifies special needs (e.g., an isolation room for infection control).
- Identifies the appropriate receiving hospital, mode, and urgency of transport, and composition of the transport team.
- Provides medical advice to practitioners at the sending hospital.
- Communicates with the receiving hospital and ensures that the receiving physician has the most current medical information.

The duties of the transport coordinating physician begin when initial contact is made by the sending physician, midwife or delegate, and only end once the infant is transferred into a physician's care at the receiving hospital.

Responsibilities of the transport coordinating (logistics) centre

The transport coordinating (logistics) centre is responsible for organizing and coordinating the mechanics of transfer within regional/provincial/territorial resources. Centre personnel:

- Determine, with the transport coordinating physician, the level of patient need and the most appropriate mode of transport.
- Mobilize and coordinate vehicular transportation.
- Stay in close communication with the transport team regarding logistical issues.
- Records calls.

The centre also collects standardized data such as dispatch and transport times—including mobilization, response, and stabilization—to benchmark performance and improve system function and standards across transport programs.

Responsibilities of the transport team

Upon arrival at the sending hospital, the transport team assumes care of the patient and updates the transport coordinating physician regarding the infant's clinical status.

Pretransport stabilization improves infant outcomes and is a focus of the transport team. They review and optimize the infant's condition and management before leaving to minimize the need for unnecessary interventions en route. They try to anticipate potential complications of transporting a sick infant based on the particular mode of transport used and ensure the infant is as stable and safe as possible for transport. They manage the transition between environments, including movement, noise and vibration levels, lighting, environmental temperature, and changes in speed. Knowledge of flight physiology is key when transporting by air.

At the sending hospital, the transport team should discuss stabilization steps with the transport coordinating physician, who retains responsibility for their medical and administrative actions.

Pretransport stabilization should be a proactive process. For example, the team may:

- Electively intubate and ventilate, to ensure supports are in place should respiratory function deteriorate during transport.
- Adjust the transport ventilator based on clinical findings, blood gas readings, and radiographs.
- Drain a pneumothorax, when clinically indicated and when the infant is to be transported by air.
- Retape or replace existing catheters to ensure adequate intravenous access during transport.
- Obtain essential blood work (e.g., blood gases and glucose).
- Check medications and prepare medications that may be needed in transit.
- Consider thermal controls (e.g., avoiding hypothermia in preterm infants or maintaining therapeutic hypothermia in term infants with hypoxic ischaemic encephalopathy).
- Minimize the infant's anxiety and discomfort by using (for example) noise reduction earmuffs, an air foam mattress, a warming mattress, blankets, or a gel pillow.

In most Canadian settings, the transport team also obtains consents for transport, admission, and care at the receiving hospital, and for the transfusion of blood products, before leaving the sending hospital.

Shared responsibilities

Medical responsibility for the infant's care rests with the sending hospital until their call is placed to the transport coordinating centre. From that moment and until the transport team arrives, responsibility is shared by the sending hospital and the transport coordinating physician. When the transport team arrives, they take primary responsibility for the infant's care, in collaboration with the transport coordinating physician and supported by the sending physician and team. The local health care team remains responsible for providing support, space, and equipment, as needed. When the infant leaves the sending hospital, the transport coordinating physician and the transport team assume responsibility for care until the infant arrives at the receiving hospital, where care of the infant is formally handed over to the receiving physician.

> Timely and constructive feedback is essential for building and maintaining an effective, collaborative, and educational transport network.

Communicating with the family

Most parents understand when circumstances determine that their sick infant must be transported to another hospital to receive a higher level of care. Every effort should be made to keep parents informed of an infant's condition and transport arrangements. It is important to provide parents the opportunity to be with their infant while preparations for transport are in progress.

Parents should be encouraged to take photos or record a video before departure.

It is not always possible for a parent to accompany their infant during transport. Separation should always be minimized, especially when an infant's condition is critical. Such cases may involve facilitating a mother's early discharge or transferring her to the receiving hospital or a facility nearby.

Because breast milk is important for infant health, consider initiating discussions around early pumping or the option for donor breast milk (if appropriate), and obtain parental consent for the latter when a mother's own milk is not expected to be available.

The transport team should introduce themselves to parents and explain their role before leaving the sending hospital. The team is responsible for explaining the infant's care en route, answering parents' questions, securing consents as needed, and providing information about the receiving hospital (e.g., contact numbers and names, directions to the NICU and accommodation and unit policies, such as breastfeeding and visiting). Personnel from the sending hospital should participate in these discussions. A designated transport team member is responsible for informing the family when their infant arrives at the receiving hospital.

Responsibilities of the receiving physician

A physician at the receiving hospital must be identified and accept responsibility for the infant after transfer. On arrival, the receiving physician or a delegate assumes medical care and communicates the infant's medical status to the sending physician and team as well as the infant's family.

Annexed to this chapter are examples of a NICU Telephone Consultation form and a Neonatal Transfer Record. Consult your regional maternal/neonatal transport system for the forms used in your area.

[insert Facility logo here]

NICU Telephone Consultation

Patient Name: _____ M F I	Date: _____ Start Time: _____ End Time: _____
Health card #: _____	Phone #: _____
Patient DOB: _____ Birth Time: _____	MD: _____ Ph#: _____
GA: _____ BW: _____ Day of Life: _____ Current Weight: _____	Hospital: _____
Presenting Problem(s): _____	Hospital Level: _____ Patient Level: _____ Case #:: _____

Primary Survey

HR: _____ BP: _____ RR: _____

Temp: _____ FiO2: _____ SpO2: _____

Resp Distress: Ø Mild Mod Sev

CPAP: _____ cm H₂O ETT: _____ cm

Vent: PIP: _____ PEEP: _____

Cap Refill: _____ sec

Pulses: _____ Fem: _____

4 Limb BPs: RA: _____ LA: _____
              RL: _____ LL: _____

SpO2: pre: _____ post: _____

Pale ☐ Pink ☐ Alert ☐ Active ☐

Seizures: _____

Glucose: _____

D%W: _____ Rate: _____ mL/hr

Feed: _____ mL every _____ hr

Breast   EBM   Donor   Formula

GIR: _____ mg/kg/min

Bili: _____ mmol/L DAT: _____

IV Access Type:

PIV ☐ UV ☐ (Low___) UA ☐

Other: _____

Problem List   Working Diagnosis
 ☐ Respiratory: _____
 ☐ Cardiovascular: _____
 ☐ Neurology: _____
 ☐ Surgical: _____
 ☐ Fluid and Glucose: _____
 ☐ Jaundice: _____
 ☐ Thermoregulation: _____
 ☐ Infection: _____

History

Maternal Age: _____ G__ T__ P__ A __L__ ROM: _____ min / hrs Fetal Distress: _____ Vag ☐ C/S ☐

ANCS: _____ MgSO4: _____ DCC: _____ sec   Mat Antibiotics: _____

GBS: _____ HIV: _____ Hep B: _____ VDRL: _____ Rubella: _____ HSV: _____ Blood type: _____

Maternal medications: _____

Cord pH: _____ O2: _____ CO2: _____ HCO3: _____ BD: _____   Active ☐ Responsive ☐ Flat ☐

APGARS ___@ 1, ___@ 5, ___@10 Meconium: yes ☐ no ☐   Chorioamnionitis: : yes ☐ no ☐

Resus: Max FiO2 _____ CPAP ☐ PPV ☐ Max PIP: ___/PEEP: ___ ETT ____ Compressions: _____ min

Epi ETT x ____ Epi IV x _____ Age HR >100 ____ First Breath _____ Regular Breathing _____ (min of age)

Narrative:

Lab Results:

pH ____ PCO2 ____ HCO3 ____ BD ____ Lactate ____ Time ____	**Level of Risk:** RED ☐ YELLOW ☐ GREEN ☐
pH ____ PCO2 ____ HCO3 ____ BD ____ Lactate ____ Time ____	CONSULT ☐
Antibiotics: _____ Given on/at: _____	TRANSFER ☐ Life or Limb ☐ <4h ☐ <12 h ☐

Sending Facility/MD: _____ Receiving Facility/MD _____ Receiving Unit: _____
Transport Team: _____ Time notified: _____ Mode of Transfer: _____

Office Use Only: CNTN: _____ Billed ☐ Recorded Call ☐ Attending Physician: _____

PHYSICIAN SIGNATURE	PRINTED NAME OF PHYSICIAN	YR	MO	DAY	TIME

Neonatal Transfer Record

<table>
<tr><td>1. Surname
   Given Name</td><td>Date/Time of Birth</td><td>Gestational
Age at Birth

weeks/days</td><td>Post Menstrual
Age

weeks/days</td><td>Birth Weight

/grams</td></tr>
<tr><td></td><td>Sex ☐ M ☐ F ☐ Unk.</td><td colspan="3">Neonatal Daily Classification</td></tr>
<tr><td>Sending Facility</td><td>Attending MD/RM</td><td colspan="2">Discharge Diagnosis</td><td>Today's Weight

/grams</td></tr>
<tr><td>Receiving Facility</td><td>Receiving Physician</td><td colspan="3">Maternal / Birth History</td></tr>
<tr><td>G T P A L</td><td>APGAR Scores</td><td colspan="3"></td></tr>
</table>

2. Parent or Guardian Name(s)

Newborn Exposure to (check if positive)
☐ HIV ☐ Hep B ☐ Hep C ☐ Substance
☐ GBS ☐ ARO ☐ HPV ☐ Other (specify)

Current Isolation Status

Hometown of Baby | Contact Number | Language Preferred

☐ Photos of Baby to Mother
☐ Mom Expressing Breast Milk

3. Vital Signs

	HR	RR	SpO₂	BP	T
Time:				/M	

4. Assessments

Respiratory: Airway: ☐ ETT # _____ @ _____ cm Date/Time: _____ Extubated Date/Time: _____ ☐ LMA # _____

Current Ventilator Settings: Mode: _____ FiO₂: _____ Rate: _____ Pressure: _____ I:T _____ VT: _____

Non-Invasive Respiratory Support: ☐ CPAP ☐ LFNP ☐ HFNP ☐ Other (specify) _____ Setting: _____ FiO₂: _____ Date Initiated: _____

Surfactant ☐ Date: _____ # of Doses _____ ☐ Caffeine Discontinued Date: _____

Date and Time of last ☐ ABG ☐ CBG: _____ Results: pH _____ pCO₂ _____ pO₂ _____ HCO₃ _____ BD or BE _____

Cardiovascular | **Neurology**

GI/GU/Other

5. Intake

☐ PVAD (PIV) ☐ PICC Type: _____ at _____ cm ☐ CVAD (CVC) Type: _____

☐ UAC at _____ cm ☐ UVC at _____ cm # of lumens: ☐ 1 ☐ 2 ☐ 3 Other: _____

Total Fluids Order (including feeds)	mL/kg/day	Site/Route	Rate
Infusion #1 Solution/Dose			
Infusion #2 Solution/Dose			
Infusion #3 Solution/Dose			
Infusion #4 Solution/Dose			
Infusion #5 Solution/Dose			

Feeding: Type ☐ EBM ☐ Donor Human Milk
☐ Human Milk Substitute (specify)

Additives

Method: ☐ BR ☐ B ☐ OG ☐ NG Date Inserted and Location of Tube
☐ NJ ☐ G-tube ☐ GJ-tube
/cm depth

Amount	Frequency	Syringe pump over _____ minutes
Last Fed	☐ Feeding Concerns (specify) _____	
	☐ Infant Feeding Assessment Tool Attached	

6. Output Last Void: | Last Stool: | Additional Losses (e.g., blood from lab tests)

7. Medications: Name / Dose / Route / Frequency ☐ Medication record attached

1.	Last Given	Next Due	4.	Last Given	Next Due
2.			5.		
3.			6.		

8. Treatments +/or Investigations ☐ Abnormal Lab Values +/or Blood Culture Results attached

9. Screening

☐ CCHD Screen Done   Date: _____   ☐ Passed

Follow-up: _____

☐ Eye Exam Done   Date of Last Exam: _____   Due: _____

Results: _____

☐ Hearing Screen Done   Date: _____   ☐ Passed

Follow-up: _____

☐ Phototherapy   Date Discontinued: _____

☐ Newborn Screen Done (blood spot card)   Date: _____
☐ Repeat Newborn Screen Needed   Date: _____
Immunizations: ☐ Provincial Immunization Record Attached
RSV Prophylaxis Candidate: ☐ Yes ☐ No
RSV Prophylaxis Date Given: _____   ☐ Not Given

10. Consultants   ☐ Social Work, Name: _____   Contact: _____   ☐ SLP   ☐ OT   ☐ PT

☐ Child Protection Agency, Name: _____   Contact: _____   ☐ Dietitian   ☐ LC   ☐ Other:

11. Complex Care / Teaching

Parent Teaching: Basic Care for Baby: ☐ Bath ☐ Diaper Change ☐ Temperature ☐ Cuddle ☐ Skin-to-Skin ☐ Feeding ☐ Safe Sleep Positions/Environment

☐ Complex Care Involvement/Teaching (specify): ☐ RSV Screening/Teaching ☐ Purple Crying ☐ Biliary Atresia ☐ Maintenance of Milk Supply ☐ Safe Storage and Handling of Human Milk

Other: _____

_____

_____

_____

12. Additional Information (including socioeconomic issues / needs)

_____

_____

_____

_____

_____

_____

13. Transfer Checklist (if applicable   * indicates mandatory)

☐ Physician Discharge Order

☐ Copy of Chart (refer to Guide for Completion)*

☐ Copy of MAR*

☐ Signed Transfusion Consent

☐ Discharge Summary from Sending Facility*
   ☐ Mother ☐ Baby

☐ 2 ID Bands on Baby*

☐ ID Bands Checked with RN/Transport Team*

☐ Parents Notified of Transfer*

☐ Parents to Accompany
   ☐ Mother ☐ Partner

☐ Pumping Initiated _____ (date)

☐ Report Given to Receiving Facility

Acute Transfer

☐ Maternal Blood

☐ Cord Blood

☐ Placenta

☐ Baby's Blood Culture

☐ Other Lab Work

☐ Vitamin K administered

☐ Erythromycin administered

Repatriation Transfer

☐ EBM double checked and in cooler

☐ Personal Belongings

☐ Medications

Environment for Transfer	**Incubator Temperature and Humidity**	☐ Dressed
☐ Incubator ☐ Car Seat ☐ Other (specify)		☐ Covered

☐ **Care Transferred to Infant Transport Team**	☐ **Ambulance Transfer with** ○ MD ○ RN

14. Nurse(s) Completing Form

Printed Name	Signature	Date	Time
Printed Name	Signature	Date	Time
Printed Name	Signature	Date	Time

Baby Left Sending Hospital: _____
Date   Time

Transport: Case 1—Should he stay, or should he go?

A late preterm infant is born in your community hospital and needs no resuscitation at birth. His gestational age is 35 w and his birth weight is 2500 g.

The ACoRN Primary Survey shows the infant to have no Alerting Signs except for risk for hypoglycemia, risk for jaundice, and at increased risk for temperature instability.

You encourage the mother to breastfeed early and to keep the baby skin-to-skin. Plans are made to check blood glucose at 2 h of age, and to check and plot bilirubin levels before discharge.

At 2 h of age, the baby's blood glucose is 1.8 mmol/L and, despite management with measured feeds and dextrose gel, fails to normalize and remains less than 2.6 mmol/L.

At 4 h of age, the blood glucose level has risen to 3.3 mmol/L with the help of a peripheral venous infusion of 4 mL/kg/h of D10W. The ACoRN Primary Survey shows risk for jaundice and an increased risk for temperature instability. The infant's axillary temperature is now 37.0°C.

You do not have a dedicated nursery in your community hospital.

1. **What factors determine Level of Risk for this infant in your centre? Tick all that apply.**
   - ☐ Stable, needing observation but a low level of intervention.
   - ☐ Expected to remain stable and well.
   - ☐ Needs a level of care that does not exceed site capabilities.
   - ☐ Stable but needs a higher level of observation or intervention.
   - ☐ Expected to remain stable but his clinical trajectory may worsen.
   - ☐ Unstable or unwell, needing higher level of observation and/or intervention.
   - ☐ Likely to become unstable or unwell.
   - ☐ Needs a level of care that exceeds site capabilities.

2. **What Level of Risk would you assign this infant?**
   - ☐ Green   ☐ Yellow   ☐ Red

3. **Staff working in every health care facility should know how to access the regional maternal/neonatal transport system. Enter the phone number that applies to your region, below:**

   _____

4. **The SBARR Communication Tool is used to organize communication and direct specific attention to the needs of the patient and care providers. SBARR stands for:**
   - ☐ The **S** is for stability
   - ☐ The **B** is for background
   - ☐ The **A** is for assessment
   - ☐ The **R** is for recommendation
   - ☐ The **R** is for resources available
   - ☐ The **S** is for situation
   - ☐ The **B** is for birth date
   - ☐ The **A** is for acuity
   - ☐ The **R** is for retrieval
   - ☐ The **R** is for readback/response

5. **You call for a consult and arrange for neonatal transport. Present this infant's case information below in SBARR format.**

Item	Verbalize	Description
S	'This is my chief concern.'	A one-line descriptor of the situation and whether the infant is stable or unstable
B	'I want you to know.'	Date and time of birth, gestational age and birth weight, condition. State the ACoRN Problem List and describe positive findings in the Primary Survey, Sequences, Focused History and Physical Exam.
A	'This is the infant's condition.'	Working diagnosis. Stable/unstable. Risk level assessment.
R	'I need.'	Consult only? Or transfer need? Identify how long care needs can be sustained in the sending hospital.
R	'Are there any questions?'	Caller responds to questions, referring to the NICU Telephone Consultation form (page 343).

Bibliography

Akl N, Coghlan EA, Nathan EA, Langford SA, Newnham JP. Aeromedical transfer of women at risk of preterm delivery in remote and rural Western Australia: Why are there no births in flight? Aust N Z J Obstet Gynaecol 2012;52(4):327–33.

Bashshur RL, Shannon GW, Bashshur N, Yellowlees PM. The empirical evidence for telemedicine interventions in mental disorders. Telemed J E Health 2016;22(2):87–113.

Demaerschalk BM, Raman R, Ernstrom K, Meyer BC. Efficacy of telemedicine for stroke: Pooled analysis of the Stroke Team Remote Evaluation Using a Digital Observation Camera (STRokE DOC) and STRokE DOC Arizona telestroke trials. Telemed J E Health 2012;18(3):230–7.

Fanaroff J, Fanaroff A. Klaus and Fanroff's Care of the High-Risk Neonate. Philadelphia, PA: W.B. Saunders; 2012.

Fang JL, Collura CA, Johnson RV, et al. Emergency video telemedicine consultation for newborn resuscitations: The Mayo Clinic experience. Mayo Clin Proc 2016;91(12):1735–43.

Ge WJ, Mirea L, Yang J, Bassil KL, Lee SK, Shah PS; Canadian Neonatal Network. Prediction of neonatal outcomes in extremely preterm neonates. Pediatrics 2013;132(4):e876–85.

Hohlagschwandtner M, Husslein P, Klebermass K, Weninger M, Nardi A, Langer M. Perinatal mortality and morbidity. Comparison between maternal transport, neonatal transport and inpatient antenatal treatment. Arch Gynecol Obstet 2001;265(3):113–9.

Jaimovich DG, Vidyasagar D. Handbook of Pediatric and Neonatal Transport Medicine, 2nd ed. Philadelphia, PA: Hanley & Belfus; 2002.

Kim JH, Unger S, Canadian Paediatric Society, Nutrition and Gastroenterology Committee. Human milk banking. Paediatr Child Health 2010;15(9):595–8.

Kollée LA, Brand R, Schreuder AM, Ens-Dokkum MH, Veen S, Verloove-Vanhorick SP. Five-year outcome of preterm and very low birth weight infants: A comparison between maternal and neonatal transport. Obstet Gynecol 1992;80(4):635–8.

Kroenke K, Krebs EE, Wu J, Yu Z, Chumbler NR, Bair MJ. Telecare collaborative management of chronic pain in primary care: A randomized clinical trial. JAMA 2014;312(3):240–8.

Ramnarayan P. Measuring the performance of an inter-hospital transport service. Arch Dis Child 2009;94(6):414–6.

Webb CL, Waugh CL, Grigsby J, et al. Impact of telemedicine on hospital transport, length of stay, and medical outcomes in infants with suspected heart disease: A multicenter study. J Am Soc Echocardiogr 2013;26(9):1090–8.

Weingarten CT. Nursing interventions: Caring for parents of a newborn transferred to a regional intensive care nursery——A challenge for low risk obstetric specialists. J Perinatol 1988;8(3):271–5.

Whyte HEA, Jefferies AL; Canadian Paediatric Society, Fetus and Newborn Committee. The interfacility transport of critically ill newborns. Paediatr Child Health 2015;20(5):265–75: www.cps.ca/en/documents/position/interfacility-transport-of-critically-ill-newborns

Answer key: Transport Case 1—Should he stay, or should he go?

1. **What factors determine Level of Risk for this infant in your centre?**
   - ☐ Stable, needing observation but a low level of intervention.
   - ☐ Expected to remain stable and well.
   - ☐ Needs a level of care that does not exceed site capabilities.
   - ✓ Stable but needs a higher level of observation or intervention.
   - ☐ Expected to remain stable but his clinical trajectory may worsen.
   - ☐ Unstable or unwell, needing higher level of observation and/or intervention.
   - ☐ Likely to become unstable or unwell.
   - ✓ Needs a level of care that exceeds site capabilities.

2. **What Level of Risk would you assign the infant?**
   - ☐ Green　　　✓ Yellow　　　☐ Red

3. **Staff working in every health care facility should know how to access the regional maternal/neonatal transport system. Enter below the phone number that applies to your region, below:**

   Regional or provincial/territorial-specific phone number: _____

4. **The SBARR Communication Tool is used to organize communication and direct specific attention to the needs of the patient and care providers. SBARR stands for:**

☐ The **S** is for stability	✓ The **S** is for situation
✓ The **B** is for background	☐ The **B** is for birth date
✓ The **A** is for assessment	☐ The **A** is for acuity
✓ The **R** is for recommendation	☐ The **R** is for retrieval
☐ The **R** is for resources available	✓ The **R** is for readback/response

5. **You call for a consult and arrange for neonatal transport. Present this infant's case information below in SBARR format.**

Item	Verbalize	Description and example
S—situation	'This is my chief concern.'	*I am calling about a 4-h-old 35 week gestation infant with hypoglycemia. The infant is stable now.*
B—background	'I want you to know'	*35 week gestation male, BW 2500 g, now 4 hours of age with ACoRN Alerting Signs in Fluid and Glucose, Jaundice, and Thermoregulation Sequences.* *His blood glucose at 2 h of age was 1.8 mmol/L. Despite management with measured feeds and dextrose gel, the glucose remained less than 2.6 mmol/L. A PIV of D10W at 4 mL/kg/hr was initiated, resulting in a blood glucose of 3.3 mmol/L. He does not appear jaundiced at this time. Axilla temperature is 37°C.*
A—assessment	'This is the infant's condition.'	*The infant is stable now, but we cannot sustain his level of care (PIV). Risk level is yellow as we are a community hospital without a dedicated nursery.*
R—recommendation	'I need.'	*Please send the transport team ASAP*
R—readback/response	'Are there any questions?'	*Do you have any questions?*

Support

Educational objectives

Upon completion of this chapter, you will be able to:

- Understand that infants experience stress and pain.
- Recognize signs of infant stress and pain.
- Provide supportive strategies to reduce infant stress and pain.
- Identify supports that families may need during stabilization.
- Recognize that members of the health care team require support to function effectively.
- Describe the behavioural skills that are essential for health care teams to perform optimally.
- Identify opportunities to improve supportive care.

Key concepts

1. Support begins at first contact with the infant and family and is an integral part of successful stabilization.
2. The infant's circle of care includes the family and health care team members.
3. Infant pain can have detrimental physiological consequences and should be assessed frequently and managed promptly.
4. Minimizing extraneous stimulation in an unstable infant's environment helps to reduce morbidity.
5. Team members may experience distress before, during, or after resuscitating or stabilizing a sick infant.
6. The decision to revise the goals of care and provide palliative or comfort care is usually reached in consultation with parents and based on the likelihood of an infant's death or survival with a poor quality of life.
7. The objective of palliative care is to move from active life-sustaining care to actively providing comfort care to the infant and the family.
8. Regular debriefing can help health care teams to improve care delivery by reinforcing what went well and exploring opportunities for improvement.

Skills

- Pain assessment and evaluation of pain management strategies
- Timely provision of nonpharmacological and pharmacological pain management

Support is an overarching component of Acute Care of at-Risk Newborns (ACoRN), permeating the whole program. It is for this reason that support forms the 'cap' over all the sequences in the Primary Survey.

Support is an integral part of the ACoRN Process, beginning at the time of first contact with the infant and family, and ending at discharge. Support of the infant includes controlling the environment, avoiding sensory overload, managing stress and pain, promoting supportive touching, skin-to-skin care, and family-centred approaches to stabilization. Support for families involves open dialogue and collaborative decision-making. Each patient and family unit is unique and has unique needs for support. Support is also about team performance, education, and the recognition and management of stress.

The goal of developmentally supportive care is to:

"Provide a structured care environment which supports, encourages and guides the developmental organization of the premature and/or critically ill infant. Developmental care recognizes the physical, psychological and emotional vulnerabilities of premature and/or critically ill infants and their families and is focused on minimizing potential short- and long-term complications associated with the hospital experience" (Coughlin M, Gibbins S, Hoath S. Core measures for developmentally supportive care in NICUs. J Adv Nurs 2009:65(10):240).

Developmental care involves the infant, the family, and members of the health care team.

Supporting the infant

Infants communicate their tolerance for caregiving activities and environmental stimulation through autonomic, motor, and nonverbal behavioural cues and responses. These signs, considered together, indicate the infant's level of stability and stress. Care that is sensitive and responsive to signs of infant stress can improve morbidity rates and shorten hospital stays significantly.

Assessing and managing infant stress

The health care team must make every effort to attend to an infant's stress cues, understanding that a newborn's ability to deal with sensory stimuli is limited and depends on several factors, including gestational age. Strategies include minimizing the impacts of noise and light and avoiding poor positioning and overhandling. Sensory overload can disrupt transition and the infant's sleep–wake cycle, increase heart rate and the need for respiratory support, and decrease oxygen saturation. Care should be paced in response to infant stability and stress cues.

Watching for and responding to early indicators of infant stability or stress are essential for providing optimal care. Table 12.1 lists signs to watch for when assessing a newborn's tolerance of interventions and environmental stimuli.

Developmentally supportive care includes minimizing the impacts of noise, light, and other environmental factors (see Figure 12.1), intervening carefully, and providing care mindfully to enhance an infant's normal physiological and neurobehavioural functioning. Parents can assist other members of the infant's care team by identifying cues, mitigating stress, and participating in developmentally supportive care.

Whenever possible, use the following seven strategies to help minimize infant stress:

1. Offer opportunities for skin-to-skin contact and breastfeeding.

Table 12.1.
Infant stability and stress cues

System	Stability cues	Stress cues
Autonomic	• Stable vital signs • Good colour • Feeding tolerance	• Change in pattern/rate of respiration • Tachycardia/bradycardia • Desaturation • Colour change (pale/mottled/dusky) • Tremors • Gagging/spitting up
Motor	• Hand to face or mouth • Hand or foot clasping • Grasping • Leg or foot bracing • Rooting/sucking • Flexed posture	• Frowning/facial grimacing • Truncal arching • Finger splaying or 'saluting' • 'Airplane' posture (arms rigidly extended like airplane wings) • Flaccidity • Averting gaze • 'Sitting on air' (lying supine with hips fully flexed and knees extended)
Behavioural	• Definite sleep state • Able to maintain a quiet alert state • Attention to caregiver • Attention to stimuli in environment • Rhythmical, robust crying • Self-soothing/consolability • Shiny-eyed alertness • Looking around	• Diffuse sleep or awake states • Panicked/worried alertness • Glassy-eyed appearance • Strained alertness • Fussing/crying • Staring • Looking away • Roving eye movements

2. Reduce noise levels:
   • Avoid loud jarring noises (e.g., snapping incubator portholes shut).
   • Avoid unnecessary noise (e.g., do not talk needlessly near the radiant warmer or over the infant, and do not use the incubator as a writing surface or a place to put supplies).
3. Reduce light exposure:
   • Shade the infant's eyes from direct light.
   • Partially cover the incubator and reduce ambient light when not involved in direct care.
   • Cycle light exposure to mimic day/night environments.
4. 'Nest' the unwell newborn to limit motor movement (Figure 12.2):
   • Flex upper and lower limbs and place them close to the trunk.
   • Surround with rolled towels or positioning aids to 'contain' the infant and limit motor movement.

Care should always be individualized. Interventions that work for one infant may not work for another. There are times when an infant will display stress cues despite supportive care. It is important to note infant responses and communicate interventions that decrease stress cues to colleagues.

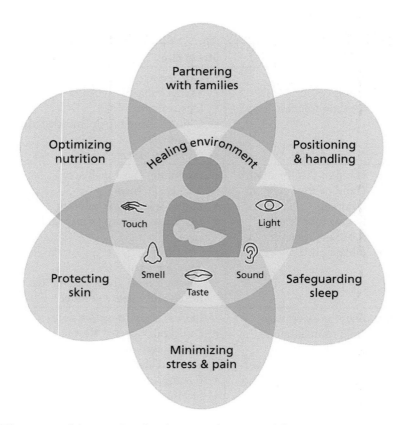

Figure 12.1. The neonatal integrative developmental care model.

Source: Altimier L, Phillips R. The neonatal integrative developmental care model: Advanced clinical applications of the seven core measures for neuroprotective family-centred care. Newborn and Infant Nursing Reviews 2016;16. Reproduced with permission.

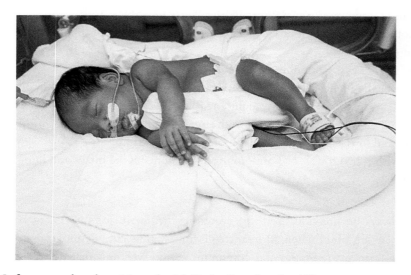

Figure 12.2. Infant nested and positioned with limbs flexed and midline.

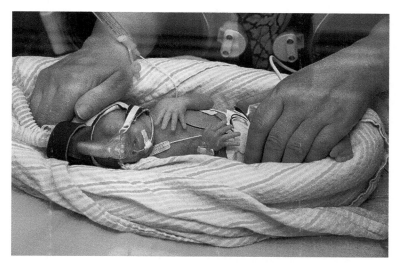

Figure 12.3. Infant contained by caregiver's hands.

5. Promote self-soothing:
   - Position the infant to allow hands to touch mouth or face.
   - Provide non-nutritive sucking (the infant's finger or thumb or a soother, if parents agree).
   - Handle the infant gently.
   - Avoid sudden postural changes.
   - Provide 'boundaries' with gentle, firm containment.
   - Limit stimulation of the infant (e.g., touching and providing containment rather than stroking the infant; Figure 12.3).
6. Adjust caregiving routines to the infant's sleep–wake cycle.
7. Pace caregiving routines based on infant responses (signs of stress).

In critical situations, it is not always possible to pause and respond to infant distress. However, every attempt should be made to provide positional support and comfort during and following stabilization. Whenever possible, an infant should be given time to recover from a stressful or painful procedure.

Assessing and managing infant pain

Stress and pain exist within a continuum in infants. Even when born extremely preterm, infants can experience stress and pain from routine caregiving, medical procedures, surgical interventions, or an underlying medical condition. Historically, stress and pain have been underrecognized and under-treated in the newborn. Infant stress and pain management should be a priority and a therapeutic goal in neonatal care.

Pain can contribute to severe short- and long-term physiological and behavioural consequences, including death, poor neurologic outcomes, and abnormal pain responses later in life. Pain should be anticipated, prevented whenever possible and, when present, minimized.

Physiological signs of infant pain include:

- Increased heart rate,
- Increased or irregular respiratory rate,
- Increased blood pressure,
- Decreased oxygen saturation, and
- Diaphoresis (in the term infant).

Behavioural signs of infant pain include:

- Strained crying,
- Posturing,
- Restlessness,
- Diminished responsiveness,
- Clenching or splaying of fingers and toes, and
- Changes in facial expression (e.g., brow-bulging or eye-squeezing).

Signs of pain vary depending on gestational age and clinical status. Based on their physiological development, extremely preterm infants appear to show a less robust behavioural response to pain or may not be able to demonstrate a pain response at all. This does not mean, however, that they do not feel pain. Infants who are ventilated, kept immobile for medical reasons, or are neurologically depressed are difficult to accurately assess for pain.

All infants should be provided with nonpharmacological pain management strategies, and some will require pharmacological interventions.

While an in-depth discussion of pain assessment and management is beyond the scope of ACoRN, monitoring indicators during stabilization using a validated pain assessment tool is recommended. Consult local regional or provincial/territorial referral hospitals for guidance.

Whenever possible, use the following nonpharmacological strategies to help minimize infant pain or distress:

- Skin-to-skin ('kangaroo') care
- Breastfeeding during a painful procedure (e.g., a heel poke for blood work)
- Holding or swaddling
- Facilitated tucking
- Nesting
- Providing nonnutritive sucking (the infant's finger or thumb, or a soother, if parents agree)
- Reducing stimulation (e.g., unnecessary noise and frequent handling)

Moderate to severe pain warrants the use of pharmacological agents (analgesics) *in conjunction with* supportive care measures. Many centres administer oral sucrose to help reduce procedural pain, such as intravenous (IV) starts and phlebotomy. Where this practice is supported, each use should be recorded as with any medication.

Always consider administering an analgesic to reduce pain associated with invasive medical procedures. When an infant receives a pharmacological agent to manage pain, monitoring is required to determine efficacy and the need to adjust dosing.

Morphine and fentanyl are the most common narcotic analgesics used in neonatal care. Pharmacological effects of bolus dosing are described in Table 12.2. For additional information on specific management, including dosages, see Appendix C, Medications, and consult your local referral centre.

Table 12.2.
Morphine versus fentanyl boluses in the unstable infant

Salient effects	Morphine	Fentanyl
Onset	5 to 10 min	3 to 5 min
Duration of action	60 to 120 min	30 min
Cardiovascular stability	Variable	Yes
Sedation	More sedative effect	Less sedative effect
Chest wall rigidity	No	Yes, with rapid administration

When administering analgesics, it is essential to have resuscitation equipment on hand, to monitor the infant closely for respiratory depression (including apnea), and to ensure that a skilled practitioner is present who can evaluate responses to treatment, manage the airway as needed, and deal with other complications and side effects if they arise.

Supporting parents

Parents are active participants in their infant's care, and their presence and involvement are essential throughout their infant's stay in hospital. Including parents in care is empowering because it recognizes and reinforces their contributions to infant well-being.

When their infant is unwell or at risk, parents may experience emotional stress, which can complicate the bonding process. Attentive communication, listening, and collaborative decision-making are essential when working with families. Parents can often help members of the infant's care team to mitigate stress and provide supportive care.

No matter how well-prepared parents are for the possibility that their infant may need medical care, the first time they see their infant attached to a monitor, even when ventilatory support is not required, can be overwhelming. They will need help and support from members of the health care team to see beyond the machinery and refocus on their infant. When resuscitation and stabilization are needed, parents may have limited opportunity to see their infant at birth, although their presence during both processes should be encouraged. Parents should be able to see, touch, and talk to their infant as soon as possible.

Parents need ongoing information about their infant's plan of care. It is important to understand and address parents' needs and questions in a manner that is timely, clear, sensitive, and honest. If possible, both parents should be present for significant conversations, which should also occur in a quiet, private space, and ideally include health team members identified by the family. A trained interpreter is essential when parents are not fluent in the language of health care providers. Relying on a family member to translate is not recommended because they are also experiencing stress and may wish to 'shield' parents from news that is upsetting or worrisome. Active listening and allowing for silence are as important as the information relayed. Parents should never feel that conversations were rushed.

Parental response to conversations depends on many factors, such as personal coping strategies, the ability to absorb information under stress, other life pressures, extended family support, and whether an infant can be cared for locally or must be transferred. Most parents will understand the need to transport their sick newborn to a facility where a higher level of care is available. In these situations, every effort should be made to keep them fully informed of transport arrangements (for details, see Chapter 11, Transport) and to keep mother and infant together.

Parents need to know that the health care team sees their infant as an individual. Team members should use the infant's name and the appropriate gender pronoun during discussions, keeping focus on the infant rather than on their condition, technologies, or procedures involved. It is important, however, to explain technical terms and describe procedures as they arise during the course of care.

Supporting the family includes asking what they need or want to help them cope with their infant's resuscitation and/or stabilization. Information should be provided both in anticipation of the parents' needs and in response to their questions and reviewed as often as they request.

Parental participation in care builds a sense of belonging, alleviates fear, and improves patient care. Parents not only observe what is being done for their infant but are also able to provide care themselves and witness the infant's responses to care. Also, being present for and witnessing the level of effort and care involved in saving or stabilizing their infant may help to ease the grieving process, in the event that the infant dies. Strategies that help parents cope with their infant's hospitalization include:

- Skin-to-skin care,
- Providing breast milk and/or breastfeeding,
- Gentle touching, with containment,
- Talking, reading, or singing to the infant,
- Participating in health care team discussions, and being as 'present' during care as possible,
- Learning about the infant's specific care and condition,
- Keeping a journal or scrapbook, and
- Connecting with parents who have had similar experiences.

Health care providers have a crucial role to play in supporting parents as integral members of the infant's health care team.

Palliative care and infant death

Sometimes, infants are born with conditions that do not respond to resuscitation and stabilization. The decision to revise the goals of care and provide palliative or comfort care is usually reached in consultation with parents and based on the likelihood of an infant's death or survival with a poor quality of life. The objective of palliative care is to move from active life-sustaining care to actively providing comfort care to the infant and family.

In these situations, expert opinion on prognosis will guide parental counselling. It is especially important that the family continue to be supported when palliative care is chosen for an infant. Parental feelings of guilt and regret should be acknowledged. The health care team can help by approaching the situation in a nonjudgemental way and being willing to explore the family's values and beliefs and share in the bereavement experience with the family. Every situation is unique, and every family has different needs. However, team members can help prepare parents for the dying process by initiating a discussion of how their infant will be cared for, including pain management. Parents also need to know that it can be difficult to predict how soon an infant will die following withdrawal of life-sustaining interventions. When duration of survival is uncertain, preparing parents for the possibility of a lengthy survival is important.

Tissue and organ donation may be possible, depending on eligibility criteria (e.g., gestational age and birth weight) and local transplantation services. Be sure to ask parents whether such procedures might fit with their beliefs and values.

Team members can help support the family by:

- Encouraging parents to see, touch, bathe, and hold their infant, if they choose to do so.
- Facilitating religious or cultural observances.
- Offering parents the opportunity to call in supportive family, friends, or spiritual advisors.
- Photographing the infant before and after death, with the parents' permission. Photographs of the infant with the family can also be a meaningful way to acknowledge the importance of the infant in the family.
- Providing hand or footprints or casts, with the family's permission.
- Encouraging the family to take as much time as they wish with their infant.
- Dressing the infant in a special outfit.
- Offering a bereavement kit, with resources and information for families. Kits are available from many tertiary care centres.
- Discussing opportunities to donate breast milk, if possible.

Be guided by, and sensitive to, the family's responses when offering any of these options. For example, some families may decline photographs and/or mementos, based on religious beliefs. Others may decline because they feel overwhelmed by the situation. For these families, and because such requests are time-sensitive, health care professionals may wish to suggest taking photographs and/or hand or foot print casts, but archive them until the family has had a chance to process the offer and decide whether they would like to accept these mementos.

If life-sustaining interventions are withdrawn prior to transport, the health care team must support each other in addition to the family.

Providing end-of-life care can be an intense experience for the health care team. All members who have interacted with the infant or the family should receive collegial support. Formal supportive measures may be needed in any clinical setting and can be supported by hospice care staff, spiritual counsellors, social workers, and human resource personnel.

While many aspects of perinatal loss are beyond the scope of ACoRN, detailed guidance and consultative services can and should be sought from your level 3 centre, as needed.

Supporting the health care team

Providers with diverse experience and expertise work together as an interprofessional health care team to resuscitate, stabilize, care for, and transport unwell infants. The demands placed upon each member of the team will vary by situation. For the individual and the team to function effectively, they require support, in the form of training, opportunities to practice, role clarification, and emotional advocacy.

Support is about ensuring that teams are prepared, equipped, and able to perform when called to stabilize a newborn. The unique challenges associated with perinatal adaptation mean that, in addition to good team dynamics, specific knowledge and skills are needed. These skills need to be acquired and practiced, using evidence from the literature and from observation of how experienced teams perform. Well-designed and validated cognitive aids in the form of algorithms are useful to support clinical learning and decision-making, leading users through complex and time-critical series of tasks. However, they need to be supported by background knowledge to allow clinical teams to navigate the variability encountered in the clinical setting.

Clinical teams are dynamic, vary in size, and include care providers with different levels of expertise and experience. Optimal teamwork maximizes performance and supports team cohesion while distributing cognitive and clinical tasks among team members. Skills include:

- Anticipating and planning,
- Knowing your environment and equipment,
- Communicating effectively,
- Assigning roles, including the leadership role,
- Distributing workload optimally,
- Allocating attention wisely,
- Obtaining and using all available information,
- Maximal use of available resources,
- Calling for help early, and
- Maintaining professional behaviour.

Team members may experience distress before, during, or after resuscitating or stabilizing a sick infant, especially when:

- Teamwork, leadership, and/or communication is suboptimal.
- Urgent care situations arise infrequently in their clinical setting.
- Expertise and resources are limited.
- There is lack of experience managing acute cases.
- Feelings of inadequacy arise during the provision of care.
- An infant's condition deteriorates rapidly.
- Immediate access to consulting specialists is lacking.

Debriefing and reflection after stressful events provide opportunities for peer support, teambuilding, education, and systems improvement.

Learning from practice

Resuscitation and stabilization processes require effective team dynamics. Every clinical experience—and especially the acute but rare event—is an opportunity for staff to learn in practice and from each other, as a team. Case review and debriefing can help the team to recognize what went well (called a 'plus') and which areas (if any) may need improvement (called a 'delta'). Debriefing in a positive, constructive team learning environment builds confidence.

A post-event debriefing (Figure 12.4) is a facilitated reflection and discussion of actions and thought processes that promotes reflective learning, proactive problem-solving, and improved clinical performance. Post-event debriefings should never be a critique of individuals. A debriefing focuses on a specific event and includes input from all team members, including the transport team if possible. Each individual brings different ideas and perspectives into review. Noting suggestions during debriefings can help to guide or improve policies, procedures, or training (Table 12.3). While lack of time and facilitation are often seen as barriers to debriefings, keeping these sessions focused, short (10 to 15 min), and structured can be very effective.

Introduction and shared mental model

"We are going to do a quick debrief of that event. It should take only a few minutes. The goal is to improve our performance as a team and the care we provide. Let's start with a description of the key clinical events."

- *Review the clinical events and establish a shared mental model of what happened.*

What went well, and what did not ('plus/delta')?

"Okay team, let's talk about our performance. What went well, and what didn't go so well?"

- *Did the team follow established guidelines and protocols? If not, why?*
- *Were there any technical, equipment, or procedural issues? If so, what?*
- *Discuss 2 to 3 key behavioral skills* relevant to the situation. How was team performance in these areas?*

What will the team do differently next time?

"How can we do better next time?"

- *Discuss changes in team performance that will be implemented in the future, based on discussion above.*
- *Identify the individual(s) responsible to follow up on issues discussed.*

Follow up issues?

"What issues, if any, should be deferred for a more in depth discussion at a later time?"

- *Record issus to be followed up later.*

Conclusion

"Thank you for taking time to participate in this debriefing."

*Key Behavioural Skills:
Knowledge of environment
Anticipation and planning
Leadership
Communication
Delegation of workload
Attention allocation
Use of available information
Use of available resources
Calling for help when needed
Professional behaviour

Figure 12.4. Post-event debriefing.

Source: Reprinted by permission from Springer Nature. Journal of Perinatology. Sawyer T, Loren D, Halamek LP. Post-event debriefings during neonatal care: Why are we not doing them, and how can we start? 2016.

Debriefings must follow local policies governing information-sharing and privacy. In cases where more formal reviews are required by a hospital's quality assurance program, these proceedings are medico-legally protected. Post-event debriefings are also different from meetings intended to assist staff with managing an emotionally taxing incident, a process known as 'critical incident stress management'.

Table 12.3.
Documenting items for follow-up

Anticipation/preparation	
Personnel	
Supplies and equipment	
Communication	
Between team members	
Between teams	
With family members	
Objective assessment of care	
As per the ACoRN framework and sequences	
Recommendations	
Equipment and supplies	
Practice and procedures	
Dissemination	
Staff education/skill maintenance	
Next steps	
Task completion	
Reassessment and refinement	

Institutional policies should facilitate a local culture that fosters debriefing by:

- Actively encouraging post–event debriefing.
- Training health care providers in debriefing.
- Providing procedural guidance and policies on debriefing that have been approved by risk management.
- Evaluating debriefing activities regularly.
- Providing private spaces to ensure debriefings can be conducted confidentially.

Support: Case 1—Managing a stressful experience

A baby boy was born at 32 weeks gestation 45 min ago. This is the first time you are taking care of a baby this small. He has moderate in-drawing, is tachypneic, and requires 40% oxygen to maintain SpO2 levels at 90% to 95%. The capillary glucose is 2.6 mmol/L. The ACoRN Primary Survey, consolidated Core Steps and Problem List have been completed. This baby's Problem List includes Respiratory, Fluid and Glucose, Jaundice, Thermoregulation and Infection, and your team has worked through the prioritized sequences down to Next Steps. You are completing your 'to-do' list. A colleague is trying to insert an IV line. You are told the baby may need to be intubated and given surfactant. The care team has designated this baby as 'Red' for Level of Risk. The physician is speaking with the transport coordinating physician at your regional level 3 centre for further advice and transport.

You take a moment to reflect on how your team functioned during the stabilization of this baby.

1. What does a team need to function optimally? Tick all that apply.
- ☐ Specific background knowledge and skills.
- ☐ Well-designed cognitive aids in the form of algorithms.
- ☐ Opportunities to practice.
- ☐ Teamwork, role clarification, and emotional advocacy.
- ☐ Leadership.
- ☐ Clear, easy communication.
- ☐ The distribution of clinical and cognitive load among the team members.
- ☐ The maximum possible number of health professionals in the room at all times.
- ☐ The development of each team member so that they are able to perform multiple necessary tasks simultaneously.

The baby is lying on a radiant warmer in the brightly lit nursery. There is a blood pressure cuff around his left arm and a pulse oximeter probe on his right wrist. Several of your colleagues are helping with the various tasks that need to be completed. There are loud voices in the background, and the radiant warmer alarm is ringing. As you place a thermometer under the baby's right axilla, he squirms and tries to raise his left hand to his mouth, but is unsuccessful. His arms and legs are fully extended. A colleague administers vitamin K intramuscularly and applies erythromycin ointment to his eyes. The baby startles with handling. A capillary blood gas and glucose are drawn via heel poke. He cries throughout the procedure. An IV is started after four attempts.

2. What signs might indicate that this baby is experiencing stress? Tick all that apply.
- ☐ Hand to face or mouth.
- ☐ Flexed posture.
- ☐ Finger-splaying.
- ☐ Brow-bulging.
- ☐ Increasing O2 saturations.
- ☐ Dry skin.
- ☐ Tremors.
- ☐ Arms extended.
- ☐ Staring or looking away.

3. Strategies to minimize pain or distress for this infant include: (Tick all that apply.)
- ☐ Holding or swaddling.
- ☐ Facilitated tucking.
- ☐ Nesting.

☐ Tapping the infant's back or chest.

☐ Facilitating non-nutritive sucking.

☐ Rubbing the infant's back.

As stabilization proceeds, it is evident that the infant needs to be transported to the nearest referral facility, which is 200 km away. The transport team is due to arrive in 90 min.

4. **What might you do to support the parents at this time? Tick all that apply.**

   ☐ Ask what the physician has told them.

   ☐ Ask whether they have any questions.

   ☐ Ask how they feel.

   ☐ Encourage them to touch their baby.

   ☐ Ask whether they have named their baby.

   ☐ Ask how you can help.

   ☐ Send them to their room to rest.

   ☐ Ask the mother to express some breast milk in a quiet room to send with the baby.

The transport team arrives at the expected time. They introduce themselves to the parents and explain how they will provide care to their baby during transport. The team receives a report from the physician and the nurse, and assesses the infant.

Before this next assessment, the baby infant squirms slightly, splays his fingers, and pushes against the sides of the nest with his feet.

5. **How might you help to settle this baby? Tick all that apply.**

   ☐ By placing your hands gently on the infant before beginning an assessment.

   ☐ By speaking softly and pacing care in response to his behavioural cues, giving him time to recover as needed.

   ☐ By standing near the radiant warmer to engage in handover or discuss the plan of care, so the baby can hear calming voices.

   ☐ By completing one intervention at a time, to avoid overwhelming the infant.

   ☐ By tapping the mother's heart rate on the incubator wall, so the baby can hear a familiar sound.

The transport team completes their assessment. Before departing, they invite the parents to see and touch their baby again, give them the phone number of the receiving hospital, and estimate their time of arrival. After the baby's departure, your team takes a moment to perform a post-event debrief.

6. **The debrief (case review) is educational, and improves quality of care because it: (Tick all that apply.)**

   ☐ Ensures that those who have not performed well are told so.

   ☐ Allows team members to talk about how they feel about a case.

   ☐ Prompts team members to reflect on what went well and what needs to be improved.

   ☐ Provides opportunities for the team and/or individual members to discuss how to improve the flow of care and communication.

   ☐ Assists staff in managing emotionally taxing incidents.

   ☐ Identifies low performing individuals.

   ☐ Identifies needs for education and skill development or maintenance.

   ☐ Identifies whether policies, procedures, equipment, or supplies need updating.

Bibliography

Altimier L, Phillips RM. The neonatal integrative developmental care model: Seven neuroprotective core measures for family-centered developmental care. Newborn Infant Nurs Rev 2013;13:9–22.

American Academy of Pediatrics, Committee on Fetus and Newborn, Section on Anesthesiology and Pain Medicine. Prevention and management of procedural pain in the neonate: An update. Pediatrics 2016;137(2):e20154271.

Anand KJ, Campbell-Yeo M. Consequences of prenatal opioid use for newborns. Acta Paediatr 2015;104(11):1066–9.

Asmerom Y, Slater L, Boskovic DS, et al. Oral sucrose for heel lance increases adenosine triphosphate use and oxidative stress in preterm neonates. J Pediatr 2013;163(1):29–35.e1.

Barrington KJ, Batton DG, Finley GA, Wallman C; Canadian Paediatric Society, Fetus and Newborn Committee; Joint statement with the American Academy of Pediatrics. Prevention and management of pain in the neonate: An update. Paediatrics and Child Health 2007, 2017;12(2):137–8: www.cps.ca/en/documents/position/prevention-managementpain-neonate

Becker PT, Grunwald PC, Morgan J, Stuhr S. Effects of development care on behavioral organization in very-low-birthweight infants. Nursing Res 1993;42(4):214–20.

Bellù R, de Waal WK, Zanini R. Opioids for neonates receiving mechanical ventilation. Cochrane Database Syst Rev 2008;23(1):CD004212.

Byers JF. Components of developmental care and the evidence for their use in the NICU. MCN Am J Matern Child Nurs 2003;28(3):174–180.

Catlin A, Carter B. Creation of a neonatal end-of-life palliative care protocol. J Perinatol 2002;22(3):184–95.

Chaudhari S. Neonatal intensive care practices harmful to the developing brain. Indian Pediatr 2011;48(6):437–40.

Chichester M. Multicultural issues in perinatal loss. AWHONN Lifelines 2005;9(4):312–20.

Coughlin M, Gibbins S, Hoath S. Core measures for developmentally supportive care in neonatal intensive care units: Theory, precedence and practice. J Adv Nurs 2009;65(10):2239–48.

De Graaf J, van Lingen RA, Valkenburg AJ, et al. Does neonatal morphine use affect neuropsychological outcomes at 8 to 9 years of age? Pain 2013;154(3):449–58.

Discenza D. Stress in the NICU: Parental worries about outcomes. Neonatal Netw 2014;33(5):289–90.

Douglas SM, Dahnke MD. Creating an ethical environment for parents and health providers dealing with the treatment dilemmas of neonates at the edge of viability. J Neonatal Nurs 2013;19(1):33–7.

Durrmeyer X, Vutskits L, Annand KJ, Rimensberger PC. Use of analgesic and sedative drugs in the NICU: Integrating clinical trials and laboratory data. Pediatr Res 2010;67(2):117–27.

Fitzgerald M. When is an analgesic not an analgesic? (Editorial). Pain 2009;144(9).

Gardner SL, Enzman-Hines M, Dickey LA. Pain and pain relief. In: Gardner SL, Carter BS, Enzman-Hines M, Hernandez JA (eds.). Merenstein and Gardner's Handbook of Neonatal Intensive Care, 7th ed. St. Louis, MO: Elsevier, 2011.

Golinau B, Krane E, Seybold J, Almgren C, Anand KJ. Non-pharmacological techniques for pain management in neonates. Semin Perinatol 2007;31(5):318–22.

Gooding JS, Cooper LG, Blaine AI, Franck LS, Howse JL, Berns SD. Family support and family-centered care in the neonatal intensive care unit: Origins, advances, impact. Semin Perinatol 2011;35(1):20–8.

Grunau RE. Neonatal pain in very preterm infants: Long-term effects on brain, neurodevelopment and pain reactivity. Rambam Maimonides Med J 2013;4(4):e0025.

Hall RW. Anesthesia and analgesia in the NICU. Clin Perinatol 2012;39(1):239–54.

Hall RW, Anand KJ. Pain management in newborns. Clin Perinatol 2014;41(4):895–924.

Harrison D, Bueno M, Reszel J. Prevention and management of pain and stress in the neonate. Res Rep Neonatol 2015;5:9–15.

Harrison D, Reszel J, Wilding J, Stevens B. Core Measure 5: Minimizing stress and pain: Neonatal pain management practices during heel lance and venipuncture in Ontario, Canada. Newb Infant Nurs Rev 2015;15:11623.

Harvey ME, Pattison HM. The impact of a father's presence during newborn resuscitation: A qualitative interview study with healthcare professionals. BMJ Open 2013;3(3):e002547.

Hendson L, Davies D; Canadian Paediatric Society, Fetus and Newborn Committee. Supporting and communicating with families experiencing a perinatal loss: www.cps.ca/en/documents/position/perinatal-loss.

Holsti L, Grunau RE, Shany E. Assessing pain in preterm infants in the neonatal intensive care unit: Moving to a 'brain-oriented' approach. Pain Manag 2011;1(2):171–9.

Holsti L, Grunau RE. Consideration for using sucrose to reduce procedural pain in preterm infants. Pediatrics 2010;125(5):1042–7.

Ionio D, Colombo C, Brazzoduro V, et al. Mothers and fathers in NICU: The impact of preterm birth on parental distress. Eur J Psychol 2016;12(4):604–21.

Jenkins D, Harigopal S, Paterson L, Boyd M. Guideline for Family Centred Developmental Care. Sunderland, UK: The Northern Neonatal Network, 2014.

Kenner C, Boykova M. Families in crisis. In: Verklan MT, Walden M (eds.). Core Curriculum for Neonatal Intensive Care Nursing, 5th ed. St. Louis, MO: Mosby-Elsevier, 2015.

Kenner C, McGrath JM, eds. Developmental Care of Newborns and Infants: A Guide for Health Professionals, 2nd ed. St. Louis, MO: Mosby, 2010.

Lago P, Frigo AC, Baraldi E, et al. Sedation and analgesia practices at Italian neonatal intensive care units: Results from the EUROPAIN study. Ital J Pediatr 2017;43(1):26.

Lemyre B, Moore G; Canadian Paediatric Society, Fetus and Newborn Committee. Counselling and management for anticipated extremely preterm birth. Paediatr Child Health 2017: www.cps.ca/en/documents/position/managementanticipated-extremely-preterm-birth.

Mancini A, Uthaya S, Beardsley C, Wood D, Modi N. Practical guidance for the management of palliative care on neonatal units. London, UK: Chelsea and Westminster Hospital, 2014.

Maria A, Dasgupta R. Family-centered care for sick newborns: A thumbnail view. Indian J Community Med 2016;41(1):11–5.

McNair C, Campbell-Yeo M, Johnson CC, Taddio A. Non-pharmacological management of pain during common needle procedures in infants: Current research evidence and practical considerations. Clin Perinatol 2013;40(3):493–508.

Mullan P, Kessler D, Cheng A. Educational opportunities with post-event debrief. JAMA 2014;312(22):2333–4.

Ng E, Taddio A, Ohlsson A. Intravenous midazolam infusion for sedation of infants in the neonatal intensive care unit. Cochrane Database Syst Rev 2017;1:CD002052.

Nimbalkar SM, Chaudhary NS, Gadhavi KV, Phatak A. Kangaroo mother care in reducing pain in preterm neonates on heel prick. Indian J Pediatr 2013;80(1):6–10.

Oczkowski SJ, Mazzetti I, Cupido C, Fox-Robichaud AE; Canadian Critical Care Society. Family presence during resuscitation: A Canadian Critical Care Society position paper. Can Resp J 2015;22(4):201–5.

Ramezani T, Hadian Shirazi Z, Sabet Sarvestani R, Moattari M. Family-centered care in neonatal intensive care unit: A concept analysis. Int J Community Based Nurs Midwifery 2014;2(4):268–78.

Renaud Smith J, Donze A. Patient safety. In: Verklan MT, Walden M (eds.). Core Curriculum for Neonatal Intensive Care Nursing, 5th ed. St. Louis, MO: Mosby-Elsevier, 2015.

Sawyer A, Ayers S, Bertullies S, et al. Providing immediate neonatal care and resuscitation at birth beside the mother: Parents' views, a qualitative study. BMJ Open 2015;5(9):e008495.

Sawyer T, Loren D, Halamek LP. Post-event debriefings during neonatal care: Why are we not doing them, and how can we start? J Perinatol 2016;36(6):415–9.

Symington A, Pinelli J. Developmental care for promoting development and preventing morbidity in preterm infants. Cochrane Database Syst Rev 2006;2:CD001814.

Tremblay S, Ranger M, Chau CMY, et al. Repeated exposure to sucrose for procedural pain in mouse pups leads to longterm widespread brain alterations. Pain 2017;158(9):1586–98.

Turnage Sprull C. Developmental support. In: Verklan MT, Walden M (eds.). Core Curriculum for Neonatal Intensive Care Nursing, 5th ed. St. Louis, MO: Mosby-Elsevier, 2015.

Vinall J, Miller SP, Bjornson BH, et al. Invasive procedures in preterm children: Brain and cognitive development at school age. Pediatrics 2014;133(3):412–21.

Walden M. Pain management and assessment. In: Verklan MT, Walden M (eds.). Core Curriculum for Neonatal Intensive Care Nursing, 5th ed. St. Louis, MO: Mosby-Elsevier, 2015.

Whit Hall R, Anand KJS. Physiology of pain and stress in the newborn. NeoReviews 2005;6(2):e61–8.

Whit Hall R, Anand KJS. Short- and long-term impact of neonatal pain and stress. 2005;6(2):e69–75.

Zwicker JG, Miller SP, Grunau RE, et al. Smaller cerebellar growth and poorer neurodevelopmental outcomes in very preterm infants exposed to neonatal morphine. J Pediatr 2016;172:81–7.

Answer key: Support Case 1—Managing a stressful experience

1. What does a team need to function optimally?
   - ✓ Specific background knowledge and skills.
   - ✓ Well-designed cognitive aids in the form of algorithms.
   - ✓ Opportunities to practice.
   - ✓ Teamwork, role clarification, and emotional advocacy.
   - ✓ Leadership.
   - ✓ Clear, easy communication.
   - ✓ The distribution clinical and cognitive load among the team members.
   - ☐ The maximum possible number of health professionals in the room at all times.
   - ☐ The development of each team member so that they are able to perform multiple necessary tasks simultaneously.

While it's important to have enough team members to provide adequate assessments and interventions for optimal care, too many team members can lead to a lack of role clarity, increase risk of procedures being done twice (or not at all), and be distracting when situational awareness is critical.

Where there is a lack of human resources, members of the team may need to perform a number of tasks while managing a crisis situation. However, team members are best able to contribute to the team by providing care that is consistent with their expertise and scope of practice. Attempting to perform a number of tasks simultaneously can weaken situational awareness and increase risk for error.

2. What signs might indicate that this baby is experiencing stress?
   - ☐ Hand to face or mouth.
   - ☐ Flexed posture.
   - ✓ Finger-splaying.
   - ✓ Brow-bulging.
   - ☐ Increasing O2 saturations.
   - ☐ Dry skin.
   - ✓ Tremors.
   - ✓ Arms extended.
   - ✓ Staring or looking away.

Infants who are immature or sick experience stress and pain on a continuum that can be observed through physiological and behavioural signs. Pain can have short- and long-term physiological and behavioural consequences.

Being able to place hand to face and mouth, adopting a flexed posture, stable vital signs, and alertnesss are all considered to be cues of infant stability.

3. Strategies to minimize pain or distress for this infant include:
   - ✓ Holding or swaddling.
   - ✓ Facilitated tucking.
   - ✓ Nesting.
   - ☐ Tapping the infant's back or chest.
   - ✓ Facilitating non-nutritive sucking.
   - ☐ Rubbing the infant's back.

4. What might you do to support the parents at this time?
- ✓ Ask what the physician has told them.
- ✓ Ask whether they have any questions.
- ✓ Ask how they feel.
- ✓ Encourage them to touch their baby.
- ✓ Ask whether they have named their baby.
- ✓ Ask how you can help.
- ☐ Send them to their room to rest.
- ☐ Ask the mother to express some breast milk in a quiet room to send with the baby.

The answers selected reflect ways that care providers can acknowledge an infant's importance and individuality and convey respect for parents. Directing them to 'go and rest' may be interpreted by parents as meaning they are 'in the way' and should leave their infant. And while expressing milk is an excellent way to contribute to infant care, directing the mother to 'produce' at a time of crisis may not be helpful.

5. How might you help to settle this baby?
- ✓ By placing your hands gently on the infant before beginning an assessment.
- ✓ By speaking softly and pacing care in response to his behavioural cues, giving him time to recover as needed.
- ☐ By standing near the radiant warmer to engage in handover or discuss the plan of care, so the baby can hear calming voices.
- ✓ By completing one intervention at a time, to avoid overwhelming the infant.
- ☐ By tapping the mother's heart rate on the incubator wall, so the baby can hear a familiar sound.

The baby is exhibiting stress cues and requires caregiving strategies to minimize stress. Pacing care activities, sequencing care to allow for recovery between procedures, providing opportunities for non-nutritive sucking and/or skin-to-skin care during or after care, and minimizing extraneous noise, can all assist in reducing infant stress.

6. The debrief (case review) is educational, and improves quality of care because it:
- ☐ Ensures that those who have not performed well are told so.
- ✓ Allows team members to talk about how they feel about a case.
- ✓ Prompts team members to reflect on what went well and what needs to be improved.
- ✓ Provides opportunities for the team and/or individual members to discuss how to improve the flow of care and communication.
- ☐ Assists staff in managing emotionally taxing incidents.
- ☐ Identifies low performing individuals.
- ✓ Identifies needs for education and skill development or maintenance.
- ✓ Identifies whether policies, procedures, equipment, or supplies need updating.

Post-event debriefings promote reflective learning and proactive decision-making, with the primary intent to improve team performance. They are never conducted to assess or critique an individual team member's performance.

A different form of debriefing, 'critical incident briefing', differs from a case debrief or review and is intended to assist staff in managing an emotionally taxing or high-stress situation.

Appendix A

Procedures

The procedures discussed in this appendix are:

1. Continuous positive airway pressure (CPAP)
2. Mechanical ventilation
3. Capillary blood sampling
4. Surfactant administration
5. Pneumothorax—Chest tube insertion
6. Central vascular access—Umbilical vein catheterization
7. Bowel bag application
8. Incubator and radiant warmer use
9. Thermoregulation management in hypoxic ischemic encephalopathy (HIE)

The use of aseptic techniques, precautions for infection control, and meticulous hand hygiene should be practiced during every procedure. Attention should be paid to the infant's stability and physiologic monitoring because procedures can be destabilizing. Nonpharmacologic and/or pharmacologic pain management should be considered before any intervention.

Those performing procedures should be familiar with their facility's policies, need for certification of competency, if applicable, and equipment guidelines from manufacturers.

Some procedures used in stabilization are explained in the *Textbook of Neonatal Resuscitation*, published by the American Academy of Pediatrics, American Heart Association, and Canadian Paediatric Society. Users should also refer to this reference for the following procedures:

1. Pneumothorax—chest transillumination
2. Pneumothorax—needle aspiration
3. Emergency vascular access—intraosseous vascular access

1. Continuous positive airway pressure (CPAP)

Indications
Respiratory conditions associated with decreased lung compliance, increased work of breathing, and poor oxygenation.

Goals
To stabilize the lungs, decreasing risk for atelectasis at end-expiration, and to stabilize the airways, decreasing risk for obstructive apnea.

Principles

Lungs with decreased compliance are 'stiff'. The alveoli tend to collapse, reducing overall lung volumes and producing poorly ventilated areas that cannot participate in gas exchange. As infants attempt to compensate, they can become increasingly distressed as indicated by the presence of retractions and nasal flaring. They may also try to maintain positive end–expiratory pressure (PEEP) by exhaling against a partially closed glottis, which presents as grunting.

CPAP administration maintains inspiratory and expiratory airway pressures at levels above ambient pressure throughout the respiratory cycle, with these results:

- Lung mechanics are stabilized.
- Collapse of distal airways is prevented.
- Atelectatic alveoli are opened up or recruited.
- Airway resistance is reduced.
- The volume of air remaining in the lung at the end of a normal expiration (functional residual capacity) is increased.
- Lungs become more compliant, allowing the delivery of a greater tidal volume for a given pressure.
- The work of breathing is decreased.
- Oxygenation is improved because there is greater surface for gas exchange.

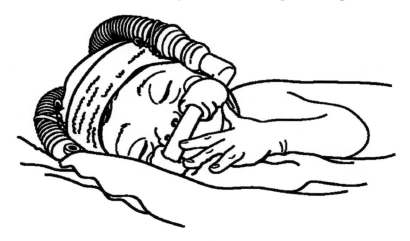

Application

The seal between nasal prongs or mask and the nares needs to be maintained for the pressure delivered by CPAP to remain constant throughout the respiratory cycle. The amount of positive pressure delivered may vary depending on whether the infant's mouth is open or closed.

An oro- or naso gastric tube should be placed to decrease gastric distension. Although nasal CPAP by itself is not a contraindication to enteral feeding, abdominal distention can decrease feeding tolerance.

Equipment

1. A source of continuous positive pressure, such as:
    a. A free flow of gas exiting through an underwater seal (bubble CPAP) or expiratory valve
    b. CPAP demand flow system
    c. Mechanical ventilator on CPAP mode
    d. A flow–inflating bag system (short-term only)
    e. T-piece resuscitator (short-term only)

2. Nasal prongs or CPAP mask (sized to the infant's nose and nares)

3. CPAP bonnet or hat (sized to the infant's head circumference)

4. A pulse oximeter and method of titrating inspired oxygen concentration

Procedure

1. Select the appropriate size mask or nasal prongs and hat.

2. Position the infant in a developmentally supportive prone, lateral, or supine position.

3. Apply nasal prongs or CPAP mask as per manufacturer's instructions or hospital policy.

4. Ensure that nasal prongs do not exert undue pressure on the nasal septum, to avoid septal erosion.

5. Set the desired initial CPAP level (usually 5 to 6 cm H2O), inspired oxygen concentration, low pressure alarm, and apnea alarm.

6. Monitor respiratory rate, work of breathing, oxygen requirements (inspired oxygen concentration and saturation), and presence/absence of apnea before and after application.

Notes

- CPAP can also be administered through an endotracheal tube whose tip is located in the posterior nasal pharynx (nasopharyngeal tube [NPT] CPAP).
  - NPTs are prone to accumulate secretions and mucous plugs, both in and around the tube. These secretions do not always clear by suctioning the NPT.
- CPAP should not be administered endotracheally in infants because the size of the endotracheal tube (ETT) is too small and the tube resistance too high for spontaneous unassisted breathing.

2. Mechanical ventilation

Indications

- Apnea
- Existing or anticipated respiratory failure
- An ACoRN Respiratory Score > 8
- An ACoRN Respiratory Score 5 to 8 with pH ≤ 7.25 or PCO2 ≥ 55
- Prolonged or ineffective manual ventilation
- Need to administer surfactant
- Diaphragmatic hernia
- Heavy sedation or paralysis as required in certain clinical conditions (e.g., persistent pulmonary hypertension [PPHN]), or surgical or radiological procedures.

Goals

To assist or take over the work of breathing, improve oxygenation and ventilation, and improve the respiratory component of acid-base balance.

Principles

A mechanical ventilator is designed to mimic the rhythmic cycle of breathing.

- To achieve inspiration, a quantity of gas is delivered to the lungs (tidal volume [V_T]) over a period of time (inspiratory time [t_I]), using sufficient pressure to expand the alveoli (peak inspiratory pressure [PIP]).
- To allow expiration to occur, the ventilator provides time for the chest wall and lung to return to resting position (expiratory time [t_E]).

- To prevent the alveoli from collapsing, distending pressure in the airway should remain positive at end expiration (PEEP).
- The number of breathing cycles/min is known as the set respiratory rate or frequency (f).
- Within a breathing cycle, the relative time spent in the process of inspiration versus expiration is known as the inspiration-to-expiration (I:E) ratio.

Application

Mechanical ventilators are classified on the basis of:

How they cycle:

- **Time-cycled ventilator modes** deliver a mandatory breath (cycle) on a set schedule, according to the respiratory rate selected.
- **Patient-triggered (synchronized) ventilator modes** deliver a breath when cued by the infant's attempt to inspire.
- **Combined modes** are patient-triggered with backup time cycling.

How they limit delivery of inspiratory gas:

- Volume-targeted ventilator modes deliver a set V_T (in mL), while the PIP varies from breath to breath depending on lung 'stiffness'.
- Pressure-targeted ventilator modes deliver a set PIP (in cm H2O), while the V_T varies depending on lung stiffness and airway resistance.

The amount of pressure required to cause inflation is referred to as 'compliance' (C). A stiff respiratory system (lung plus chest wall) is less compliant and requires a greater PIP to deliver a given V_T.

Compliance is expressed mathematically as: $\quad C = \dfrac{\text{change in volume}}{\text{change in pressure}}$

Airway resistance (Raw) is the resistance to flow of gas through the airway during inspiration and expiration. Calibre or diameter and length of the airways has a significant impact on resistance. Airways with smaller lumen resist gas flow, requiring greater pressure to push gas through the airways.

Airway resistance is expressed mathematically as: $\quad \text{Raw} = \dfrac{\text{change in pressure}}{\text{change in flow (volume/time)}}$

Conditions that decrease compliance of the respiratory system include:

- Respiratory distress syndrome,
- Meconium aspiration syndrome,
- Pneumothorax,
- Congenital thoracic dystrophies,
- Diaphragmatic hernia, and
- Other space-occupying lesions in the chest.

Clinical situations that increase airway resistance include:

- Secretions in the airways,
- Abnormally small or collapsing airways (e.g., in stenosis or malacia),
- Using an endotracheal tube that is too small, and

- Water accumulating in the ventilator circuit.

New ventilator models have made measuring V_T in newborns more accurate, but they require a high level of operator training and expertise. Be sure to consult the operating manual for the specific ventilator model in use.

Equipment

1. Neonatal ventilator and circuit tubing
2. Heated humidifier with sterile distilled water and thermostat control
3. Oxygen blender and air and oxygen hoses
4. Oxygen and medical air supply

Procedure

1. Connect the assembled circuit tubing and humidifier to the ventilator.
2. Connect the air and oxygen hoses to corresponding wall outlets.
3. Set the initial ventilator parameters (e.g., pressure-limited or volume guarantee), guided by the settings being used with the bagging system and information provided in Table A.1.

Table A.1.
Initial ventilation parameters

Parameter	Preterm or LBW infant with lung disease	Term infant with lung disease	Normal lungs (e.g., apnea but no signs of lung disease)
PIP (cm H2O)	18 to 20	20 to 25	15
PEEP (cm H2O)	5	6	4
Tidal volume (V_T)	4 to 5 mL/kg	4 to 5 mL/kg	4 mL/kg
f (per min)	40 to 60	40 to 60	30
t_I^* (sec)	0.3	0.4	0.3 to 0.4
t_E (sec)	0.7 to 1.2	0.6 to 1.1	1.6
% oxygen	Titrate as needed to maintain SpO2 90% to 95%		
Flow (L/min)	6 to 8	10 to 15	6 to 10

f: Frequency; LBW: low birth weight; PEEP: positive end-expiratory pressure; PIP: peak inspiratory pressure; SpO2: oxygen saturation; t_I: inspiratory time; t_E: expiratory time
*The t_I is initially set at 0.25 to 0.30 sec for a patient-triggered ventilator.

4. Check the integrity of the patient circuit by occluding the tubing, noting whether the PIP and PEEP settings are reached.
5. Turn the ventilator on, check all pressures, and set alarms (low and high pressure, volume, apnea, and oxygen analyzer).
6. Connect the ventilator circuit to the endotracheal tube.

7. Immediately check the infant's response to initial settings by assessing:
    a. Degree of chest expansion
    b. Quality of spontaneous respiratory effort
    c. Quality of breath sounds bilaterally, for both mandatory and spontaneous breaths
    d. Oxygen saturation (relative to inspired oxygen concentration)
    e. Tidal volume, if available, which should be between 4 mL/kg and 6 mL/kg
8. Adjust the ventilator settings according to the infant's response and Table A.2.

Table A.2.
Suggested ventilator adjustments based on infant respiratory signs

Clinical sign	Action
Poor chest expansion or decreased breath sounds	Increase PIP or V_T
Chest expansion visible and breath sounds heard	Maintain PIP or V_T
Chest appears to be over-expanding	Decrease PIP or V_T
Chest is expanding but infant is fighting the ventilator	Increase f Consider sedation
Adjust inspired oxygen concentration to maintain oxygen saturation 90% to 95%	

f: frequency; PEEP: positive end-expiratory pressure; PIP: peak inspiratory pressure; SpO2: oxygen saturation; V_T: tidal volume

9. After 15 to 30 min of mechanical ventilation, obtain arterial (PCO2, PO2, and pH) or venous/capillary (PCO2 and pH) blood gas. Make adjustments to ventilation in consultation with your referral centre.

Notes
- The requirement for high PIPs should signal the need to rule out reversible causes of inadequate chest movement (e.g., atelectasis, endotracheal tube obstruction by secretions, or pneumothorax).
- Optimal PEEP for a particular infant and condition increases lung compliance, but too much or too little PEEP can reduce compliance.
- An infant's fighting the ventilator may indicate a need to adjust the set respiratory rate to synchronize with intrinsic respiratory effort.
- Increasing t_I may improve chest expansion in bigger infants or infants with stiff lungs. To prevent air-trapping, ensure the t_E allows time for full expiration.
- The initial oxygen concentration may be high for infants with lung disease. Wean as quickly as possible while maintaining SpO2 within the target range.
- For patient-triggered ventilators, a flow sensor is required as per manufacturer instructions.

3. Capillary blood sampling

Indication
To obtain small blood samples for point-of-care or small volume laboratory testing.

Equipment
1. Warm (≤ 40°C) compress [Optional]
2. Non-latex gloves

3. Depth-restricted sterile micro lancet, tip ≤ 2 mm deep
4. Antiseptic solution or swabs
5. Sterile 2 × 2 gauze sponges
6. Small adhesive bandages
7. Blood collection device(s) appropriate for the tests ordered (e.g., capillary tubes, reagent strips, a container of ice for blood gas)

Procedure

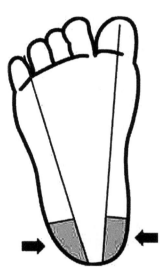

Figure A.1. Heel poke sampling area.

1. Assemble equipment and supplies.
2. If a warm compress is being used to increase regional circulation, apply it for 5 to 10 minutes. The heel should be warm at the time of puncture.
3. Consider using nonpharmacologic strategies for pain reduction as outlined in Chapter 12, Support, pages 353–56.
4. Wash hands and apply gloves.
5. Hold the infant's foot by the heel and pull the skin taut.
6. Select a sampling site in the soft lateral or medial area of the plantar surface.
7. Cleanse the site using appropriate antiseptic solution or swab, as per facility policy, and allow to air dry.
8. Using aseptic technique and standard precautions, puncture the heel with the lancet (≤ 2 mm deep).
9. Using a dry sterile 2 × 2 gauze, gently wipe away the first droplet of blood to prevent an inaccurate sample due to test interference from the alcohol.
10. Collect blood into appropriate specimen containers.
    a. When collecting capillary blood gases, fill heparinized capillary tubes without introducing air. Firmly seat both capillary tube end caps. Mix blood and anticoagulant by rolling.
11. Dry the heel with sterile gauze, apply pressure until the bleeding stops, and cover site with a small adhesive bandage.

Notes
- Review your facility's policies and certification process for capillary blood sampling.
- Venipuncture is more appropriate for the collection of larger blood samples and blood cultures.

- Potential complications include:
  - o Bruising of the infant's foot or leg from excessive squeezing.
  - o Injury to nerves, tendons, and cartilage if sampling outside the indicated areas or too deeply.
  - o Infection.
  - o Repeated punctures over the weight-bearing area of the heel can cause scar tissue to form, leading to pain, delayed walking, and/or abnormal gait.

4. Surfactant administration

Indications

- Treatment of moderate to severe respiratory distress syndrome (RDS).
- Treatment of secondary (acquired) RDS, such as in meconium aspiration syndrome (MAS), pneumonia, or pulmonary hemorrhage.
- Early treatment in newborns judged to be at high risk for developing RDS (e.g., intubated, and < 32 weeks gestational age [GA], or for whom CPAP is not effective).
- Preterm infants with RDS and inspired oxygen requirements of ≥ 30%, despite adequate CPAP.

Goal

To improve respiratory function by replacing absent or inactivated endogenous surfactant.

Principles

Surfactant is a lipid- and protein-rich material produced and secreted by pulmonary alveolar type II cells under the influence of steroids and other hormones. After birth, surfactant forms a monolayer at the alveolar–air–liquid interface, reducing surface tension in the lungs and preventing collapse. Surfactant released into lung fluid before and at birth helps alveoli to inflate and remain inflated. RDS is a primary deficiency of surfactant in newborns. A secondary deficiency of surfactant may occur with infection, meconium aspiration, or pulmonary hemorrhage. Administration is recommended within the first 2 h of life, and within a few minutes after intubation.

Use of surfactant before inter-facility transport of preterm infants requiring respiratory support is associated with lower oxygen requirements and shorter duration of respiratory support.

Application

Surfactant, in liquid form, is administered:

- Directly into the tracheobronchial tree through an ETT or other airway catheter as in less invasive surfactant administration (LISA) or minimally invasive surfactant therapy (MIST).

Refer to the product monograph and hospital policies for storage, dosing, and re-dosing recommendations. Bovine extract surfactants are generally administered at a dose of 4 to 5 mL/kg. Porcine surfactants are administered at a dose of 2.5 mL/kg.

Equipment

1. Surfactant, syringe, and 18-gauge needle, antiseptic solution or swab
2. 5 Fr feeding tube *or* ETT connector with side port
3. Mechanical ventilator, T-piece, or bagging system

Procedure

1. Before surfactant instillation:
   a. Establish cardiorespiratory and oxygen saturation monitoring.
   b. Ensure that the ETT is properly positioned.
   c. Suction the infant's airway via ETT.
   d. Position the infant supine, with head midline.
2. Warm the surfactant to room temperature by rolling the vial gently between palms. Do not use a heating device and do not shake, which creates bubbles.
3. Remove the cap and swab the top of the vial. Draw the correct dose of surfactant into the syringe.
4. Administer the dose as directed by the product monograph and hospital policies.
   a. ***ETT with side port adapter:*** Attach the syringe to the port and administer an aliquot of surfactant with each mechanical inspiration. The total dose is administered as quickly as the infant tolerates it.
   b. ***ETT without side port adapter:*** Insert the feeding tube attached to the surfactant-containing syringe into the ETT and administer the appropriate amount of surfactant as quickly as the infant tolerates it.
   c. Consult your local referral centre for guidance on LISA or MIST, as indicated.
5. Ventilate using the mechanical ventilator, T-piece, or bagging system as surfactant is administered.
6. If reflux of surfactant into the ETT occurs, stop administration and ventilate the infant until the ETT is clear of surfactant, then slowly resume administration.
7. Adjust FiO_2 as required during administration to maintain SpO_2 90% to 95%. Hypoxemia is transient. Stabilize the infant and administer surfactant more slowly.
8. Avoid suctioning the infant for 2 hours post-administration of surfactant unless absolutely indicated.

Notes

- Many infants desaturate during surfactant administration and become transiently bradycardic due to temporary airway obstruction. Hand ventilating the infant and delivering the surfactant more slowly or in aliquots may help.
- A dramatic increase in lung compliance may occur following surfactant administration. Ventilator changes (e.g., PIP and rate) should be anticipated and performed quickly, as required.
- Oxygen saturation usually improves rapidly, allowing the FiO_2 to be decreased.
- Potential complications include:
  - Obstruction of the ETT, which may necessitate suctioning or replacement.
  - Transient hypoxemia and bradycardia requiring supplemental oxygen.
  - Pneumothorax caused by rapid changes in pulmonary compliance and failure to adjust the ventilator parameters to compensate.
  - Pulmonary hemorrhage (usually a late complication).
- Health care providers administering surfactant must be:
  - Skilled in neonatal intubation,
  - Prepared to deal with rapid changes in lung compliance and oxygenation during and after this procedure, and
  - Able to manage potential complications.

5. Pneumothorax—Chest tube insertion

Indications
- Severe respiratory distress caused by pleural air or fluid.
- Significant pneumothorax in an infant requiring air transport.

Goals
To decrease respiratory distress and improve respiratory stability by evacuating free air or fluid in the pleural cavity.

Principles
Gas or fluid within the pleural cavity forms a space-occupying lesion that impedes lung expansion, limits gas exchange, and reduces venous return to the heart. A chest tube inserted between the infant's ribs and connected to an underwater seal is an effective way to drain free air or fluid from the pleural cavity.

Application
These instructions outline the procedure for inserting the chest tube system most commonly available in smaller centres (chest tubes with trocars). Some care providers may be familiar with the Seldinger technique and will use these chest tubes in accordance with manufacturer instructions.

In general, the tip of a chest tube draining air is oriented up, toward the anterior pleural space, where air is most likely to collect in an infant lying supine. The tip of a tube placed for draining pleural fluid is aimed inferiorly and posteriorly, as fluid settles in the basal region.

The point of insertion into the chest wall, in the intercostal space between the fourth and fifth rib in the mid- to anterior axillary line, is similar in both cases. Care should be taken to avoid the nipple area.

The equipment list, infant positioning, skin preparation, insertion site, and drainage systems are similar, whether the operator is inserting a chest tube for fluid or air, or using either the trocar or Seldinger technique.

Equipment
1. Sterile gloves, mask, hat, and sterile drapes (minimum in an emergency), sterile gown
2. Antiseptic solution or swabs, sterile water
3. 1 mL syringe and 27G needles to infiltrate lidocaine
4. 1% lidocaine, without epinephrine
5. Sterile hemostats, straight and curved
6. Scalpel handle and blade
7. One rubber-tipped curved forceps for each chest tube to be inserted
8. Sterile gauze (4 × 4), transparent occlusive dressing, waterproof tape, scissors
9. Chest tube with trocar (sizes 8, 10, and 12 Fr)
10. Suture kit
11. Thoracic drainage system/underwater seal device or one-way valve

Procedure
1. Prepare the thoracic drainage system as per manufacturer's instructions and connect it to wall suction *or* prepare the one-way valve for connection to the chest tube.
2. Review the infant's chest radiograph to confirm location of the pneumothorax.
3. Make sure that cardiorespiratory and saturation monitoring is in place. Ensure leads are kept well away from the chest tube insertion area.
4. Measure the length of chest tube required (usually the distance from skin incision to sternum). Note the distance on the black markings of the chest tube.

5. Position the infant with the affected side up, at a 45° to 60° angle, with a roll as back support.

6. Raise the infant's arm up over her head and locate the intercostal space between the fourth and fifth rib in the mid- to anterior axillary line. Avoid the nipple area.

7. Cleanse the area with the antiseptic solution and inject a small amount of buffered 1% lidocaine (maximum dose 0.3 mL/kg) intradermally and subcutaneously in the insertion area: just below the fourth rib.

8. Mask, scrub, and don a sterile gown, gloves, and hat.

9. Cleanse the insertion site and surrounding area with antiseptic solution. Avoid using an excess amount of antiseptic solution, which can irritate and burn immature skin. Allow the solution to dry, then wipe the area with sterile water.

10. Cover the area with sterile drapes.

11. Make a 0.5 cm-long, transverse incision along the top of the fifth rib.

12. Insert the chest tube (trocar type) using either of two techniques.

Blunt dissection method:

   a. Remove the trocar from the chest tube.

   b. Take the small curved hemostat and insert the closed tip into the skin incision.

   c. Bluntly dissect the subcutaneous tissue and slide the forceps over the fifth rib into the fourth intercostal space. Always dissect just over the top of the rib to avoid hitting the neurovascular bundle beneath each rib.

   d. Using forceps, punch through into the pleural space. A gush of air or fluid may be released.

   e. Carefully advance the chest tube (without the trocar) the determined distance, aiming anteriorly toward the infant's opposite shoulder (Figure A.2).

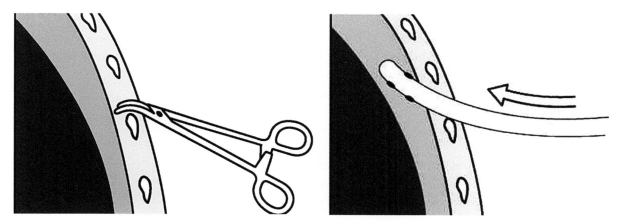

Figure A.2. Blunt method chest tube insertion.

Trocar method:

   a. Take a small piece of gauze and place around the chest tube (with trocar in place), securing it with the curved forceps cross-clamped approximately 2 cm from the tip of the tube.

   b. Take the small curved hemostat, insert the closed tip into the skin incision and bluntly dissect the subcutaneous tissue. Insert the chest tube with trocar and forceps guard into the tunnel created. Clamping the forceps across the tube with the trocar in place stops the tube from penetrating deeper than 2 cm.

   c. When the chest tube 'pops' into the pleural space, release the clamp and remove the trocar from the tip of the chest tube.

d. Carefully advance the chest tube the determined distance, aiming anteriorly toward the infant's opposite shoulder. Pull the trocar out as the chest tube advances. Condensation inside the chest tube will be seen as the trocar is removed.

13. Have an assistant attach the chest tube to the drainage system tubing or flutter valve, using a universal adapter. Tape the connection with waterproof tape.

14. Secure the chest tube with a suture through the skin, which is also tightly tied around the tube. Tape the tube in place, making sure no tension is applied to the chest tube. Protect the insertion site with a sterile, transparent dressing.

15. Turn on the wall suction. When using an underwater seal system, observe for slow bubbling in the suction control chamber.

16. Order a new chest radiograph to verify correct chest tube placement and drainage.

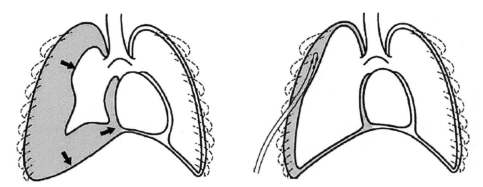

Figure A.3. Evacuation of pneumothorax by chest tube.

Notes

- To prevent infection, never leave a chest tube open to the air. A one-way valve attached to the free end of a chest tube provides optimal drainage during transport. The valve allows air and fluid to drain and stops inspired air from being drawn into the pleural space.
- Potential complications associated with chest tube insertion include:
  - Puncture of the lung,
  - Bronchopleural fistula,
  - Hemorrhage,
  - Rupture of great vessels or cardiac chambers, and
  - Subcutaneous placement of the chest tube, rather than intrathoracic.
- Health care providers performing chest tube insertion must be:
  - Skilled in neonatal airway management,
  - Prepared to deal with rapid changes in respiratory and cardiovascular function during and after this procedure, and
  - Able to manage potential complications.

For insertion of a chest tube via the Seldinger method, refer to product monograph instructions.

6. Central vascular access—Umbilical vein catheterization (UVC)

Indications

- Actual or anticipated need for volume expansion
- Ongoing intravenous (IV) infusions
- Intravascular drug administration
- Exchange transfusion
- Blood sampling during stabilization

Goal

To obtain secure central intravascular access for post-resuscitation care.

Principles

Unlike UVCs placed during resuscitation, lines placed for ongoing infusions are ideally positioned through the ductus venous with the tip lying in the inferior vena cava, just below the junction with the right atrium. UVC position must be confirmed by X-ray because up to 50% of lines inserted to a calculated depth require some repositioning.

This route is only accessible during the first few days of life.

Application

No one method of calculating depth of insertion is fail-safe. Three commonly used formulas for insertion depth are based on either linear measurements or birth weight:

Calculations for UVC insertion depth in cm:
- Umbilicus to xiphoid process (cm) + umbilical stump length (cm)
- Umbilicus to middle of inguinal crease (cm) × 2 + umbilical stump length
- (3 × weight [kg] + 9) ÷ 2

Contraindications to UVCs include:
- Omphalocele,
- Peritonitis, and
- Necrotizing enterocolitis.

Equipment

1. Antiseptic solution (2% chlorhexidine preferred)
2. Sterile drapes, surgical cap, mask, gown, and sterile gloves
3. Sterile procedure tray with forceps, dilator, scissors, and needle driver
4. Umbilical tape and sterile 2×2 gauze
5. Measuring tape (to calculate depth of insertion)
6. 3–0 silk suture
7. Curved iris forceps, if available
8. Umbilical catheters, size 3.5 F (< 1500 g) and 5.0 F (≥ 1500 g)
9. IV tubing and IV infusion pump
10. Three-way stopcock, 10 mL syringe, and sterile 0.9% NaCl
11. #10 scalpel blade

Procedure

1. If the umbilical cord is dry, it can be rehydrated prior to the procedure with a warm, moist compress.
2. Prepare the umbilical catheterization tray and necessary equipment.
3. Position the infant appropriately in a supine position.
4. Ensure cardiorespiratory monitoring (including pulse oximetry) is in place, and that leads are kept well away from the UVC insertion area.
5. Calculate the depth of insertion of the UVC.
6. Mask, hat, scrub, and don a sterile gown and gloves.
7. Have an assistant open additional equipment onto a sterile field.
8. Connect umbilical catheter, stopcock, and syringe. Flush with 0.9% NaCl. Close the stopcock to the catheter to prevent fluid loss and air entry.

9. Have an assistant hold up the umbilical cord using the cord clamp or forceps.

10. Using aseptic technique, cleanse the skin surrounding the umbilical stump as well as the stump itself with antiseptic solution. Avoid using an excess amount of antiseptic solution, which can irritate and burn immature skin.

11. Being careful to maintain sterile technique, tie umbilical tape loosely around the cord stump.

12. Grasp the cord stump with forceps and cut off the umbilical clamp with the scalpel blade, leaving about 1 to 2 cm of cord stump. Control bleeding, if necessary, by gently tightening the umbilical tape.

13. Identify the umbilical vessels. The single vein is thin-walled and easily opened; the two arteries are thick-walled, with a pinpoint opening.

14. Insert the iris forceps or dilator gently into the umbilical vein. Remove any visible clots.

15. Gently dilate the vein with forceps, as needed.

16. Turn the stopcock so that the system is open between the syringe and the catheter. Ensure that the catheter remains saline-filled and air-free before inserting it to the pre-determined depth. Do not force against resistance.

17. Aspiration of blood confirms placement within the venous system.

18. Secure the line in place with a purse-string suture through the Wharton's jelly.

19. Confirm positioning with X-ray.

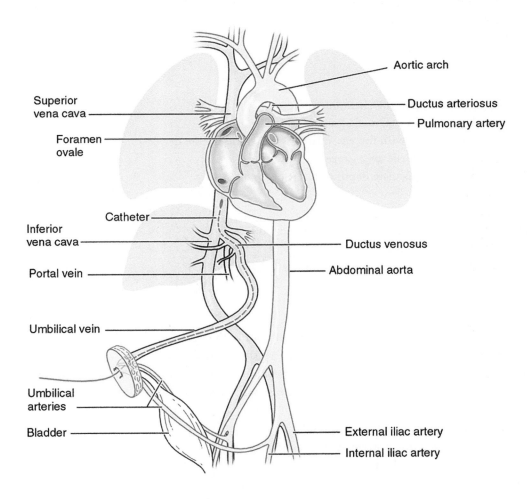

Figure A.4. Correct high-line UVC placement.

Source: Goodman DM, Green TP, Unti SM, Powell EC: *Current Procedures: Pediatrics*: www.accesspediatrics.com

20. Once correct positioning is confirmed, use bridging tapes or an umbilical line-securing device to hold the catheter in place.
21. Remove any residual antiseptic from the infant's skin with saline or sterile water.
22. Ensure that the stopcock is closed to the infant whenever disconnected. Never leave the catheter open to air, due to risk for air embolus.

Notes
- Malpositioning of the UVC within the right atrium increases the risk for complications or infections. While the vein is usually easily identified, erroneous insertion into an umbilical artery can also occur (more commonly when there is a single umbilical artery). X-ray confirmation of final positioning is mandatory for any UVC used for ongoing infusions.
- On X-ray:
  - UVC tracks immediately cephalad and to the right of the umbilicus on anteroposterior view. On the lateral view, the UVC is anteriorly placed.
  - Umbilical arterial catheters track down toward the pelvis then turn cephalad into the descending aorta on anteroposterior view. On the lateral view, the umbilical artery catheter is positioned posteriorly. (Umbilical artery catheter insertion is beyond the scope of ACoRN but is mentioned here to help providers identify a UVC that is incorrectly positioned within the umbilical artery.) AP view of normal UVC placement (left) Lateral view of normal UVC placement (right). The UAC is present in both.

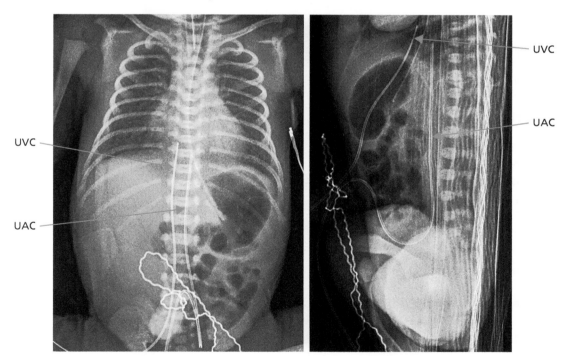

Correct UVC/UAC positioning and route of lines

- Potential complications associated with UVC insertion include:
  - Burns on the abdomen or flank due to antiseptic solution, particularly in preterm infants.
  - False lumen—no blood is aspirated.
  - Failure of catheter to pass through the ductus venosus. Reinsertion should be attempted, or the line pulled back to below the liver.
  - Misplacement within the right atrium, portal vein, or superior mesenteric vein, or extravasation into the abdominal cavity.

o Perforation of a major blood vessel or the right atrial wall.

o Blood loss with catheter dislodgement.

o Air embolism.

o Infection—use of UVCs for more than 7 days is associated with increased risk for sepsis.

o Liver abscess.

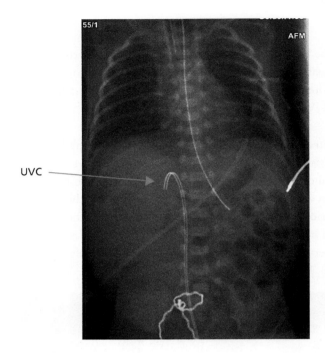

Abnormal UVC position on X-ray

7. Bowel bag application

Indications

- Gastroschisis
- Ruptured omphalocele
- Exposed abdominal viscera

Goal

To protect exposed organs from excessive water loss, minimize heat loss from evaporation, and decrease risk for infection.

Principles

Applying a transparent plastic covering or bowel bag minimizes risks for breakdown, infection, and thermal, fluid, and electrolyte losses, while providing clear visualization of the exposed bowel.

Equipment

1. Sterile bowel bag with ties
2. Non-latex sterile gloves

Procedure

1. Administer vitamin K before applying the bowel bag, which will cover the infant's lower limbs.
2. Wearing non-latex sterile gloves, open the bowel bag. Be careful to keep the inside as clean as possible.
3. Collect the exposed bowel on top of the infant's abdomen and ask an assistant to place the infant feet-first into the bowel bag and pull the bag up to ensure that the exposed organs are covered.
4. Reposition the bowel on the infant's abdomen as close to midline as possible to ensure adequate blood supply, prevent twisting and traction on the exposed viscera, and minimize risk for bowel ischemia.
5. Pull tie tapes on a bowel bag closed. They should be snug under the infant's arms to completely enclose the defect and keep tissues moist.
6. Place the infant in a supine or right-side lying position. To prevent the bowel from flopping, kinking, or twisting, support it with rolls. If the defect is large and cannot be stabilized midline, gently wrap rolled gauze around the bowel over the bowel bag. Ensure that the bowel can be visualized at all times.
7. Insert a gastric tube for drainage of swallowed air to prevent visceral distention from compromising blood flow to the bowel.

8. Incubator and radiant warmer use

Indications

Infants requiring close observation or frequent access for procedures, those unable to maintain their temperature within normal limits (e.g., preterm, small for gestational age, infants with an abdominal or neural tube defect), or infants requiring therapeutic hypothermia.

Goals

To provide environments for unwell or at-risk newborns where temperature can be maintained within normal or prescribed (i.e., as in therapeutic hypothermia) limits.

Principles

A neutral thermal environment (NTE) is defined as the environmental air temperature range in which an infant can produce heat and maintain normal body temperature with minimal metabolic expenditure and oxygen consumption.

The importance of obtaining and maintaining normothermia in the at-risk or unwell newborn cannot be overemphasized. Limited ability to regulate body temperature immediately after birth places all infants at risk for temperature instability. Providing and maintaining an NTE and monitoring infants frequently to ensure their body temperature remains within the appropriate range are essential to stabilization.

Application

Incubators are heated by circulating warm air (convection). The buffered thermal environment they provide decreases the effect of temperature fluctuations caused by changes in room temperature. Incubators operate in two modes: air temperature control or servo control (automatic).

Air temperature mode heats the air inside the incubator to a chosen temperature. Several charts have been published to guide the selection of temperature settings according to infant weight and age, with the aim of maintaining body temperature within a normal range and minimizing energy expenditure.

Table A.3 is for initial guidance only. For specific and ongoing care, always refer to the manufacturer's instructions for the equipment used in your facility.

Table A.3
Selecting initial incubator air temperature within the first 12 h post-delivery

Birth weight (grams)	Air temperature setting (°C) (double-walled, humidified incubator)
< 750	39.3 (37.5)
750 to 1000	39.0 (37.0)
1000 to 1200	37.5
1200 to 1500	36.5
1500 to 2000	35.5
≥ 2000	34.0

Source: Adapted from Jaimovich DG, Vidyasagar D. Handbook of Pediatric and Neonatal Transport Medicine, 2nd edn. Philadelphia, PA: Hanley & Belfus, 2005.

Servo control mode turns the heating element on and off automatically in response to skin temperature, based on readings from a probe that is usually set at 36.5°C.

Radiant warmers use infrared heat as their heat source. Like incubators, they function in two modes: manual and servo control (automatic). Newer radiant warmer models can also function as incubators, allowing easier access to the infant needing care.

In manual mode, the warmer continues to heat unless it is turned off, making thermal environment harder to maintain and increasing risk for overheating. Servo control mode is recommended because the warmer turns on and off in response to skin temperature (measured by a probe), making it easier to control thermal environment and decreasing risk for hypo- or hyperthermia.

Radiant heat can be blocked by blankets, sterile drapes, plastic shields, equipment, and the hands and heads of care providers. Drafts around the radiant warmer increase the risk of convective heat loss.

Radiant warmers also increase insensible water loss. Consider moving unwell and/or hypothermic infants to an incubator (or convert the warmer to incubator mode) as soon as possible, to ensure adequate thermoregulation, prevent insensible water loss, and facilitate rest. When the infant cannot be moved to an incubator, consider the following strategy to ensure temperature stability, especially for VLBW infants:

- Raise the side panels and cover the radiant warmer bed with plastic wrap. Supply warm, humidified air.
- Ensure warm humidified air is not blowing directly on the infant—water droplets may burn the skin.
- Reposition the infant carefully; disturbing the plastic wrap can cause temperatures to fluctuate.

Equipment

1. Incubator or radiant warmer
2. Servo control probe and reflective cover
3. Sterile distilled water (for humidity in incubator)

Procedures

Incubator:

1. Prewarm the incubator based on infant's gestational age, weight, and condition. Refer to manufacturer's instructions for information related to providing humidity and adding sterile distilled water.
2. Position the incubator away from drafts and direct sunlight, if possible.
3. Place the infant in the incubator, removing blankets and all clothing except the diaper.

4. Place the servo control probe on the upper right quadrant of the infant's abdomen, ensuring that it lies flat against the skin, and fasten with a reflective cover. If the infant is prone, place the probe on either flank (not between the scapulae) and fasten with a reflective cover. Monitor frequently to ensure the probe remains securely attached.

5. Set the alarm limits 0.5°C above and below the desired temperature range.

6. Monitor the infant's axillary temperature as ordered. Note incubator temperature at the same time.

Warming a hypothermic infant in an incubator:

1. Set incubator air temperature 1°C to 1.5°C higher than the infant's body temperature, or at 36.0°C.

2. Monitor the infant's temperature at least every 15 to 30 minutes. If the infant's temperature does not rise, check for objects, such as a blanket, that may be blocking exogenous heat. If no obstructions are found, increase the incubator air temperature every 30 minutes: first to 37.0°C, then to 38.0°C. If there is inadequate response, consider increasing the humidity level.

3. When the infant's axillary temperature reaches the normal range, the incubator setting is gradually lowered to the air temperature and humidity settings recommended for age and weight, as described above.

Radiant warmer:

1. Preheat radiant warmer according to manufacturer's instructions.
2. Position warmer away from drafts, if possible.
3. Place the infant on the warmer, removing blankets and all clothing except the diaper.
4. Place skin temperature probe on the upper right quadrant of the infant's abdomen, ensuring that it lies flat against the skin, and fasten with a reflective cover. If the infant is prone, place the probe on either flank (not between the scapulae) and fasten with a reflective cover. Monitor frequently to ensure the probe remains securely attached.
5. Set the skin probe temperature to 36.5°C.
6. Set high and low temperature alarms 0.5°C above and below the pre-set temperature.
7. Monitor the infant's axillary temperature as ordered. Note temperature of the warmer at the same time.

Warming a hypothermic infant on a radiant warmer:

1. Set warmer temperature 0.5°C higher than the infant's body temperature, in manual mode.

2. Monitor the infant's temperature at least every 15 to 30 minutes. If the infant's temperature does not rise, check for objects, such as a blanket, that may be blocking exogenous heat. If no obstructions are found, increase the warmer temperature every 30 minutes.

3. When the infant's axillary temperature reaches the normal range, the warmer should be switched to servo mode, as described above.

Notes

- **Caution:** The methods of rewarming a hypothermic infant described above should *never* be used to rewarm an infant who received therapeutic hypothermia. Rewarming following therapeutic hypothermia is outside the scope of ACoRN and occurs in tertiary settings.

- Premature infants are at high risk for evaporative loss. They require a humid environment to help manage body temperature. ELBW infants should receive humidity at approximately 70% in the first week of life to facilitate normothermia and counter high insensible water losses.

- Newer incubators have in-built humidification systems that add sterile and filtered distilled water to clean air entering the incubator. Older incubators, which provide humidity via a water reservoir, can increase risk for infection and are not recommended. Be sure to follow the manufacturer's instructions and your hospital's infection control guidelines for proper care of incubator humidification systems.
- The most common complication during rewarming is apnea. Infants need to be closely monitored, with vital signs recorded every 30 minutes.
- If an infant is hyperthermic and the incubator air temperature is on its lowest setting, consider transferring the infant to a radiant warmer or cot, to modulate temperature. Remember: air flow ceases when an incubator is turned off.
- When tracking the difference between incubator air and an infant's skin temperature, be sure to recheck that:
  - o Incubator temperature and heat output is being monitored accurately.
  - o The servo control skin probe is functioning, attached properly, and being used appropriately.
  - o Direct sunlight or phototherapy lights are not impacting incubator temperature.

9. Thermoregulation management in infants at risk for hypoxic ischemic encephalopathy (HIE)

Indication

Infants identified in the ACoRN Neurology Sequence as being **'At risk for HIE'** requiring thermo-regulatory management include those with:

- A significant perinatal hypoxic ischemic event:
  - o Fetal heart rate monitoring abnormalities.
  - o Evidence or suspicion of bleeding, cord occlusion, or cord prolapse.
  - o Infants who had respiratory depression at birth and required prolonged resuscitation.
- An Apgar score of 0 to 3 for 5 or more minutes, *or* an Apgar score of 0 to 5 for 10 or more minutes.
- An umbilical cord arterial pH less than 7.15.
- An umbilical cord arterial base deficit greater than or equal to 10 mmol/L, or lactate greater than 5 mmol/L.

The **'At risk for HIE'** Alerting Sign identifies newborns who require close observation and assessment because they are at higher risk for developing HIE. Clinical signs of end-organ perfusion problems indicate higher risk for long-term sequelae from moderate to severe HIE. Evidence of multi-system organ dysfunction in the immediate neonatal period includes:

- Neurologic dysfunction may manifest as hypotonia, seizures, coma, or abnormal activity.
- Renal dysfunction is indicated by decreased urine output, microscopic hematuria, elevation of serum creatinine, and low serum sodium.
- Hepatic injury manifests as elevated liver enzymes, abnormal clotting factors, and other abnormalities in synthetic function, such as albumin production and glucose control.
- Thrombocytopenia may accompany abnormal clotting factors.
- Signs of cardiac injury include poor contractility, low blood pressure, reduced peripheral perfusion and (occasionally) heart failure and arrhythmias.
- Significant acidosis may result in pulmonary hypertension and persistent fetal shunts, causing cyanosis.
- Gastrointestinal injury can manifest as ileus or necrotizing enterocolitis.

Goals

The goal of thermoregulatory management in infants at risk for HIE is to obtain core body temperatures in a specified target range (strict normothermia 36.5°C to 37.0°C, or therapeutic hypothermia 33°C to 34°C) by 6 hours postnatal age, to minimize the risk for long-term neurologic complications associated with HIE.

Principles

Therapeutic hypothermia is a neuroprotective intervention that has been shown to decrease mortality and severe long-term neurodevelopmental disability at 18 months when initiated in the first 6 hours postdelivery to infants with moderate and severe HIE and a GA ≥ 35 weeks.

Strict normothermia

Strict normothermia involves active thermal management to **prevent** hyperthermia in:

- All infants identified as 'At risk for HIE'.
- Infants with suspected HIE, when therapeutic hypothermia has not been, or cannot be, initiated.

The aim of strict normothermia is to maintain the infant's axillary temperature in the 36.5°C to 37.0°C range. Strict normothermia measures are taken:

- For all infants ≥ 35 weeks GA who are depressed at birth and being assessed to determine whether they meet criteria for therapeutic hypothermia, but for whom consultation with the clinical transport coordinator has not yet occurred.
- For all infants with suspected HIE who do not meet the criteria for GA, or have severe cardiorespiratory instability, or have evidence of disseminated intravascular coagulation (DIC).
- For all infants with suspected HIE who have missed the 6-hour window to initiate therapeutic hypothermia.
- In consultation with your tertiary care referral centre, when it is determined *not* to initiate therapeutic hypothermia.

Therapeutic hypothermia

Therapeutic hypothermia involves active thermal management to maintain the infant's core temperature between 33°C to 34°C. Therapeutic hypothermia is considered for infants:

- ≥ 35 weeks GA who meet either treatment criteria A or B, and also meet criteria C:
- **Criteria A**: Cord pH ≤ 7.0 or base deficit ≥16 **or**
- **Criteria B**: pH 7.01 to 7.15 or base deficit 10 to 15.9 on cord gas or blood gas within 1 h of age, **and**
  - History of acute perinatal event (such as, but not limited to, cord prolapse, placental abruption, or uterine rupture) **and**
  - Apgar score ≤ 5 at 10 min, or at least 10 min of positive-pressure ventilation

and

- **Criteria C**: Evidence of moderate (Sarnat II) or severe (Sarnat III) encephalopathy, as demonstrated either by the presence of seizures or by observing at least one sign in three or more of the moderate or severe columns of the Encephalopathy Assessment Table 5.5, page 161.

391

- Therapeutic hypothermia should only be initiated in infants who meet criteria, and only after consultation with your tertiary care centre, following a strict protocol.
- The infant's GA is ≥ 35 weeks and postnatal age is ≤ 6 hours.
- Resuscitation and stabilization procedures must be completed.
- Cardiorespiratory function, including oxygen requirement, must be stable.
- The presence and severity of coagulopathy has been determined and treatment initiated when indicated.
  - Only those infants who meet all the above conditions qualify to receive therapeutic hypothermia; otherwise infants receive strict normothermia.
  - Therapeutic hypothermia is not routinely offered to newborns < 35 weeks GA or presenting later than 6 hours post-birth because there is no evidence of benefit for these infants at the present time.

Application

Close monitoring is essential whenever therapeutic hypothermia is initiated because:

- Therapeutic hypothermia may worsen pulmonary hypertension in infants with impaired cardiorespiratory transition.
- Therapeutic hypothermia increases the risk of coagulopathy.
- Heart rate decreases during therapeutic hypothermia.
- Cardiac function and rhythms can change in infants as they are cooled. They may experience low cardiac output resulting in hypotension and/or develop arrhythmias.
- Seizure activity may occur.

Contraindications to therapeutic hypothermia include:

- Evidence of severe head trauma or intracranial bleeding.
- Coagulopathy not under control.
- Presence of a major congenital or genetic abnormality where no further aggressive treatment is planned.

Essential reasons for consulting with your tertiary referral centre/clinical transport coordinator *before* initiating therapeutic hypothermia include the following:

- Obtaining advice on all other aspects of care management
- Making sure an infant meets all criteria
- Considering the management of contraindications
- Determining absolute (versus relative) contraindications
- Evaluating the risk–benefit profile for each case
- Supportive care during therapeutic hypothermia
- Anticipating, preventing, and managing complications
- Coordinating care before and during transport.

Infants with moderate to severe encephalopathy should be triaged for transfer to a level 3 centre that is equipped to provide:

- Therapeutic hypothermia,
- Multisystem care and consultation,

- Neurological subspecialty care,
- Electroencephalogram monitoring, and
- Neonatal neuroimaging.

Equipment:

1. A rectal or esophageal temperature probe
2. A thermometer capable of reading temperatures below 33°C

Procedure:

1. Establish venous access and continuous cardiorespiratory and pulse oximetry monitoring before initiating the cooling process.
2. Restrict initial total fluid infusion rates to between 2 to 3 mL/kg/h or lower.
3. Monitor the infant's temperature continuously, using a rectal temperature probe:
   - Lubricated with water-soluble jelly,
   - Carefully inserted 5 cm into the rectum, and
   - Secured at the perineum and thigh with infant tape.

   If this mode of monitoring is not available at the sending site, use an axillary thermometer.

   Document the temperature every 15 minutes. Ensure the temperature does not fall below 33°C.
4. Initiate passive cooling:
   - Turn off the overhead warmer.
   - Remove the infant's hat and clothing.
5. Consider analgesia with low-dose morphine infusion (5 mcg/kg/h to 10 mcg/kg/h). Hypothermia in the infant may result in reduced drug clearance and increases the risk of toxic serum concentrations. Ideally, the morphine infusion rate should not exceed 10 mcg/kg/h.

   Indications for analgesia include agitation, signs of pain, or shivering.
6. Initiate treatment of seizures in all cases where seizure-like movements are observed. Phenobarbital is the first-line therapy for infants who are having seizures.
7. Discontinue therapeutic hypothermia if the infant develops any of the following complications:
   - Persistent pulmonary hypertension of the newborn (PPHN is a relative contraindication)
   - Severe, uncorrectable coagulopathy
   - Arrhythmia requiring medical treatment.
8. Therapeutic hypothermia requires specific tasks to be completed by the nursing staff and physicians caring for these infants.

Nursing care

1. Document temperature (by rectal probe or axillary thermometer), respiratory rate, and heart rate before and after cooling starts.
2. Record the time cooling was started and document the time that target temperature is obtained.
3. Document temperature (by rectal probe or axillary thermometer) every 15 minutes once cooling is initiated.
4. Document cardiorespiratory status, including saturations, every 30 minutes.
5. Review the ACoRN Primary Survey and applicable ACoRN Sequences every 30 minutes.
6. Keep a seizure log (see Chapter 5, Neurology, pages 164 and 179 for examples).
7. Monitor skin integrity.
8. Monitor the infant for pain, agitation.
9. Manage intravenous fluid infusions.

Medical care

1. Assess and track neurological findings using the Encephalopathy Assessment Table, and keep tables and results with the patient record.
2. Assess and document degree of encephalopathy. Document any discussions with your tertiary referral centre/referral centre, subspecialty consultants, and parents.
3. Document cord blood gases and/or a blood gas with lactate within 1 hour of age.
4. Document the presence of seizures, treatment approach, and effectiveness.
5. Record cardiorespiratory status at initiation of therapeutic hypothermia and ensure documentation occurs every 30 minutes.
6. Note the date and times that therapeutic hypothermia was ordered and initiated.
7. Ensure the infant has adequate pain management. Record signs of agitation or pain, the time that morphine infusion is initiated, and signs of treatment effect.
8. Determine coagulation status (platelet count, international normalized ratio, and partial thromboplastin time).

Notes

- Regional practice varies considerably across Canada. Contact your referral centre for direction and advice.
- Cool gel packs may be recommended by some referral centres, but care must be taken to not overcool the infant or cause injury to the skin. Ice packs should never be used: they increase the risk for subcutaneous fat necrosis and cause overcooling, significantly increasing the risk for cardiac arrhythmias.
- It is critical that resuscitation, early stabilization, and a level 3 neonatal consultation be completed before initiating therapeutic hypothermia for HIE.
- Therapeutic hypothermia decreases metabolic activity and alters metabolism by the liver. Therefore, pharmacokinetics may be significantly altered during the cooling process.

Bibliography

American Physiological Society and ACCP-ATS Committee on Pulmonary Nomenclature. Respiratory Care standard abbreviations and symbols. Respiratory Care 1997;42(6):637–42: http://www.rcjournal.com/guidelines_for_authors/symbols.pdf.

Edwards AD, Brocklehurst P, Gunn AJ, et al. Neurological outcomes at 18 months of age after moderate hypothermia for perinatal hypoxic ischaemic encephalopathy: Synthesis and meta-analysis of trial data. BMJ 2010;340:c363.

Goldsmith JP, Karotkin EH, Suresh G, Keszler M. Assisted Ventilation of the Neonate: An evidence-based Approach to Newborn Respiratory Care. 6th edn. Philadelphia, PA: Elsevier, 2016.

Gomella TL, Cunningham MD, Eyal FG. Neonatology: Management, Procedures, On-call Problems, Diseases and Drugs. 7th edn. New York, NY: McGraw-Hill Education, 2013.

Jacobs SE, Berg M, Hunt R, Tarnow-Mordi WO, Inder TE, Davis PG. Cooling for newborns with hypoxic ischemic encephalopathy. Cochrane Database Syst Rev 2013;(1):CD003311.

Jacobs SE, Morley CJ, Inder TE, et al. Whole-body hypothermia for term and near-term newborns with hypoxic ischemic encephalopathy: A randomized controlled trial. Arch Pediatr Adolesc Med 2011;165(8):692–700.

Jacobs SE, Tarnow-Mordi WO. Therapeutic hypothermia for newborn infants with hypoxic-ischaemic encephalopathy. J Paediatr Child Health 2010;46(10):568–76.

Jobe AH. Pulmonary surfactant therapy. N Engl J M 1993;328(12):861–8.

Lean WL, Dawson JA, Davis PG, Theda C, Thio M. Accuracy of five formulae to determine the insertion length of umbilical venous catheters. Arch Dis Child Fetal Neonatal Ed 2018;104(2):F165–69.

Lemyre B, Chau V; Canadian Paediatric Society, Fetus and Newborn Committee. Hypothermia for newborns with hypoxic ischemic encephalopathy. Paediatr Child Health 2018;23(4):285–91: https://www.cps.ca/en/documents/position/hypothermia-for-newborns

London Health Sciences Centre. Capillary blood sampling: For use with newborns and older infants; self-directed learning package. Revised September 2010: https://www.lhsc.on.ca/critical-care-trauma-centre/procedure-blood-gas-sampling

MacDonald MG, Ramasethu J, Rais-Bahrami K, eds. Atlas of Procedures in Neonatology, 5th edn. Philadelphia, PA: Lippincott, Williams and Wilkins, 2013.

Morley CJ, Davis PG. Continuous positive airway pressure: Scientific and clinical rationale. Curr Opin Pediatr 2008;20(2):119–24.

New Zealand Child and Youth Clinical Networks. Newborn Services Clinical Guideline. Umbilical artery and vein catheterization. November 3, 2018. https://www.starship.org.nz/guidelines/umbilical-artery-and-vein-catheterisation-in-the-neonate/

Ng E, Shah V; Canadian Paediatric Society, Fetus and Newborn Committee. Guidelines for surfactant replacement therapy in neonates. Paediatr Child Health 2021;26(1): https://www.cps.ca/en/documents/position/guidelines-for-surfactant-replacement-therapy-in-neonates.

Polin RA, Carlo WA; American Academy of Pediatrics, Committee on Fetus and Newborn. Surfactant replacement therapy for preterm and term neonates with respiratory distress. Pediatrics 2014;133(1):156–63.

Shankaran S, Abbot R, Laptook MD, et al. Whole-body hypothermia for neonates with hypoxic-ischemic encephalopathy. N Engl J Med 2005;353(15):1574–84.

Shah PS. Hypothermia: A systematic review and meta-analysis of clinical trials. Semin Fetal Neonatal Med 2010;15(5):238–46.

Sinkin RA, Chisholm CA, Niermeyer S, et al. Perinatal Continuing Education Program Book III: Neonatal Care. 3rd edn. Elk Grove Village, IL: American Academy of Pediatrics, 2016.

Thoresen M. Supportive care during neuroprotective hypothermia in the term newborn: Adverse effects and their prevention. Clin Perinatol 2008;35(4):749–63.

Thoresen M. Hypothermia after perinatal asphyxia: Selection for treatment and cooling protocol. J Pediatr 2011;158(2 Suppl):e45–9.

Wachtel EV, Hendricks-Muñoz KD. Current management of the infant who presents with neonatal encephalopathy. Curr Probl Pediatr Adolesc Health Care 2011;41(5):132–53.

Winnipeg Regional Health Authority. Neonatal clinical practice guideline: Mechanical ventilation of newborns. December 2015. http://www.wrha.mb.ca/extranet/eipt/files/EIPT-.35-21.pdf.

Appendix B

Interpretation of Investigations

The investigations discussed in this appendix are:

1. Blood gases
2. Complete blood count and differential (CBCD)
3. Chest radiograph (CXR) interpretation

1. Blood gases

Goal

To determine adequacy of respiratory function (oxygenation and ventilation) and acid-base status to guide diagnosis and management.

Principles

- **pH** estimates the total blood acid load. It is a measured value that reflects the balance between dissolved CO_2 (respiratory component) and serum acids and bases (metabolic components), such as lactic acid.
- **PCO2** is an indicator of the adequacy of ventilation: how well the lung is removing CO_2 from the blood.
- **PaO2** (arterial PO2) indicates how well the lungs are transferring oxygen to blood (oxygenation) in relation to % inspired oxygen.
- **SpO2** is the percentage of oxygen-saturated hemoglobin relative to total hemoglobin (unsaturated + saturated) in blood. SpO2 can be used as a continuous estimate of oxygenation.
- **Base deficit (BD)** estimates how much metabolic acid is present in the blood. Base excess, the negative value of BD, and bicarbonate are also used to describe acid-base status.
- **pH ≤ 7.25** with PCO2 >/= 55 indicates poor ventilation (respiratory acidosis).
- **pH ≤ 7.25** and BD > 4 to 6 (metabolic acidosis) is due either to an excessive loss of bicarbonate ion or to an elevated lactic or other organic acid and indicates need to measure the anion gap and the arterial or venous lactic acid levels.

Application

Arterial, venous, or capillary blood samples are nearly equally useful for determining PCO2, pH, and BD. The choice of sample depends on ease of access and the purpose of investigation. An arterial blood gas sample is needed to determine a PaO2 value (oxygenation). Capillary and venous samples are not appropriate for assessment of PaO2. The use of pulse oximetry has reduced the need to measure arterial PaO2 to assess oxygenation.

When arterial sampling is not possible or desirable, capillary sampling is most commonly used in newborns. The accuracy of capillary blood gas pH depends on perfusion at the sample site. The heel is often used for infant samples (see Appendix A.3). A sample taken from a poorly perfused site results in a falsely low pH value. Warming the heel to promote vasodilation and arterial flow (arterialization) can minimize this effect. For infants whose peripheral perfusion is poor, an arterial or venous sample will give a better estimate of acid base status.

In infants requiring stabilization, the individual parameters on the blood gas can be high, low, or within a normal range (Table B.1).

In acute respiratory illness, blood gases are considered satisfactory when the pH is 7.25 to 7.40 and the PCO2 is 45 to 55 mmHg.

Table B.1.
Interpretation of blood gas values

	Low	Normal range	High
pH	< 7.35 acidosis	7.35 to 7.45	> 7.45 alkalosis
PCO2	< 35 mmHg hypocapnia respiratory alkalosis hyperventilation	35 to 45 mmHg	> 45 mmHg hypercapnia, respiratory acidosis hypoventilation
Base deficit	< 0 mmol/L metabolic alkalosis, too much buffer	0 to 4 mmol/L	> 4 mmol/L metabolic acidosis, too little buffer
PaO2	< 50 mmHg hypoxemia	50 to 80 mmHg	> 80 mmHg hyperoxemia

Interpretation

1. Determine whether the pH is normal, low (acidosis) or high (alkalosis).
2. Determine whether the PCO2 is normal, low, or high.
3. Determine whether the base deficit is normal, low, or high.
4. Determine the primary type of acidosis or alkalosis (Table B.2).
5. Assess whether oxygenation (SpO2 or arterial PaO2) is normal, high (hyperoxemia), or low (hypoxemia).

Table B.2.
Interpretation of primary type of acidosis or alkalosis

pH	PCO2	Base deficit	Interpretation
Decreased	Increased	Normal	Respiratory acidosis
Decreased	Normal	Increased	Metabolic acidosis
Increased	Decreased	Normal	Respiratory alkalosis
Increased	Normal	Decreased	Metabolic alkalosis

Notes

- Most acid-base problems in newborns are caused by inadequate lung function, which leads to respiratory acidosis.
- For infants with metabolic acidosis, the goal is to treat the underlying cause, which is often poor end-organ perfusion secondary to cardiovascular insufficiency.
- Although treatment generally aims for blood gas values in the normal range, acceptable levels of PCO2 and PaO2 may be higher or lower depending on an infant's condition or clinical status.

2. Complete blood count and differential (CBCD)

Goal

To interpret hematologic indices on the complete blood count (CBC) and differential in at-risk or unwell infants.

Principles

- CBC consists of red blood cells (RBC) and white blood cells (WBC), and platelets. A CBC and differential includes a count of the subsets of WBC involved in immune function (see Table B.3 for early normal ranges).
- RBC contain hemoglobin, which carries almost 98% of the oxygen contained in blood. Hemoglobin concentration (g/L) measures hemoglobin per volume of blood. The hematocrit measures the relative volume (L/L) of red cells in a spun sample of whole blood.
- WBC are key indicators of immune system function.
- Platelets are clotting agents.

Application

Arterial, venous, or capillary blood samples can be used for CBC analysis. The hematocrit is higher in capillary samples than in venous or arterial blood.

- A CBC for hemoglobin and hematocrit should be checked in infants who are pale or plethoric, or when blood loss is suspected.
- A CBCD should be performed when infection is suspected.
- A CBC for platelet count should be ordered when bleeding or infection are investigated.

Interpretation

Hemoglobin and hematocrit

Values vary with postnatal and gestational age (GA). Hemoglobin and hematocrit normally increase in the first 12 h post-birth, then gradually decline. By 4 weeks, hemoglobin in a term baby drops to a mean of 110 g/L (and as low as 70 g/L in low birth weight infants).

Preterm infants have lower hemoglobin at birth.

- The hemoglobin (g/L) for infants born at 23 to 31 weeks GA on day 1 ranges from 145 ± 16 to 162 ± 17 (mean ± SD).
- The corresponding hematocrit (L/L) is 0.435 ± 0.042 to 0.48 ± 0.05.

Table B.3.
Normal CBC ranges for term infants in the first 12 h post-birth (capillary samples)

CBC indices	Mean value ± SD	Range
Hemoglobin (g/L)	193 ± 22	150 to 220
Hematocrit (L/L)	0.61 ± 0.074	0.45 to 0.66
Total WBC ($\times$ 10^9/L)	24.0 ± 6.1	16.2 to 31.5
Total neutrophil count ($\times$ 10^9/L)	15.6 ± 4.7	6.0 to 26.0
Immature neutrophil count (bands) ($\times$ 10^9/L)	2.5 ± 1.8	0.7 to 4.3
Immature-to-total neutrophil (I:T) ratio	0.16 ± 0.10	0.05 to 0.27
Platelets ($\times$ 10^9/L)		150 to 350

White blood count (WBC)

The WBC count also increases over the first 12 h post-birth, then declines. The normal range in the first month is 5 to 15 × 10⁹/L. WBC counts obtained in the first few days post-birth are usually analyzed manually because historically, automated counts are less reliable.

In infants with bacterial sepsis, the WBC can be high, low, or even normal. The neutrophil count may be elevated, decreased, or show a rise in immature neutrophils or bands, with an increase in the I:T ratio (left shift). Some jurisdictions no longer report immature neutrophils or bands. Instead they report immature granulocyte. The normative values are represented in Table B.4.

Table B.4.
Normal values for IG cells and IG % during the first 90 days

CBC indices	Median value ± SD	5th - 95th percentiles
	0 to 48 h of age	
Immature granulocyte (IG) count, (cells/μL)	539 ± 270	50 to 1460
Immature granulocyte (IG) percent (IG%)	1.99 to 1.7	0.5 to 6.2
	Beyond 48 h of age	
IG count (cells/μL)	308 ± 70	10 to 613
IG percent (%)	1.62 ± 0.7	0.2 to 4.2

Findings suggestive of a bacterial infection include:

- Leukopenia (WBC < 5 × 10⁹/L)
- Neutropenia (< 2 × 10⁹/L). Neutropenia in newborns is significant and may be the first clue to infection.
- IG% > normative range
- I:T ratio > 0.25

Platelets

Bleeding time is prolonged in thrombocytopenic infants, particularly in those with platelet counts below 100 × 10⁹/L. Thrombocytopenia can have many causes, including sepsis, coagulation disorders, and infection.

Notes
- The interpretation of a CBCD should take the infant's clinical circumstances into account. The WBC, differential count, I:T ratio, and IG% are not highly sensitive or specific predictors of early-onset bacterial sepsis. The decision to initiate antibiotic therapy is clinical and should not be delayed while waiting for laboratory results in an unwell infant.
- Stress can cause an increase in the neutrophil count, with steroid-induced demargination of mature neutrophils.
- Infants born to mothers with HELLP syndrome (hemolysis, elevated liver enzymes, low platelets), or with marked intrauterine growth restriction may have neutropenia and thrombocytopenia lasting for several days.

3. Chest radiograph (CXR) interpretation

Goal

To assist in identification of common neonatal respiratory or cardiac conditions.

Principles

When a radiograph is taken, X-rays pass through intervening tissues to reach the film or digital recorder. The more X-rays that are able to pass through, the darker the area will appear on the image. If an object has little density, such as an aerated lung, most of the X-ray beam will pass through and the image appears black. If an object is dense, such as a bone, fewer X-rays reach the film and the image appears white.

Application

Anatomic structures seen on a radiograph can be identified by their characteristic density. There are five radiographic densities in order of increasing brightness: air, fat, fluid, bone, and metal. The lungs appear dark ('air density') because they are air-filled, while heart tissues, which are largely composed of water, look brighter ('fluid density').

Interpretation

1. Check labels for the infant's name, date and time of imaging, and positional (right/left) markers.
2. Assess the general quality of the radiograph.
   - Is the image centred? (Medial ends of the clavicles should be equidistant from the spinous processes of vertebrae.)
   - Is the image over- or underexposed?
3. Identify medical equipment on the radiograph, such as:
   - ECG leads.
   - An ETT: Note placement and position of the tube tip in relation to head position and the carina.
   - Umbilical lines (UAC or UVC): Note placement and location of catheter tips.
   - Oro- or nasogastric or chest tube: Note placement and location of catheter tips.
   - Servo-control temperature and/or transcutanious CO_2 probe, as applicable.
4. Identify the anatomic structures seen, starting from the centre of the radiograph and working outward.
5. Look for abnormalities in each of the following zones (Figure B.1):

Mediastinum

- Trachea, left and right main bronchi
- Aortic arch and descending aorta
- Left and right pulmonary arteries
- Heart shadow site, size and shape, right and left heart borders, cardiothoracic ratio (usually < 0.6)
- Thymus
- Esophagus (not normally seen unless containing a radio-opaque oro- or nasogastric tube)

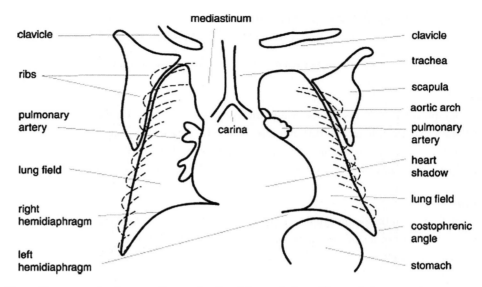

Figure B.1. Zones to check on radiograph. (See Normal chest X-ray, facing page.)

Lung fields

- Lung tissue should fully extend to the chest wall.
- Most conditions affecting lung tissue displace air in the alveoli, and common descriptors of radiographic findings include 'streaky', 'grainy', 'patchy', 'bubbly', 'fluffy', 'hazy', 'dotty', and 'white-out'. It should be noted whether these findings are focal or diffuse.
- Horizontal fissure separating the right upper and middle lobes
- Pulmonary vascular pattern

Chest wall

- Bones, including clavicles and twelve pairs of ribs
- Soft tissues

Diaphragms

- Is the right hemi-diaphragm upwardly displaced by the liver?
- On inspiration, both hemidiaphragms are usually located at the level of the ninth rib.
- Costophrenic angles should appear sharply defined.
- Check under the diaphragm for free air.

Upper abdomen

- Check position of the stomach bubble.

Notes

Three abnormal observations to check for are:

1. Lung markings:
   - Absent (pneumothorax)
   - Reduced (cyanotic congenital heart disease)

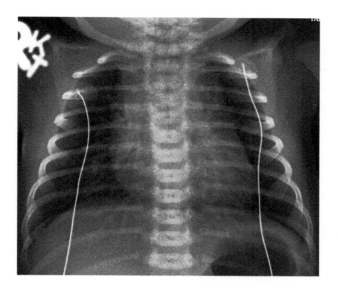

Normal chest X-ray

- Increased (pulmonary edema)
- Diffuse (respiratory distress syndrome)
- Focal (pneumonia)
2. Heart shape or size
    - Small (hypovolemia)
    - Normal
    - Large (cardiac disease)
3. Incorrect placement of endotracheal tube and lines

See examples of radiographs for common neonatal respiratory, cardiac, and surgical conditions in their respective chapters.

Bibliography

Alur P, Devapatla SS, Super DM, et al. Impact of race and gestational age on red blood cell indices in very low birth weight infants. Pediatrics 2000;106(2 Pt1):306–10.

Banerjee AK. Radiology made easy. 2nd edn. London, U.K.: Cambridge University Press, 2006.

Brouillette RT, Waxman DH. Evaluation of the newborn's blood gas status: National Academy of Clinical Biochemistry. Clin Chem 1997;43(1):215–21.

MacQueen BC, Christensen RD, Yoder BA, et al. Comparing automated vs. manual leukocyte differential counts for quantifying the 'left shift' in the blood of neonates. J Perinatol 2016;36(10):843–8.

Manroe BL, Weinberg AG, Rosenfeld CR, Browne R. The neonatal blood count in health and disease: I. Reference values for neutrophilic cells. J Pediatr 1979;95(1):89–98.

Martin RJ, Fanaroff AA, Walsh M. Neonatal-perinatal medicine: Diseases of the fetus and infant. 9th edn. St. Louis, MI: Saunders/Elsevier, 2011.

Mouzinho A, Rosenfeld CR, Sanchez PJ, Risser R. Revised reference ranges for circulating neutrophils in very-low-birth-weight infants. Pediatrics 1994;94(1):76–82.

Ouellette H, Tétreault P. Clinical radiology made ridiculously simple. 2nd edn. Miami, FL: Medmaster, 2015.

Shapiro BA, Penuzzi WT, Templin R. Clinical application of blood gases. 5th edn. Toronto, Ont.: Mosby, 1994.

Appendix C

Medications

Medications discussed in this appendix:

1. Acyclovir
2. Adenosine
3. Alprostadil (Prostaglandin E1)
4. Ampicillin
5. Cefotaxime
6. Cloxacillin
7. 40% dextrose oral gel
8. Dopamine
9. Fentanyl
10. Gentamicin/Tobramycin
11. Glucagon
12. Hydrocortisone
13. Metronidazole
14. Morphine
15. Phenobarbital
16. Phenytoin
17. Premedication before intubation
18. Vancomycin

Disclaimer: This appendix identifies common drugs used during neonatal stabilization. Information is based on available literature and clinical experience and should always be used in conjunction with clinical expertise, medical judgment, and applicable local guidelines. For any reader who is unfamiliar with a drug, expert consultation and reference to the official product monograph before administration is recommended. As research and clinical experience evolve, changes in the drug therapies summarized here may be necessary. Specific dosages and dosing intervals included herein may differ from local practice and consultation with your tertiary referral centre is recommended to discuss regional guidelines.

A general note on drug administration and dosing: Renal function and clearance of antibiotics are influenced by both gestational and postnatal age. For infants more than 7 days old, the postmenstrual age (PMA) should be considered in the dosing schedule.

For infants whose PMA is not known, base the dosing schedule on body weight categories, which approximate PMA.

1. Acyclovir: Antiviral agent

Indications: Treatment of herpes simplex virus (HSV) and varicella-zoster infections.

Supplied: 50 mg/mL vials. Do not refrigerate: Drug may precipitate.

Administration: Recommended intravenous (IV) concentrations are 7 mg/mL for central access and 5 mg/mL for peripheral access, infused over 1 to 2 h.

Dosing:

Table C.1.
Dosing schedule for acyclovir

Indications		Dose (mg/kg/dose)	Duration (days)
Herpes simplex virus	Central nervous system/disseminated	20	21
	Limited to skin, eyes, or mouth	20	14
Varicella-zoster		15	14

Table C.2.
Dosing intervals for acyclovir

Postmenstrual age (weeks) and body weight (g)	Interval (h)
< 32 or < 1200	q12h
≥ 32 and ≥ 1200	q8h

For infants with renal impairment, consider extending the dosing interval because acyclovir is renally cleared. Consult a pharmacist when renal impairment is suspected. It is important to maintain adequate hydration to avoid renal precipitation of acyclovir. Ensure a urine output of > 1 mL/kg/hr.

Precautions/adverse effects:
- Transient renal dysfunction associated with rapid infusion or large doses
- Phlebitis at IV site, due to this drug's high pH
- Reversible neutropenia (absolute neutrophil count < 1×10^9/L)

Monitoring:
- Test serum creatinine and urea at least twice weekly during therapy.
- Complete blood count (CBC) with differential weekly. Consider dose reduction if absolute neutrophil count is < 0.5×10^9/L.
- Monitor injection site for extravasation during infusion.

Treatment notes: Draw blood or cerebrospinal fluid sample for HSV polymerase chain reaction testing.

2. Adenosine: Antiarrhythmic agent

Indication: Treatment of supraventricular tachycardia.

Supplied: 3 mg/mL vials. Do not refrigerate: Drug may precipitate.

Administration: For initial dose, dilution to 0.3 mg/mL with 0.9% NaCl is recommended. To ensure accurate dose and rapid delivery, maintain the dose volume between 0.2 mL to 1 mL.

Central administration by rapid IV push is followed by a 0.9% NaCl flush to ensure delivery of dose to the heart.

Dosing: Initial dose is 0.05 mg/kg, which may be increased by 0.05 mg/kg every 2 min, up to a maxiumum of 0.3 mg/kg/dose.

Precautions/adverse effects:
- Contraindications: Second- or third-degree atrioventricular block or sick sinus syndrome
- Flushing, hypotension, dysrhythmia

Monitoring:
- Continuous heart rate (HR) monitoring.
- Blood pressure (BP) before and immediately following administration, and ongoing until the infant is stable.
- A defibrillator, and personnel familiar with its use at the bedside during administration, should be available.

Treatment notes:
- Vagal manoeuvres should be attempted before administering adenosine.
- Consultation with a paediatric cardiologist is strongly suggested before administering adenosine.
- Start electrocardiogram (ECG) monitoring before initiating treatment.
- Half-life is < 10 seconds.
- Clinical effects occur rapidly and may not be sustained.

3. Alprostadil (Prostaglandin E1)

Indications: To maintain a patent ductus arteriosus (PDA) in suspected or diagnosed 'duct-dependent' congenital heart disease, including:
- Obstruction to pulmonary blood flow with right-to-left shunts (e.g., tricuspid or pulmonary atresia)
- Obstruction to systemic blood flow (e.g., hypoplastic left heart syndrome or aortic stenosis)
- Mixing of pulmonary and systemic circulations (e.g., transposition of the great arteries)
- Persistent pulmonary hypertension of the newborn (PPHN), to reduce right ventricular afterload.

Supplied: 500 mcg/mL ampules. Must be refrigerated.

Administration: Dilute with D5W or NS to 5 mcg/mL. Fresh infusions should be prepared q24h and administered in either a peripheral or central venous line.

Dosing:

Initial infusion rate: 0.05 to 0.1 mcg/kg/min. Higher infusion rates are not more effective and are associated with more adverse effects.

Preparation of infusion:

> **Step 1:** Dilute alprostadil to a 5 mcg/mL concentration:
> Add 1 mL of 500 mcg/mL alprostadil to 99 mL of D5W or NS
> Final concentration = 5 mcg/mL

> **Step 2:** Infusion rate $(mL/h) = \dfrac{dose(mcg/kg/min) \times wt(kg) \times 60(min/h)}{concentration\ of\ alprostadil(mcg/mL)}$

In consultation with a paediatric cardiologist, titrate to response, 0.005 to 0.01 mcg/kg/min. Infusions as low as 0.001 mcg/kg/min have been used (balancing oxygenation and adverse effects). Continue the infusion at the lowest rate that maintains oxygenation effectively, and maintain consultation with referral centre.

Example: 3200 gm infant, starting dose 0.05 mcg/kg/min

$$\text{Infusion rate (mL/h)} = \frac{0.05 \times 3.2 \times 60}{5\,mcg/mL} = 1.9\,mL/h$$

Precautions/adverse effects: Risk for apnea, hypotension and cutaneous flushing, bradycardia or tachycardia, fever, diarrhea, inhibition of platelet aggregation, or seizure-like activity.

Monitoring: Closely monitor respiratory, pre- and post-ductal oxygen saturation, HR and rhythm, BP, and temperature. SpO2 and PaO2 will rise and colour will improve if the infant is responding to therapy.

Treatment notes: Expect maximum effect 15 to 30 minutes after infusion begins in cyanotic congenital heart disease, and in 1.5 to 3 h in acyanotic congenital heart disease. Ongoing management requires discussion with a paediatric cardiologist.

If prostaglandin E1 is discontinued, the ductus arteriosus will begin to close within 1 to 2 h after the drug is stopped.

4. Ampicillin: A semisynthetic penicillin with broad-spectrum bactericidal action

Indication: Treatment of infections due to Group B *Streptococcus* (GBS), *Listeria monocytogenes*, *Enterococcus fecalis*, and susceptible *Escherichia coli* species. Commonly used for broad-spectrum coverage conjunctively with an aminoglycoside or cephalosporin until a pathogen is identified.

Supplied: Powder in 250 mg and 500 mg vials. Reconstitute using sterile water for injection.

Administration: IV administration is preferred but may be delivered intramuscularly (IM). Recommended IV concentration is 50 mg/mL, to a maximum of 100 mg/mL. Recommended IM concentration is 250 mg/mL.

A slow IV push over 5 minutes must not exceed a rate of 100 mg/min.

Dosing: 50 mg/kg/dose. For GBS meningitis, some experts recommend doubling the dose to 100 mg/kg/dose, to a maximum of 300 mg/kg/day. Increase the dosing interval for cases of severe renal failure.

Table C.3.
Ampicillin dosing

Postmenstrual age (weeks)	Use body weight (g) if postmenstrual age not known	Postnatal age (days)	Interval (h)
≤ 29	< 1200	0 to 28	q12h
		> 28	q6h
30 to 36	1200 to 2000	0 to 7	q12h
		8 to 28	q8h
		> 28	q6h
≥ 37	> 2000	0 to 7	q8h
		> 7	q6h

Precautions/adverse effects:
- Do not mix ampicillin and aminoglycosides (amikacin, gentamicin, and tobramycin) in the same line or administer concurrently. Flush the IV line well between medications or separate administration times by at least 1 hour.
- Hypersensitivity reactions are rare in neonates.

Monitoring: With prolonged therapy (over 14 days), monitor serum creatinine, urea, CBC with differential, aspartate aminotransferase (AST), and γ-glutamyl transferase (GGT) every 2 weeks.

Treatment notes: Clearance is primarily renal and increases with postnatal age. Dosage interval needs to be adjusted over time.

5. Cefotaxime: Preferred third-generation cephalosporin in neonates

Indications: Treatment of neonatal sepsis and meningitis caused by susceptible gram-negative organisms.

Supplied: Powder in 500 mg vials. Reconstitute using sterile water for injection.

Administration: The recommended concentration for IV infusion is 100 mg/mL over 20 min.

Dosing: 50 mg/kg/dose. Increase dosing interval for cases of severe renal impairment.

Table C.4.
Cefotaxime dosing

Postmenstrual age (weeks)	Use body weight (g) if postmenstrual age not known	Postnatal age (days)	Interval (h)
≤ 29	< 1200	0 to 28 > 28	q12h q8h
30 to 36	1200 to 2000	0 to 7 > 7	q12h q8h
≥ 37	> 2000	0 to 7 > 7	q12h q8h

Precautions/adverse effects:
- Do not mix cefotaxime and vancomycin in the same line or administer concurrently. Flush the IV line well between medications or separate administration times by at least 1 hour.
- Adverse reactions are rare.
- Resistance may develop during treatment for some gram-negative infections.

Monitoring: With prolonged therapy, monitor serum creatine, urea, CBC with differential, aspartate aminotransferase, and γ-glutamyl transferase.

Treatment notes: When renal function or urine output is a concern, or monitoring aminoglycoside levels is difficult, cefotaxime may be substituted for an aminoglycoside (e.g., gentamicin) for broad-spectrum coverage.

6. Cloxacillin: A penicillinase-resistant penicillin

Indications: To treat neonatal infections caused by penicillinase-producing staphylococci (e.g., *Staphylococcus aureus*).

Supplied: Powder in 500 mg vials. Reconstitute using sterile water for injection.

Administration: The recommended concentration for IV infusion is 100 mg/mL over 20 min.

Dosing: 25 mg/kg/dose. Increase to 50 mg/kg/dose for meningitis. No dosage adjustment is required for cases with renal impairment.

Table C.5.
Cloxacillin dosing

Postmenstrual age (weeks)	Use body weight (g) if postmenstrual age not known	Postnatal age (days)	Interval (h)
≤ 29	< 1200	0 to 28 > 28	q12h q6h
30 to 36	1200 to 2000	0 to 7 8 to 28 > 28	q12h q8h q6h
≥ 37	> 2000	0 to 7 > 7	q8h q6h

Precautions/adverse effects:

- Do not mix cloxacillin and aminoglycosides (amikacin, gentamicin, and tobramycin) in the same line or administer concurrently. Flush the IV line well between medications or separate administration times by at least 1 hour.
- Risk for phlebitis, tissue irritation, interstitial nephritis, or hypersensitivity rash.

Monitoring: With prolonged therapy, monitor CBC, platelet count, urinalysis, urea, serum creatinine, and liver enzymes.

7. 40% dextrose oral gel: An antihypoglycemic agent

Indications: Treatment of acute hypoglycemia. The goal is to stabilize blood glucose in infants experiencing transient, asymptomatic hypoglycemia, to raise blood glucose levels in infants who are unwell, have symptomatic hypoglycemia, or should not be fed when access to IV dextrose is delayed.

Supplied: Dextrose in the form of gel with approximately 40% carbohydrate. Tube sizes vary.

Administration: Intrabuccal only.

Dosing: 0.5 mL/kg/dose, administered with breastfeeds or supplemental measured feeds.

Precautions/adverse effects: There is no available evidence to guide use beyond two doses.
Monitoring: Recheck blood glucose 30 min post-feed, as per the ACoRN Fluid and Glucose Sequence.

Treatment notes: Commercial products may not have internal consistency with regard to dextrose concentration.

8. Dopamine: A vasopressor and inotrope

Indications: In neonates, dopamine is used primarily to increase BP by raising systemic vascular resistance through peripheral vasoconstriction.

To treat hypotension caused by hypovolemia, a volume expander should be administered first to correct hypovolemia *before* starting dopamine therapy.

Supplied: Ready-to-use concentrations of 1600 mcg/mL and 3200 mcg/mL in D5W. Only the 1600 mcg/mL concentration is used for neonates. Solutions must be protected from light.

Administration: Syringe preparation (withdraw from 1600 mcg/mL premixed minibag):

- For rates less than 0.1 mL/h, use 3 mL syringe
- For rates of 0.1 mL/h or greater, use 20 mL syringe

Deliver a continuous IV infusion through a central venous line (preferred) or peripheral line with a syringe pump. A central line is preferred because it is more secure and avoids potentially severe complications associated with peripheral line extravasation.

Dosing:

Initial dose: 5 mcg/kg/min to 10 mcg/kg/min.

Maintenance infusion: Titrate gradually up to a maximum of 20 mcg/kg/min, balancing desired cardiovascular effects (BP and HR) with adverse effects.

Dopamine's pharmacological action is variable and unpredictable in immature neonates.

- For dopaminergic effect: renal vasodilation—2 to 4 mcg/kg/min (this pharmacologic effect is extrapolated from adult data)
- For beta-1 effect: chronotropic (increased heart rate): 5 to 10 mcg/kg/min
- For alpha effect: vasoconstriction (increased blood pressure): > 10 mcg/kg/min

$$\text{Infusion rate mL/hr} = \frac{\text{dose}(\text{mcg/kg/min}) \times \text{weight}(\text{kg}) \times 60}{\text{concentration of infusion solution}(\text{mcg/mL})}$$

Precautions/adverse effects:
- To prevent an inadvertent dopamine bolus and sudden increases in BP, do not use the dopamine infusion line to administer other medications.
- Use high doses with caution in persistent pulmonary hypertension of the newborn (PPHN).
- The commercial preparation of dopamine contains sodium bisulfite, which has been reported in rare cases to cause anaphylaxis.
- Some infusion pumps may deliver an undesirable pulsatile flow instead of steady fluid. Check the manufacturer's instructions for minimum fluid flow rate and adjust the concentration to achieve the appropriate minimum infusion rate.
- Risk for atrial and ventricular arrhythmias, hypertension, increased pulmonary artery pressure, tissue sloughing following extravasation, or peripheral circulatory impairment.

Monitoring:
- Continuous HR monitoring.
- BP monitoring, preferably via arterial line, otherwise every 15 minutes.
- Assess circulation (skin colour, capillary refill time, temperature of extremities, and pulses), urinary output.
- Check the IV site for signs of extravasation.

Treatment notes:
- If infused peripherally, white tracking due to peripheral vasoconstriction may appear along the course of the vein.

9. Fentanyl: An opioid analgesic

Indications: Treatment for pain and as premedication for painful procedures (e.g., intubation). Fentanyl is the preferred opioid analgesic for infants with compromised cardiovascular function.

Supplied: 50 mcg/mL

Administration: IV delivery

Dosing:
- Fentanyl is more potent than morphine. A clinical ratio of 10 to 15:1 (morphine: fentanyl) is generally applied for dose conversion (i.e., 10 mcg to 15 mcg morphine = 1 mcg fentanyl) when used as a continuous infusion. For intermittent dosing, a conversion ratio of 100:1 (morphine:fentanyl) is used for dose conversion.
- Analgesia: 0.5 to 4 mcg/kg/dose, slowly over 3 to 10 min q2 to 4 h, as required.

- Continuous infusion: 0.5 to 5 mcg/kg/h—usually 2 mcg/kg/h—with a loading dose of 1 to 2 mcg/kg slowly over 3 to 10 min.

Precautions/adverse effects:
- Ensure that resuscitation equipment (i.e., suction apparatus, a mask, positive pressure delivery system, and an oxygen source) is immediately available.
- The narcotic antagonist naloxone (Narcan) can be used to reverse respiratory depression associated with fentanyl use. The naloxone dose is a 0.1 mg/kg IV push or IM. Consider repeating in 3 to 5 min if there is no response. Naloxone should never be given to infants with neonatal abstinence syndrome (NAS) or neonatal opioid withdrawal (NOW), or whose mothers have a history of opioid use, because it may precipitate severe withdrawal symptoms, including seizures.
- Risk for: respiratory depression, apnea, chest wall rigidity and laryngospasm (especially with rapid administration and a large dose, which can be reversed with naloxone), bradycardia (with rapid IV injection), decreased gastrointestinal motility (i.e., delayed gastric emptying, constipation, ileus), or urinary retention.

Monitoring: Continuous cardiorespiratory monitoring, urine output, and sedation/pain relief levels.

10. Gentamicin/Tobramycin: Aminoglycoside antibiotics

Indications: For treatment of infections with aerobic gram-negative bacilli, including *Pseudomonas, Klebsiella, E. coli, Proteus*, and *Serratia*.

Supplied: As an injectable solution. The paediatric solution of 10 mg/mL is recommended.

Administration: IV infusion over 30 min. IV is preferred but may be given IM.

Dosing: Gentamicin dosing regimens vary greatly among centres. One possible dosing suggestion is listed below. Providers are advised to confirm dosing guidelines with their regional referral centre.

Table C.6.
Gentamicin/Tobramycin extended interval dosing

Postmenstrual age (weeks)	Postnatal age (days)	Dose (mg/kg)	Interval (h)
≤ 29	0 to 7 days	5	1 dose only, then do levels
	≥ 8 days	4	1 dose only, then do levels
30 to 34	0 to 7 days	4.5	q36h
	≥ 8 days	4	q24h
≥ 35	All infants	4	q24h

Source: Young TE, Mangum OB. Neofax: A Manual of Drugs Used in Neonatal Care. Edn 23. Thomson Reuters/PDR Network, 2010.

Precautions/adverse effects
- Dosage must be adjusted in cases of renal insufficiency.
- Do not mix ampicillin and gentamicin or tobramycin in the same line or administer concurrently. Flush the IV line well between medications or separate administration times by at least 1 hour.

- Risk for: renal toxicity, vestibular and/or ototoxicity, prolonged muscle paralysis when used in conjunction with neuromuscular blocking agents, or neuromuscular weakness when given to patients with elevated magnesium or conditions that depress neuromuscular transmission.

Monitoring: When using the extended dosing schedule, follow serum levels after the first dose to determine whether the suggested dosing interval is appropriate. For infants undergoing therapeutic hypothermia, and for those with asphyxia, severe oliguria, or increased serum creatinine, results of serum drug levels should be evaluated before subsequent doses are administered.

Therapeutic serum concentrations:

- Peak 6 mg/L to 12 mg/L (post-level): Draw sample 30 min after end of 30-min infusion or 1 hour after IM injection.
- Trough < 2 mg/L (pre-level): Draw sample no more than 30 min before the dose is due.
- Assess urine output and monitor urea and creatinine.

Treatment notes:
- IM injection is associated with variable absorption, especially in infants weighing less than 1500 g.
- Clearance and serum half-life is prolonged in preterm infants and in neonates with hypoxic ischemic injury. Clearance is also decreased in infants receiving indomethacin or ibuprofen.

11. Glucagon: An antihypoglycemic agent

Indications: Treatment for persistent or acute hypoglycemia in the setting of presumed hyperinsulinism.

Supplied: 1 mg vials, for injection.

Administration: Reconstitute powder with diluent supplied to 1 mg/mL for IM injection. For IV infusion, further dilute to 40 mcg/mL by adding 1 mL of 1 mg/mL glucagon to 24 mL of D5W, for a resulting total volume of 25 mL.

Dosing:
- IM dose is 30 mcg/kg/dose; repeat as required.
- Continuous infusion of 10 to 20 mcg/kg/h (0.5 to 1 mg/day) can also be considered, in consultation with your referral centre.

Precautions/adverse effects:
- Vomiting, tachycardia, ileus, hyponatremia, hypoglycemia, and thrombocytopenia

Monitoring: Monitor blood glucose at least q 30 min, initially and with each change in infusion rate.

Treatment notes:
- Critical samples including serum insulin, cortisol, and growth hormone should be drawn before starting a glucagon infusion.
- Half-life is about 5 min.
- Change solution q24h.

12. Hydrocortisone: A corticosteroid

Indications: To treat hypotension unresponsive to initial volume expansion or pressor administration, adrenal insufficiency, and persistent neonatal hypoglycemia.

Supplied: Hydrocortisone sodium succinate 100 mg vials for IV infusion.

Administration: Reconstituted concentration is 50 mg/mL. Further dilute to 1 mg/mL with 0.9% NaCl. Infuse IV over 5 min.

Dosing: Conversion from IV dose to PO dose is 1:1.

Table C.7.
Hydrocortisone dosing based on indication

Indication	Dose (mg/kg)	Interval (h)
Neonatal hypotension (volume and pressor-resistant)	1	q6 to 12h
Neonatal hypoglycemia	1 to 2	q8h
Physiological replacement	0.3 to 0.4	q12h
Stress dose (acute adrenal insufficiency)	1 to 2	q12h
Congenital adrenal hyperplasia*	0.4 to 0.6	q8h

*Fludrocortisone is also needed. An endocrinologist should be consulted.

Precautions/adverse effects:
- Draw blood cortisol level before starting therapy.
- Risk for fluid and electrolytes imbalances, hyperglycemia, adrenal suppression and growth failure (with long-term use), or increased risk of spontaneous bowel perforations when infant is also receiving indomethacin/ibuprofen.

Monitoring: Serum electrolytes and blood glucose at least once daily.

Treatment notes: It may take 2 to 3 h to observe BP response.

13. Metronidazole: An antibiotic

Indication: Treatment for suspected or proven infections with anaerobic bacteria, most often abdominal sepsis.

Supplied: 5 mg/mL premixed bag.

Administration: Infused IV over 60 min.

Dosing: No dosing adjustments for renal impairment. Decrease dose and/or frequency empirically for infants with hepatic impairment (specific dosing guidelines are not available).

Table C.8.
Metronidazole dosing

Weight	Age	Dosing
< 1200 g	0 to 28 days	Loading dose: 15 mg/kg Maintenance dose: 7.5 mg/kg/dose q48h
1200 to 2000 g	0 to 7 days	Loading dose: 15 mg/kg Maintenance dose: 7.5 mg/kg/dose q24h
	> 7 days	Loading dose: 15 mg/kg Maintenance dose: 7.5 mg/kg/dose q12h
> 2000 g	0 to 7 days	Loading dose: 15 mg/kg Maintenance dose: 7.5 mg/kg/dose q12h
	> 7 days	15 mg/kg/dose q12h
Any weight	> 28 days (all infants)	15 mg/kg/dose q12h

Some centres do not use loading doses but initiate metronidazole at maintenance dose only.

Precautions/adverse effects:
- Diarrhea and vomiting
- Rash
- Brownish discolouration of urine from drug metabolites

Monitoring: None required for IV administration.

Treatment note: Usually reserved for infants with signs of peritonitis (e.g., severe necrotizing enterocolitis) or needing abdominal surgery.

14. Morphine: An opioid analgesic

Indications: Treatment for pain, as premedication for painful procedures (e.g., intubation), and to treat withdrawal in infants with neonatal abstinence syndrome (NAS) or neonatal opiate withdrawal (NOW).

Supplied: As injectable solutions: 2 mg/mL, 10 mg/mL, 15 mg/mL. As oral solution: 1 mg/mL.

Administration: IV, IM, subcutaneously, or PO.

Dosing:

For pain management: 50 to 100 mcg/kg/dose IV over at least 5 minutes q3 to 4 h, as needed. Same dose may be given IM or subcutaneously. For continuous IV infusion: 5 to 20 mcg/kg/h and titrate as needed.

To treat NAS/NOW: Dosage and weaning schedules vary. Consult your referral centre and refer to applicable guidelines.

Precautions/adverse effects:

- Ensure that resuscitation equipment (i.e., suction apparatus, a mask, positive pressure delivery system, and an oxygen source) is immediately available.
- The narcotic antagonist naloxone (Narcan) can be used to reverse respiratory depression associated with morphine use. The naloxone dose is 0.1 mg/kg IV push or IM. Consider repeating in 3 to 5 min if there is no response. Naloxone should never be given to infants with NAS or NOW, or whose mothers have a history of opioid use, because it may precipitate severe withdrawal symptoms, including seizures.
- Risk for: respiratory depression, apnea, hypotension, decreased gastrointestinal motility (delayed gastric emptying, constipation, ileus), or urinary retention.

Monitoring:

- Continuous cardiorespiratory monitoring, urine output, and sedation/pain relief levels.
- Observe for abdominal distention and ileus.

15. Phenobarbital: A barbiturate anticonvulsant

Indication: To treat neonatal seizures.

Supplied: 30 mg/mL solution for injection, or as a 5 mg/mL elixir, for oral administration.

Administration: IV route preferred but can be given PR or IM in an emergency.

Dosing:

- **Loading dose (IV):** 20 mg/kg slow IV infusion (maximum rate for IV infusion is 1 mg/kg/min).
- Administer repeat doses of 10 mg/kg at 20- to 30-min intervals, up to a total maximum loading dose of 40 mg/kg.
- **IV maintenance dose** 24 h after loading dose: 1.5 to 2.5 mg/kg/dose q12h, or 3 to 5 mg/kg/q24h (maximum rate for IV infusion 1 mg/kg/min).
- **Oral maintenance dose** 24 to 48 h after loading dose: 1.5 to 2.5 mg/kg/dose q12h or 3 to 5 mg/kg/q24h.

Adverse effects/precautions:

- Lethargy and sedation
- Serum half-life varies from 40 h to 200 h in neonates.
- Serum levels can increase with concomitant use of phenytoin (see following text).
- Rapid administration and high doses can cause respiratory depression, apnea, or hypotension.

Monitoring:

- Cardiorespiratory status, including BP.
- Observe for continuation or suppression of seizures.
- Determine clinical correlation with electroencephalogram for seizures.

- Maintenance: Trough serum levels are recommended before the third dose after starting or changing the maintenance dose, then twice weekly until levels are stable.
- Recommended therapeutic range is 65 to 170 μmol/L.
- Check IV site for signs of extravasation and phlebitis.

Treatment notes:
- Phenobarbital is 50% to 70% metabolized by the liver and 20% to 40% eliminated by the kidneys.
- Alkalinization of urine may enhance elimination of phenobarbital.
- Approximately each 10 mg/kg dose will increase blood concentration by 40 μmol/L.
- In neonates with hypoxic ischemic encephalopathy who are undergoing therapeutic hypothermia, elimination of phenobarbital may decrease and a lower maintenance dose of 3 mg/kg/day should be considered.

16. Phenytoin: A sodium channel-blocking anticonvulsant

Indication: Treatment for persistent seizures that are refractory to maximum phenobarbital doses.

Supplied: As 50 mg/mL ampoules for IV administration. Also, as a 6 mg/mL suspension for oral use. Keep at room temperature and shake well before each use.

Administration: IV, PO. **Do not** give IM.

The recommended concentration for IV administration is 10 mg/mL diluted with NS (solution is stable for up to 2 h at room temperature). Phenytoin is unstable and can crystallize in solution. To prevent infusing crystallized phenytoin into the line, a 0.22 micron in-line filter should be attached during IV administration.

Dosing:
- **Loading dose (IV)**: 20 mg/kg by slow IV infusion (maximum rate of 1 mg/kg/min).
- **IV maintenance dose**: 2 to 4 mg/kg/dose q12h by slow IV infusion.
- **Oral maintenance dose**: 2 to 4 mg/kg/dose PO q12h starting 24 h after last loading dose.
- A higher oral dose may be necessary due to variable absorption of this drug. Adjust dose according to serum levels.

Precautions/adverse effects:
- A standard concentration of 10 mg/mL in NS (versus 50 mg/mL) for all dose volumes decreases the potential for adverse reactions (e.g., hypotension) when administered too quickly.
- When administered in conjunction with phenobarbital, serum levels of phenytoin may increase or (more usually) decrease. Monitor phenytoin levels closely when an infant is receiving both medications.
- Acute effects following IV administration may include hypotension, bradycardia, ventricular arrhythmias, vasodilation, venous irritation, pain, thrombophlebitis, and skin rash. Observe the IV site carefully. Extravasation may cause tissue inflammation and necrosis.
- Long-term phenytoin use has been associated with hepatitis, gingival hyperplasia, hyperglycemia, and osteoporosis.

Monitoring:

- Monitor serum phenytoin levels closely when an infant is receiving phenobarbital and phenytoin.
- Maintenance: Trough serum levels are recommended before the third dose after starting or changing the maintenance dose, then twice weekly until levels are stable.
- Recommended therapeutic range is 40 μmol/L to 80 μmol/L.
- Continuous cardiorespiratory monitoring and BP measurement with IV administration.

Treatment notes:

- Phenytoin can interact with many other medications that are metabolized in the liver.
- The 10 mg/mL dilution in NS must be used within 2 h after preparation.

17. Premedication before intubation

Premedication before elective or semi-urgent laryngoscopy and intubation involves three drugs: an analgesic, an anticholinergic, and a neuromuscular blocking agent. Their combined effects, sedation and muscle paralysis, help to:

- Reduce an infant's physiological stress response.
- Make the vocal cords easier to see, facilitating intubation.

Administration: Morphine (100 mcg/kg) or fentanyl (2 mcg/kg) can be used for analgesia.

- There is extensive experience with morphine use in newborns, but the action onset for morphine is slower than for fentanyl.
- Fentanyl's action onset is fast, but there is risk for adverse effects such as chest wall rigidity and laryngospasm. Both effects can be prevented by administering fentanyl slowly (over 3 to 5 min).

A neuromuscular blocking agent (e.g., succinylcholine) should only be administered by care providers who are familiar with its use and skilled in neonatal intubation. When this is not possible, administering fentanyl is not recommended and morphine should be used for analgesia.

Administer morphine (or fentanyl) first. Allow 5 to 10 min for sedation/analgesia to take effect. Then administer atropine (observe the infant for increased HR), followed approximately 30 to 60 sec later by succinylcholine. The action onset for succinylcholine is approximately 45 to 60 sec.

Dosing:

Table C.9.
Premedications for intubation

Class	Agent	Dose and route	Action
Analgesic	Morphine	100 mcg/kg IV	Pain relief
	Fentanyl	2 mcg/kg IV	
Anticholinergic	Atropine	20 mcg/kg IV	Prevents reflex bradycardia
Neuromuscular blocking agent	Succinylcholine	2 mg/kg IV	Induces paralysis, facilitates visualization

Precautions/adverse effects

- Ventilation must be supported until the effect of succinylcholine has dissipated.
- Ensure that resuscitation equipment (i.e., suction apparatus, a mask, flow-inflating bag or T-piece resuscitator, and an oxygen source) is immediately available.
- Multiple or prolonged attempts to intubate can cause hypoxia and bradycardia. If the infant develops these signs, stop intubation and provide positive pressure ventilation.

Monitoring

- HR, pulse oximetry.
- Colour cycling of colorimetric CO_2 detector and bilateral breath sounds on auscultation to confirm intubation is successful.

Treatment notes

- Administering premedication should not delay emergent intubation when the risk of waiting outweighs the need for pain management.
- When the infant's anatomy is unusual or there is concern that the airway cannot be managed by bag-and-mask ventilation (e.g., in a paralyzed infant), modify the premedication regimen. In both scenarios, give morphine and atropine but not succinylcholine.

18. Vancomycin: A glycopeptide antibiotic

Indications: To treat sepsis and meningitis caused by methicillin-resistant *Staphylococcus aureus* and *Staphylococcus epidermidis*.

Supplied: As 500 mg vials of powder. Reconstitute using sterile water for injection.

Administration: Recommended concentration for IV infusion is 5 mg/mL, delivered by syringe pump over 60 min.

Dosing: Vancomycin dosing regimens vary greatly among centres. One possible dosing suggestion is listed below. Providers are advised to confirm dosing guidelines with their regional referral centre.

Administer 15 mg/kg/dose for both sepsis and meningitis. Adjust levels to upper end of therapeutic range for both peak and trough when treating meningitis.

Table C.10.
Vancomycin dosing

PMA (weeks)	Postnatal age (days)	Interval (h)
< 27	< 28	q24h
27 to 30	< 28	q18h
31 to 36	< 28	q12h
≥ 37	0 to 7	q12h
	> 7	q8h
All infants	> 28	q8h

Precautions/adverse effects:
- Nephrotoxicity
- Ototoxicity
- Neutropenia
- Rapid infusion can cause a diffuse red rash and hypotension ('red man' syndrome).

Monitoring:

Serum levels: Measure trough (pre-) levels after the second or third dose for neonates who do not have signs of renal disease and when duration of treatment is longer than 3 days. Peak (post-) levels are recommended when treating meningitis.

Optimal serum concentration: Peak (sample taken 60 min post 1-hour infusion) 25 mg/L to 35 mg/L; trough (sample taken within 30 min before the next dose) 5 mg/L to 15 mg/L.

Treatment note:

Do not mix vancomycin and cefotaxime in the same line or administer them concurrently. Flush the IV line well between medications or separate administration times by at least 1 hour.

Bibliography

Barrington KJ; Canadian Paediatric Society, Fetus and Newborn Committee. Premedication for endotracheal intubation in the newborn infant. Paediatr Child Health 2011;16(3):159–64.

Bradley JS, Nelson JD, eds. Nelson's pocket book of pediatric antimicrobial therapy. 20th edn. Elk Grove Village, IL: American Academy of Pediatrics, 2014.

Carbajal R, Eble B, Anand KJ. Premedication for tracheal intubation in neonates: Confusion or controversy? Semin Perinatol 2007;31(5):309–17.

Cherry J, Demmler-Harrison G, Kaplan S, Steinbach W, Hotez PJ. Feigin and Cherry's Textbook of Pediatric Infectious Diseases. 8th edn. New York, NY: Elsevier, 2017 Children's Hospital of Eastern Ontario (CHEO). Neonatal Drug Therapy Manual: https://outreach.cheo.on.ca/manual/1274.

Children's Hospital of Eastern Ontario (CHEO). Neonatal Drug Therapy Manual: https://outreach.cheo.on.ca/manual/1274

Harris DL, Weston PJ, Signal M, Chase JG, Harding JE. Dextrose gel for neonatal hypoglycemia (the Sugar Babies Study): A randomised, double-blind, placebo-controlled trial. Lancet 2013;382(9910):2077–83.

Hudak ML, Tan RC; American Academy of Pediatrics Committee on Drugs, Committee on Fetus and Newborn. Neonatal drug withdrawal. Pediatrics 2012;129(2):e540–60.

Jobe AH. Pulmonary surfactant therapy. N Engl J M 1993;328(12):861–8.

Lacaze T, O'Flaherty P; Canadian Paediatric Society, Fetus and Newborn Committee. Management of infants born to mothers who have used opioids during pregnancy. Updated October 2019: www.cps.ca/en/documents/position/opioids-during-pregnancy

Narvey MR, Marks SD; Canadian Paediatric Society, Fetus and Newborn Committee. The screening and management of newborns at risk for low blood glucose. Paediatr Child Health 2019 24(8):536–44.

Ng E, Shah V; Canadian Paediatric Society, Fetus and Newborn Committee. Guidelines for surfactant replacement therapy in neonates. Paediatr Child Health (in press).

Oei J, Hari R, Butha T, Lui K. Facilitation of neonatal nasotracheal intubation with premedication: A randomized controlled trial. J Paediatr Child Health 2002;38(2):146–50.

Smyth J, McDougal A, Vanderpas E, eds. Neonatal drug dosage guidelines. Vancouver, BC: Children's and Women's Health Centre of British Columbia, 2015.

Sweet CB, Grayson S, Polak M. Management strategies for neonatal hypoglycemia. J Pediatr Pharmacol Ther 2013; 18(3):199–208.

Young TE, Mangum OB. Neofax: A Manual of Drugs Used in Neonatal Care. Edn 23. Montvale, NJ: Thomson Reuters/PDR Network, 2010.

Zhang J, Penny DJ, Kim NS, Yu VYH, Smolich JJ. Mechanisms of blood pressure increase induced by dopamine in hypotensive preterm neonates. Arch Dis Child Fetal Neonatal Ed 1999;81:F99–104.

Index

Tables, figures and boxes are indicated by *t, f* and *b* following the page number